Hybrid Cardiac Imaging for Clinical Decision-Making

Francesco Nudi • Orazio Schillaci
Giuseppe Biondi-Zoccai
Ami E. Iskandrian
Editors

Hybrid Cardiac Imaging for Clinical Decision-Making

From Diagnosis to Prognosis

Springer

Editors
Francesco Nudi
Service of Hybrid Cardio Imaging
Madonna della Fiducia Clinic
Rome, Lazio, Italy

Giuseppe Biondi-Zoccai
Department of Medical-Surgical
Sciences and Biotechnologies
Sapienza University of Rome
Latina, Lazio, Italy

Orazio Schillaci
Department of Biomedicine
and Prevention
University of Rome Tor Vergata
Rome, Lazio, Italy

Ami E. Iskandrian
Division of Cardiovascular Disease
University of Alabama at Birmingham
Birmingham, AL, USA

ISBN 978-3-030-99390-0 ISBN 978-3-030-99391-7 (eBook)
https://doi.org/10.1007/978-3-030-99391-7

This Springer imprint is published by the registered company Springer Nature Switzerland AG
The registered company address is: Gewerbestrasse 11, 6330 Cham, Switzerland

For Raffaele, Alessandro, Andrea, and Isabella, my cardinal points.

Foreword

Towards a One-Stop Shop for the Heart

The Hidden Organ

The heart is the hidden organ: Indeed, ancient physicians only had indirect access to the heart by feeling the pulse. In particular, Chinese medicine made a sophisticated art out of that. In Western medicine, it took centuries after William Harvey's seminal discovery of the circulation[1] to actually see a heart without vivisection. It took almost three centuries until on November 8, 1895, Wilhelm Röntgen discovered X-rays allowing to visualize at least the shadow of the heart.[2] Only 6 years later, he was awarded the Nobel Prize in Physics in 1902; he would have deserved the one in medicine as well. However, chest X-rays only allowed for measurements of the size of the heart, usually expressed as the cardiac-thoracic ratio, but provided no information on its function. Nevertheless, they for the first time and for decades thereafter gave important clinical information for practicing physicians about the cardiac size in patients with heart disease.

From X-Rays to Coronary Angiography

In 1929, Werner Forssmann performed a seminal experiment on himself that today would not be approved by any ethical committee but made history:[3] He introduced a ureter catheter through the cubital vein of his left arm into the left atrium without any side effects and documented it in a chest X-ray. Although initially this did not advance medicine, it demonstrated the feasibility of catheterizing the heart without risking feared deadly arrhythmias.

[1] Harvey W.S.: De motu cordis. Referenced after: William H. Harvey: An anatomical disputation concerning the movement of the heart and blood in living creatures. By G. Whitteridge Blackwell Scientific, Oxford, U.K. 1976.

[2] Wilhelm Conrad Röntgen: Ueber eine neue Art von Strahlen. Vorläufige Mittheilung. 2d Edition, Würzburg, FRG 1896.

[3] Forssmann W.: Die Sondierung des rechten Herzens. Klin. Wochenschr. 1929;8: 2085–2087.

This stimulated André F. Cournand and Dickinson W. Richards to develop clinically cardiac catheterization to allow for measurements of pressures and flow throughout the circulation—and rightly so the two with Werner Forssmann received the second Nobel Prize, this time in Medicine and Physiology. On October 30, 1958, Mason Sones, then chief of the Cardiac Laboratory at the Cleveland Clinic in Ohio, USA, inadvertently pioneered coronary angiography when, upon injecting contrast, his catheter slipped from the aortic root into the right coronary artery and provided the first coronary angiogram. The anxiously awaited ventricular fibrillation did—against the paradigm of the day—not take place, although the patient experienced a vagal reaction, which upon coughing passed swiftly. In line with Louis Pasteur's saying: "*Le hazard ne touche que l'ésprit préparé*" Sones immediately realized the importance of his mistake and introduced coronary angiography into clinical practice.[4] This for the first time provided a precise image of coronary anatomy and in turn allowed for coronary bypass surgery that René Favaloro pioneered in 1968 at the same institution.[5]

Radioisotopes

Almost at the same time of Röngten's discovery, i.e., in 1896 Henri Becquerel discovered that uranium-emitted penetrating rays similar to X-rays.[6] A few years later, Marie and Pierre Curie reported that ^{229}Thorium was also radioactive, and proposed two new elements, i.e., Polonium and Radium—discoveries that earned another three Nobel prizes. In the 1920s, radioisotopes started to be used in cardiology, but it took a few decades until ventricular function could be quantified using first pass and equilibrium techniques. In 1973, myocardial stress perfusion imaging was introduced using ^{43}Potassium, followed by using new tracers, mainly ^{201}Thallium. However, Thallium was associated with significant radiation and hence ^{99m}Technetium-labeled agents became popular. While radiation remains a disadvantage of myocardial perfusion imaging, it has—due its longtime use—the most solid long-term outcomes data of all imaging modalities. Of note outcome prediction of SPECT myocardial perfusion imaging could be further improved after CT attenuation correction[7]—the first step towards hybrid imaging.

[4] Sones FM Jr, Shirey EK. Cine coronary arteriography. Mod Concepts Cardiovasc Dis. 1962;31:735–738.

[5] René Favoloro:

[6] Henri Becquerel: Sur les radiations émises par phosphorescence. In: Comptes Rendus de l'Académie des sciences. 1986;122:420–421.

[7] Aju P. Pazhenkottil*, Jelena-Rima Ghadri*, Rene N. Nkoulou, Mathias Wolfrum, Ronny R. Buechel, Silke M. Küest, Lars Husmann, Bernhard A. Herzog, Oliver Gaemperli, and Philipp A. Kaufmann: Improved Outcome Prediction by SPECT Myocardial Perfusion Imaging After CT Attenuation Correction. J Nucl Med 2011; 52:196–200.

Echocardiography

However, radiation remained an issue and hence echocardiography, using ultrasound technology initially developed for navigation of ships, was another breakthrough in imaging. In 1953, the Swedish physician Inge Edler and his physicist friend, Hellmuth Hertz, marked the beginning of this new diagnostic noninvasive technique by applying ultrasound to the heart, initially to study mitral stenosis and mitral regurgitation prior to surgery.[8] Soon, however, the technology evolved beyond M-mode recordings and 2D echocardiography was developed, followed by color flow by Doppler and color flow technology and eventually 3D echocardiography[9]—today echocardiography is the new stethoscope and because of its versatility the working horse of clinical cardiology.

Beyond Röntgen

In 1971, Sir Godfrey N. Hounsfield, working at EMI in Hayes, Middlesex in the United Kingdom, brought Röntgen's X-rays at a new level when he developed Computer Tomography (CT), initially to scan the brain of a woman with cerebral cyst[10] which earned him in 1979 together with Allan MacLeod Cormack also a Nobel Prize in Medicine. To visualize the beating heart and in particular continuously moving coronary arteries was however a real challenge: Indeed, it took more than 20 years until single-slice helical CT systems were widely introduced. Ever since, CT coronary angiography impressively developed with ever-increasing image quality allowing for a precise visualization of coronary anatomy in a noninvasive manner. This revolutionized the diagnosis of coronary artery disease, particularly since the radiation exposure could be markedly reduced.

Magnets for the Heart

Finally, in the 1980s magnetic resonance imaging (MRI) was introduced and applied first to non-moving organs such as the brain and most organs of the body—a well-deserved Nobel Prize followed for the pioneers Paul C. Lauterbur and Peter Mansfield in Medicine and Physiology and one in Chemistry for Richard R. Ernst for the discovery of NMR spectroscopy. Also here, the moving heart was a challenge, but eventually this was achieved by many today allowing for an assessment of cardiac structure and function as well as tissue texture with an unprecedented precision. Furthermore, gadolinium contrast allowed for the quantification of myocardial perfusion at rest

[8]Edler I, Lindstrom K. The history of echocardiography. Ultrasound Med Biol 2004;30:1565–644.

[9]Harvey Feigenbaum. Evolution of echocardiography. Circulation 1996;93:1321–7.

[10]Hounsfield GN. Computerized transverse axial scanning (tomography). 1. Description of system. Br J Radiol 1973;46:1016–22.

and during stress and as such to diagnose ischemia. Indeed, perfusion cardiac MRI proved non-inferior to intracoronary FFR[11] and at least as sensitive and specific and possibly superior to single-photon emission computed tomography (SPECT) in detecting coronary ischemia.[12] Furthermore, cardiac MRI detects myocardial edema[13] and using late gadolinium enhancement (LGE) the amount of scar in the heart muscle in myocarditis[14] and ischemic cardiomyopathy. The assessment of fibrosis and scars is becoming increasingly important to assess the risk of arrhythmias in heart failure.

SWOT

How can we perform a Strengths, Weaknesses, Opportunities and Threats (SWOT) analysis? As impressive the development of all these different imaging modalities was, each of them had advantages and disadvantages. Indeed, angiography of cardiac chambers in the coronary arteries is a rather invasive technique, while echocardiography, being the most easily available imaging modality, is prone to imprecision due to operator skills, specific patient properties, and limitation in picture resolution. Computer tomography, on the other hand, is primarily providing structural information, much less so functional insights into the performance of the heart, except with significant radiation exposure. Finally, magnetic resonance imaging requires significant resources in terms of personnel, equipment, and magnetic isolation of rooms. Also, cardiac MRI, in spite of all developments, has not evolved into a one-stop shop providing structure function, as well as coronary anatomy.

Although all cardiac imaging modalities have their strengths, on their own they all also have their downsides. Most and foremost, X-rays and radioisotopes can damage tissues and DNA even at small dosages and hence repetitive examinations are or should be performed with caution, particularly in the

[11]Robert Manka, Ingo Paetsch, Sebastian Kozerke, Marco Moccetti, Rainer Hoffmann, Joerg Schroeder, Sebastian Reith, Bernhard Schnackenburg, Oliver Gaemperli, Lukas Wissmann, Christophe A. Wyss, Philipp A. Kaufmann, Roberto Corti, Peter Boesiger, Nikolaus Marx, Thomas F. Lüscher, Cosima Jahnke: Whole-heart dynamic three-dimensional magnetic resonance perfusion imaging for the detection of coronary artery disease defined by fractional flow reserve: determination of volumetric myocardial ischaemic burden and coronary lesion location. Eur. Heart J. 2012;33:2016–2024.

[12]John P Greenwood, Neil Maredia, John F Younger, Julia M Brown, Jane Nixon, Colin C Everett, Petra Bijsterveld, John P Ridgway, Aleksandra Radjenovic, Catherine J Dickinson, Stephen G Ball, Sven Plein. Cardiovascular magnetic resonance and single-photon emission computed tomography for diagnosis of coronary heart disease (CE-MARC): a prospective trial. Lancet 2012; 379:453–60.

[13]Robert Manka, Sebastian Kozerke, Andrea K Rutz, Christian T Stoeck, Peter Boesiger and Juerg Schwitter: A CMR study of the effects of tissue edema and necrosis on left ventricular dyssynchrony in acute myocardial infarction: implications for cardiac resynchronization therapy Journal of Cardiovascular Magnetic Resonance 2012;14:47.

[14]Jan Berg, Jan Kottwitz, Nora Baltensperger, Christine K. Kissel, Marina Lovrinovic, Tarun Mehra, Frank Scherff, Christian Schmied, Christian Templin, Thomas F. Lüscher, Bettina Heidecker, Robert Manka: Cardiac Magnetic Resonance Imaging in Myocarditis Reveals Persistent Disease Activity Despite Normalization of Cardiac Enzymes and Inflammatory Parameters at 3-Month Follow-Up, Circ. Heart Fail. 2017;10:e00426.

young. The lack of radiation is a major advantage of echocardiography and cardiac MRI (although the effects of magnetic forces on DNA have been discussed controversially in the literature).[15]

On the other hand, the disadvantage of echocardiography is its operator-dependence and varying image quality depending on the patient, while MRI provides consistently high imaging quality, but is logistically cumbersome. CT coronary angiography provides structure of the coronary arteries, but not function (except CT FFR that is in development).[16] In contrast, stress-echocardiography, particularly with contrast, provides indirect evidence of ischemia as reflected by new wall motion abnormalities during exercise or pharmacological stress, while cardiac MRI and myocardial perfusion imaging directly measure myocardial perfusion, with positron emission tomography (PET) with either H_2O or NHR as the gold standard.

The Whole is More Than Its Parts

So why not combine different imaging modalities with complementary strength? With all these advantages and limitations of different imaging modality, the concept of hybrid imaging was an important next step. The first attempts have been successfully made by combining CT coronary angiography and PET.[17] And indeed, both in coronary artery disease, heart failure, and congenital heart disease, the new hybrid technology provided incremental diagnostic value, [18] albeit at the costs of increased radiation exposure. For centers without a cyclotron, SESTAMIBI-CT was introduced as well.[19] More recently, PET and MRI were combined providing impressive tissue

[15]Juhani Knuuti, Antti Saraste, Marko Kallio, Heikki Minn: Is cardiac magnetic resonance imaging causing DNA damage? Eur Heart J. 2013;34:2337–2339.

[16]Carlos Collet, Yoshinobu Onuma, Daniele Andreini, Jeroen Sonck, Giulio Pompilio, Saima Mushtaq, Mark La Meir, Yosuke Miyazaki, Johan de Mey, Oliver Gaemperli, Ahmed Ouda, Juan Pablo Maureira, Damien Mandry, Edoardo Camenzind, Laurent Macron, Torsten Doenst, Ulf Teichgräber, Holger Sigusch, Taku Asano, Yuki Katagiri, Marie-angele Morel, Wietze Lindeboom, Gianluca Pontone, Thomas F Lüscher, Antonio L Bartorelli, Patrick W Serruys. Coronary computed tomography angiography for heart team decision-making in multivessel coronary artery disease. Eur. Heart J., 2018;39:3689–3698.

[17]Pazhenkottil, Aju P., Nkoulou, Rene N., Ghadri, Jelena-Rima, Herzog, Bernhard A., Küest, Silke M., Husmann, Lars, Wolfrum, Mathias, Goetti, Robert, Buechel, Ronny R., Gaemperli, Oliver, Lüscher, Thomas F., Kaufmann, Philipp A. Impact of cardiac hybrid single-photon emission computed tomography/computed tomography imaging on choice of treatment strategy in coronary artery disease. Eur. Heart J. 2011;32:2824–2829.

[18]Thomas F. Lüscher: Imaging as a basis of clinical decision-making in congenital and coronary disease and heart failure. Eur. Heart J. 2016;37:1171–1173.

[19]Aju P. Pazhenkottil*, Dominik C. Benz*, Christoph Gräni, Michael A. Madsen, Fran Mikulicic, Elia von Felten, Tobias A. Fuchs, Beatrice Hirt Moch, Julia Stehli, Thomas F. Lüscher, Oliver Gaemperli, Ronny R. Buechel, Philipp A. Kaufmann. Hybrid SPECT Perfusion Imaging and Coronary CT Angiography: Long-term Prognostic Value for Cardiovascular Outcomes. Radiology 2018; 288:694–702.

characterization for use initially in oncology and later also in cardiology.[20,21] The last step was then combining 3D-strain echocardiography with coronary CT.[22] Thus, we are getting closer to a "one-stop shop" providing cardiac structure, function, and myocardial perfusion with an ever-increasing sensitivity, specificity, and image quality.

It took 12 Nobel laureates to get us where we are today—an impressive journey within a century!

The Seminal Textbook

It is very timely and a great achievement by the editors of this textbook, *Hybrid Cardiac Imaging for Clinical Decision Making—From Diagnosis to Prognosis*, Francesco Nudi, Orazio Schillaci, Giuseppe Biondi-Zoccai, and Ami E. Iskandrian to provide a comprehensive overview of this exciting development in cardiac imaging. The book starts with a more technical section on the specialists' perspectives with 11 chapters dedicated to all imaging modalities and their combination and is then followed by the second section on imaging in clinical practice with 7 chapters providing insights into the practical use and value of each of the combined imaging techniques. As such this remarkable textbook provides a timely and comprehensive update of emerging imaging technologies for the specialist and the clinician—it's truly a must for cardiologist who want to be at the forefront of cardiac imaging.

London, January 8, 2021.

Thomas F. Lüscher

Royal Brompton and Harefield Hospitals
Heart Division and Imperial College
National Heart and Lung Institute, London, UK

Center for Molecular Cardiology
University of Zurich, Zurich, Switzerland

[20] Robert Manka, Felix P. Kuhn, Silke M. Kuest, Oliver Gaemperli, Sebastian Kozerke, Philipp A. Kaufmann. Hybrid cardiac magnetic resonance/computed tomographic imaging: first fusion of three-dimensional magnetic resonance perfusion and low-dose coronary computed tomographic angiography. Eur Heart J. 2011;32(21):2625

[21] von Spiczak, Jochen; Manka, Robert; Gotschy, Alexander; Oebel, Sabrina; Kozerke, Sebastian; Hamada, Sandra; Alkadhi, Hatem(2018). Fusion of CT coronary angiography and whole-heart dynamic 3D cardiac MR perfusion: building a framework for comprehensive cardiac imaging. International Journal of Cardiovascular Imaging, 34(4):649–660.

[22] Aju P Pazhenkottil, Felix C Tanner, Ronny R Buechel, Andreas A Giannopoulos, Philipp A Kaufmann, Michel Zuber. Cardiac hybrid imaging combining 3D-strain echocardiography with coronary computed tomography angiography. Eur. Heart J. Volume 2019;40:395–396.

Preface

Cardiac imaging has a pivotal role in the prevention, diagnosis, and treatment of ischemic heart disease. *Hybrid Cardiac Imaging for Clinical Decision-Making* is a readable, practical, and comprehensive guide to this new subspecialty, which is able to provide a noninvasive assessment of coronary anatomy and myocardial perfusion, from diagnosis to prognosis. The hybrid imaging approach helps to identify the most appropriate treatment strategy with or without coronary revascularization and might translate into lower morbidity and mortality, impacting clinical decision-making in a large percentage of patients, with an important added clinical value. Therefore, in the time of personalized and precision medicine, cardiac hybrid imaging offers robust assessment of myocardial ischemia, which can be used to guide individual risk stratification and direct treatment decision-making. Including both technical and clinical aspects, the text provides core knowledge essential for those practitioners from any background, whether at a basic or advanced level, with cutting-edge coverage of multimodal cardiac imaging ideal for nuclear medicine physicians, cardiologists, and radiologists. The updated information contained in this title are vitally important and useful to both trainees and existing practitioners: cardiac imaging techniques and hybrid imaging are advancing and changing so rapidly that concise and pertinent information are absolutely necessary and helpful; all these areas are well addressed in the text. It is hoped that this book will help readers be better equipped for the full understanding and utilization of these fascinating new imaging methods, useful for offering to patients the best treatment options in the third millennium medicine scenario.

Rome, Italy — Francesco Nudi
Rome, Italy — Orazio Schillaci
Latina, Italy — Giuseppe Biondi-Zoccai
Birmingham, AL, USA — Ami E. Iskandrian

Terminology

The following terms will be used within this book:

- The term "multiparametric" is used when multiple imaging parameters from one modality are acquired within the same examination. As an example, coronary CT angiography and dynamic stress CT perfusion can be acquired within a single examination on the same CT scanner.
- The word "multimodal" refers to different imaging modalities that are combined for a common diagnostic purpose. For instance, coronary CT angiography and cardiac MRI stress perfusion are acquired in two independent examinations but assess complementary diagnostic aspects of the same pathology in the same patient (i.e., coronary artery disease).
- "Hybrid" imaging describes the possibility to acquire two different modalities at the same time and in the same scanner. This technique is often used in nuclear imaging, i.e., by combining CT with single-photon emission tomography or CT with positron emission tomography. In a wider sense, some authors also use the term as a synonym for "multimodal" imaging.
- Image "fusion" refers to postprocessing techniques that fuse image data from different modalities and/or parameters into one common image by means of co-registration and subsequent two-dimensional overlay or three-dimensional rendering.

Contents

Part I Specialists' Perspectives to Hybrid Cardiac Imaging

1 **Hybrid Cardiac Imaging for the Clinical Cardiologist** 3
Samia Massalha and Ora Israel

2 **Hybrid Cardiac Imaging for the Cardiologist with Expertise in Echocardiography** 29
Eugenio Picano and Paul Leeson

3 **Hybrid Cardiac Imaging for the Specialist with Expertise in Cardiac Magnetic Resonance** 39
Jannike Nickander and Martin Ugander

4 **Hybrid Imaging Using Single Photon Emission Computed Tomography** 55
G. Ross Farris, Ami E. Iskandrian, Fadi G. Hage, and Pradeep Bhambhvani

5 **Hybrid Cardiac Imaging for the Specialist with Expertise in Computed Tomography** 75
Jochen von Spiczak, Robert Manka, and Hatem Alkadhi

6 **Hybrid Cardiac Imaging for the Invasive Cardiologist** 93
Enrico Romagnoli, Francesco Burzotta, Cristina Aurigemma, and Carlo Trani

7 **Hybrid Cardiac Imaging for the Interventional Cardiologist** . . 117
Niya Mileva, Sakura Nagumo, Jeroen Sonck, and Carlos Collet

Part II Hybrid Imaging in Clinical Practice

8 **Systematic Review of Hybrid Cardiac Imaging** 131
Susanna Breviario, Davide Tore, Ovidio De Filippo, Gaetano Maria De Ferrari, Paolo Fonio, Fabrizio D'Ascenzo, and Alessandro Depaoli

9 **Hybrid Cardiac Viability Assessment** 147
Kenji Fukushima and Michinobu Nagao

10 Hybrid Cardiac Imaging in Clinical Practice: From Diagnosis to Prognosis and Management 173
Cigdem Akincioglu and Saurabh Malhotra

11 Clinical Cases of Hybrid Cardiac Imaging 191
Kenji Fukushima and Michinobu Nagao

12 Hybrid Cardiac Imaging: The Role of Machine Learning and Artificial Intelligence 203
Jan-Walter Benjamins, Ming Wai Yeung, Alvaro E. Reyes-Quintero, Bram Ruijsink, Pim van der Harst, and Luis Eduardo Juarez-Orozco

Introduction

Hybrid imaging was born with the goal of becoming the cornerstone of diagnostic tests for primary and secondary prevention in the different stages of coronary heart disease: from the onset to the progression, to the fearful complications.

The opportunity for imaging experts is to broaden their skills and bring the diagnostic exam closer to the clinical setting, using algorithms that integrate in first place the variables of the patient's clinical history with the result of the diagnostic test and subsequently the result of the exam with the prognosis and therefore the therapeutic choice. The evolution of technology and computing power that has become available in recent years will increasingly integrate the benefits of processes that use expert systems, artificial intelligence, and machine learning with the aim of supporting the interpretative and decision-making process of the medical doctor (Fig. 1).

The best approach is the preliminary understanding of the clinical-anamnestic context in which the hybrid examination is performed. The more complete and detailed the group to which a patient belongs, using clinical and diagnostic variables, the more precise the "starting prognosis" and the homogeneity of the patients with respect to the events will be. An example of this methodology is the warranty period, i.e., foreseeing a temporal phase of clinical stability. It has been widely shown that, within the same results of a diagnostic test, the clinical variables, even age alone or a single cardiovascular risk factor, can determine different warranty periods.

And it is also common knowledge nowadays, as further confirmation, that in important trials, such as Courage, the use of multiple diagnostic variables, in the latter case myocardial perfusion, substantially changed the results regarding the prognostic benefit between Revascularization Therapy and Optimal Medical Therapy (Fig. 2).

The promise of hybrid imaging is also to be less dependent on the anatomical–functional examinations used, precisely because the acquisition of a "double" result, coupled with the specific experience of a center, will compensate for any limitations of the single examination and the qualitative differences of the available equipment, keeping in mind that more recent technologies allow a dramatic decrease in radiation absorbed dose (Fig. 3). Each center will therefore decide, based on its own procedures and organization, which information, anatomical or functional, to acquire first.

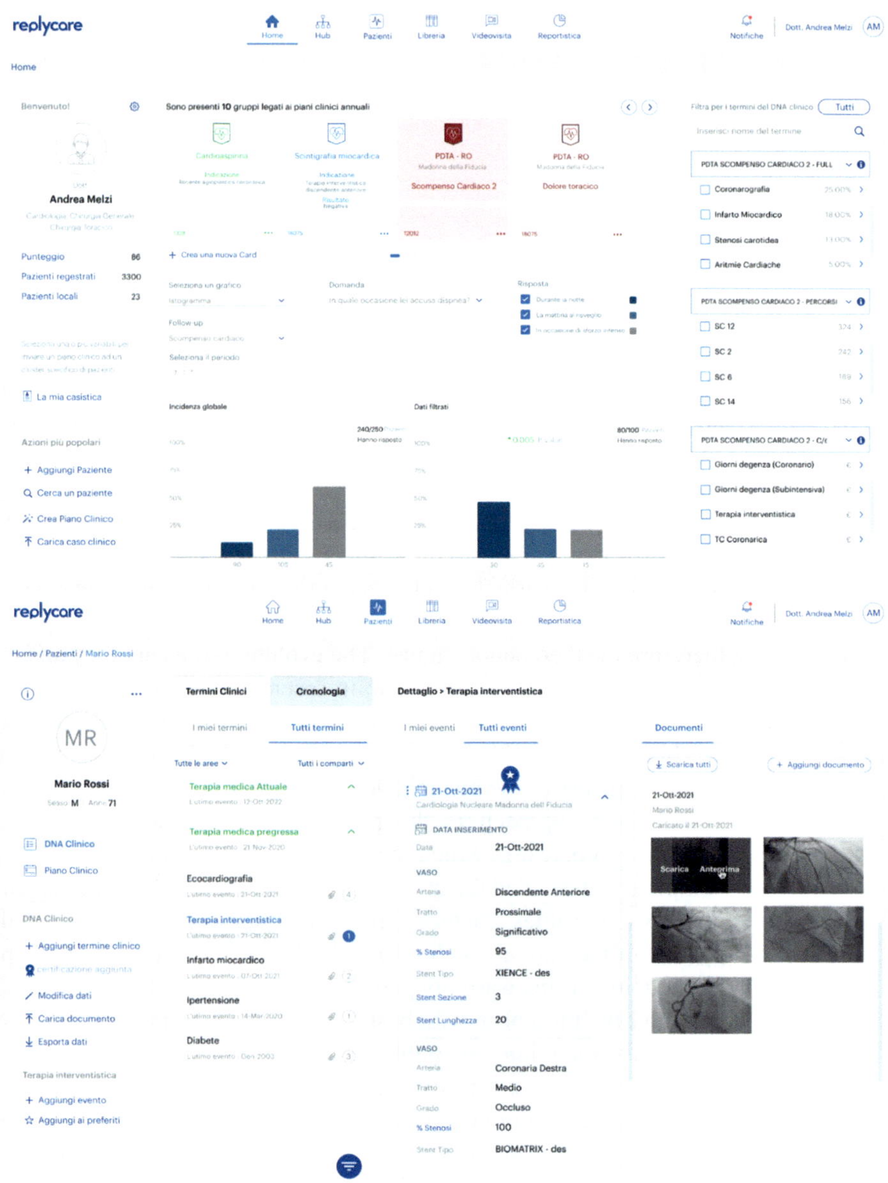

Fig. 1 Leveraging artificial intelligence to improve medical decision-making

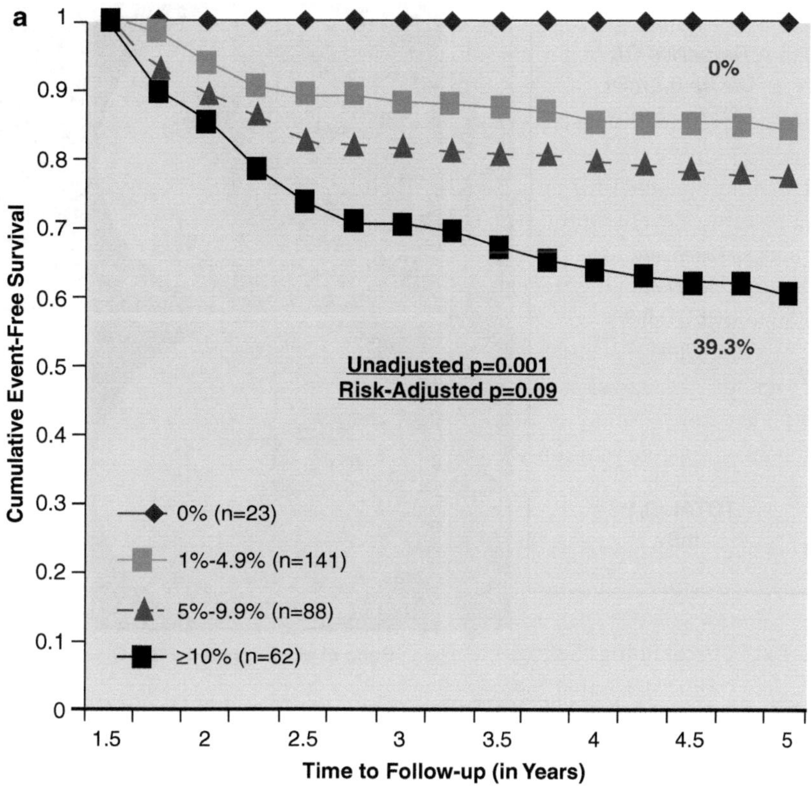

Fig. 2 Optimal medical therapy with or without percutaneous coronary intervention to reduce ischemic burden (Shaw et al.—Circulation 2008)

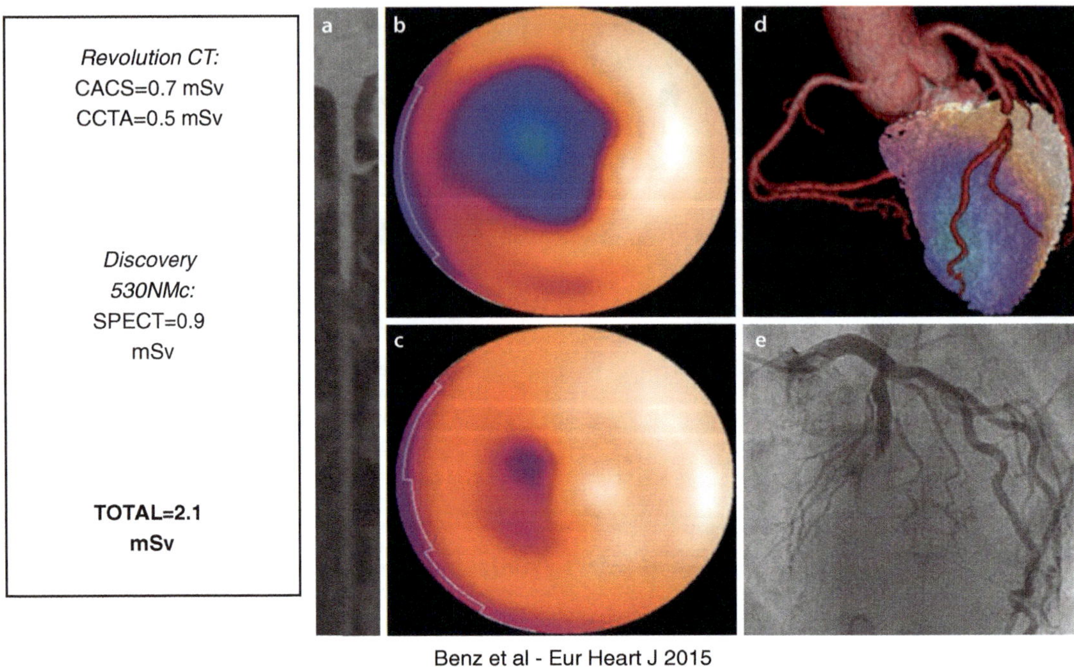

Fig. 3 Promise of hybrid SPECT/CT (Benz et al.—Eur Heart J 2015). (**a**) CT Scan angiography. (**b**, **c**) Stress rest perfusion SPECT. (**d**) 3D rendering of CT Scan angiography.(**e**) coronary angiography

Definition of Hybrid Imaging

Hybrid imaging in its most essential definition is the representation in a single image of anatomical (CT Angiography) and functional (SPET, PET, ECHO, CT, MNR) data. Currently, this definition finds concrete application in oncological imaging, but the situation is somehow different in cardiological imaging where it is not essential to have actually integrated images, but it is perfectly adequate to have them "side by side." Indeed, the CT images that are used for fusion, using a dedicated software, are often incomplete and not the most detailed. The exams, anatomical and functional, must necessarily be performed in different time phases as the preparation protocol is different for the two exams, in particular as regarding beta blockers, that have to be suspended for the functional exam and to be at full dose for the anatomical one.

An important aspect is the relationship between the coronary vessels and the myocardial regions. The correlation is high for the left descending anterior artery: if an alteration of a functional variable is detected in any anterior-septal-apical region, the direct involvement of the left descending anterior artery is remarkably granted. Instead, a more or less extensive alteration in the infero-postero-lateral region may depend on a stenosis affecting the circumflex or right coronary artery based on the quality of the native vessels and their dominance. In these cases, an anatomical-functional analysis allows the physician to cross-check and control this variable (Fig. 4). In fact, knowing the coronary anatomy of the individual patient, the relationship between the site of the stenosis and the dependent myocardial region is almost always possible; this fact has allowed us to combine since a long time, in our mind, the data of an invasive coronary angiography with the results of the functional examination.

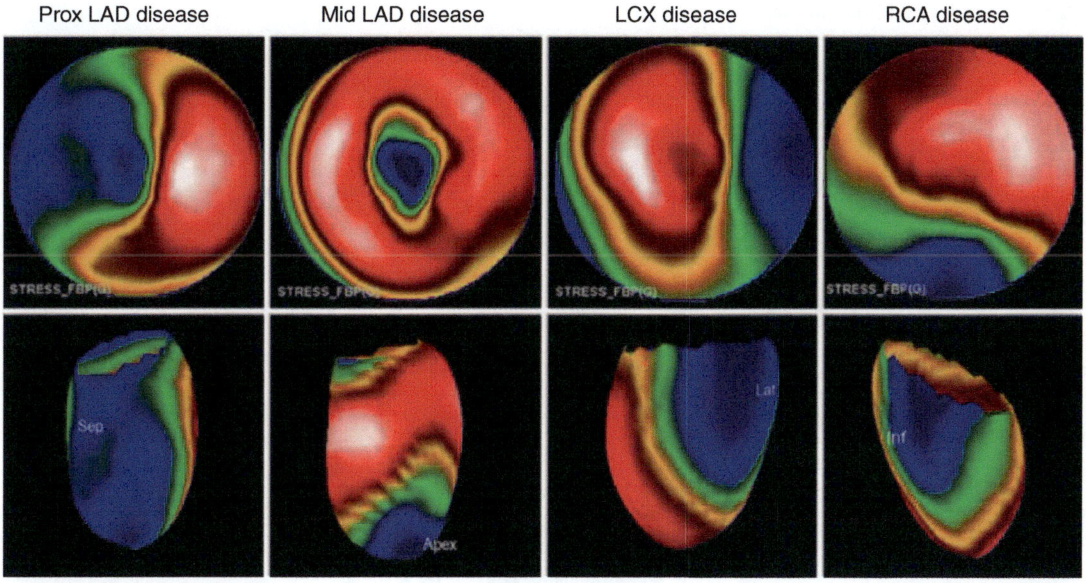

Fig. 4 SPECT imaging: a novel and clinically relevant segmentation approach (Nudi F, et al.—J Nucl Cardiol 2014)

Anatomical Imaging

At present for noninvasive evaluation of coronary arteries, both in the literature and in clinical practice, CT scan is the standard, while waiting for the MRI to possibly improve. CT scan has been used for years to correct the attenuation allowing to differentiate artifacts from real lesions. Furthermore, the usefulness of the Agatston calcium score for risk stratification, low (<100), intermediate (101–399), high (≥400), is widely demonstrated.

Nowadays, the technological advancements grant images with high spatial and temporal resolution, with an increasing reliability in term of quantification of the stenosis. In addition, more recently, CT itself provides functional information on myocardial stenosis and perfusion.

In some studies, CT scan has been compared to invasive coronary angiography, confirming the low correlation index between coronary stenosis (anatomical data), on the one hand and myocardial ischemia (functional data), on the other. Assuming a good relationship between noninvasive and invasive angiographic anatomical data, given the same stenosis (even significant ones), FFR and CFR may be, to varying degrees, reduced or completely normal (Fig. 5).

This finding depends on a set of factors that affect coronary resistance in the epicardial tract and/or in the microcirculation: anatomical aspects such as the site, the diameter and the length of the stenosis, the presence of in series stenosis, an intra-myocardial bridge, as well as the vasomotor tone, a compensatory remodeling of the plaque, and the collateral circulation. Furthermore, even in the presence of normal epicardial vessels, myocardial ischemia may be present due to alterations that can affect the microcircula-

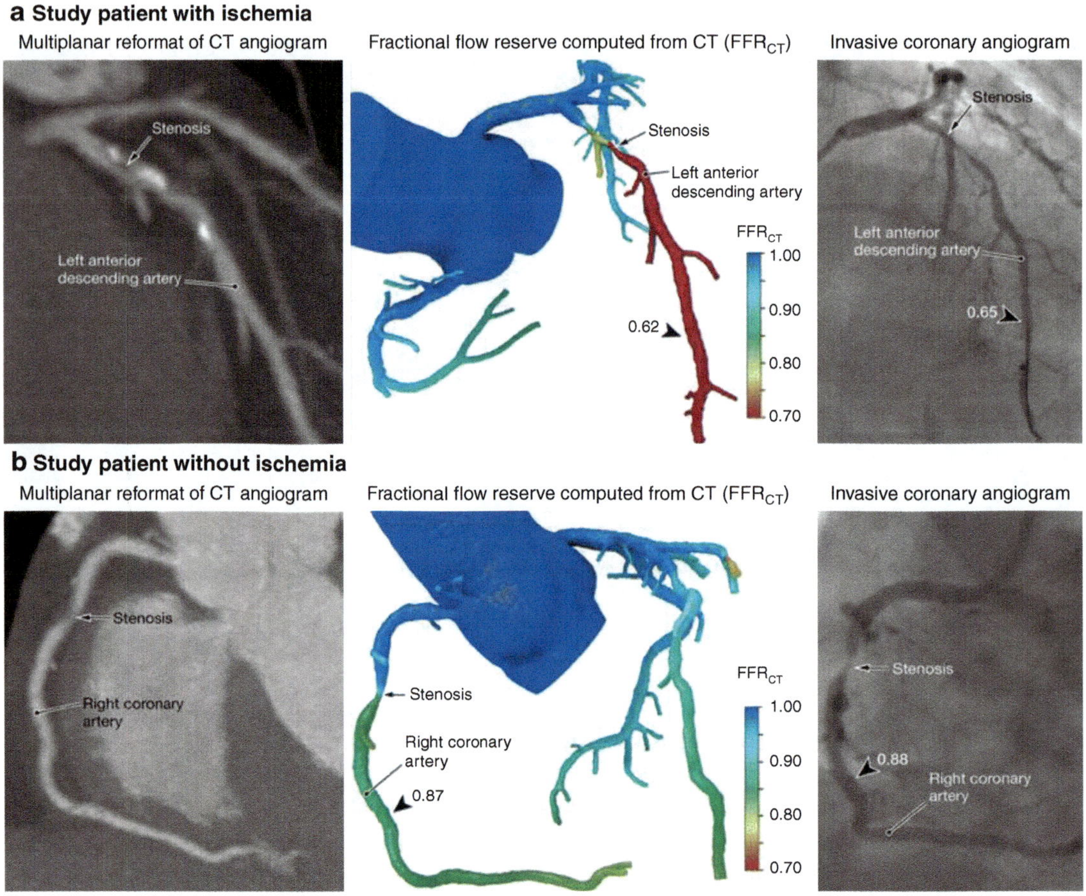

Fig. 5 Diagnostic accuracy of fractional flow reserve from anatomic CT angiography (Min JK et al.—J Am Med Assoc 2012)

tion. These include spasm, arteriolar remodeling, reduced capillary density as well as structural and/or functional coronary microvascular dysfunction, which interferes in the regulation of resistance in small vessels.

Functional Imaging

The functional data is acquired with different parameters in relation to the examination carried out, and its main advantage is that it allows a simple and accurate measurement of the effect of the possible pathophysiological alterations described above on tissue perfusion, with a high negative predictive value (VPN). The functional data has its main limit in the presence of a negative result that does not differentiate the various underlying anatomical pictures, from normal coronary arteries to the presence of an initial disease, from moderate to significant stenosis up to the occluded vessel. In all these cases, the patient cluster would be imprecise and so would the warranty period and the optimal therapeutic choice.

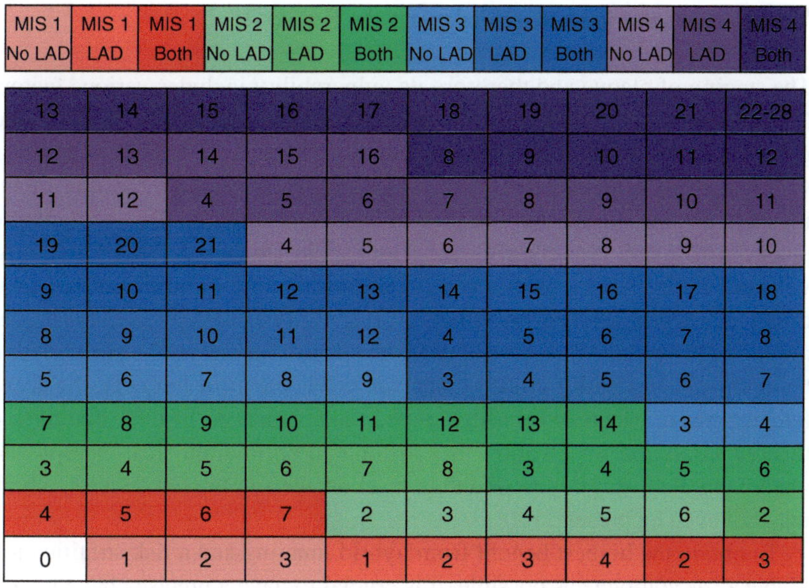

Fig. 6 Vessel-related ischemia (VRI) (Nudi F et al.—J Nucl Cardiol 2015)

A lesser yet significant problem is the possibility of underestimating the extent of multivessel coronary artery disease in cases of balanced ischemia or the degree of ischemia when using relative perfusion parameters. The study of exertional contractility and the possibility of quantitatively measuring the coronary flow (absolute myocardial blood flow expressed in mL/g/min) with PET or SPET using CZT (Calcium Zinc Telluride) technology, allow to overcome the limit described, making this test particularly advantageous in term of cost/effectiveness. The functional study also includes the identification of residual viable myocardium downstream of a stenosis with the double advantage of identifying the patient at greater risk of events when a significant share of viable myocardium is present and simultaneously in whom revascularization therapy is required. On the contrary, even in the presence of reduced ventricular function, the absence of viable myocardium contraindicates revascularization therapy, as the spontaneous adverse events would also add to the procedural ones. Another aspect to take into account is the score utilized for the evaluation of the functional data when measured with semi-quantitative parameters: hybrid imaging facilitates the identification of specific clusters with respect to the degree of regional ischemia and the coronary vessel on which it depends. Currently, the scores implemented to quantify myocardial ischemia use a rough percentage value of a total, not differentiating, for example, a mild and extensive ischemia from a severe ischemia that affects a few regions, as the score might end up being the same in both cases (Fig. 6).

Vulnerable Plaque and Vulnerable Patient

The staging of plaque and therefore its vulnerability includes various factors (fibrous cap, lipids, activated inflammatory cells, production of cytokines and growth factors, activation of macrophages). The role of hybrid imaging is very promising both in the study of inflammation, thanks to molecular imaging, and in the automated analysis of plaque using CT. The non-calcific plaque with a radiodensity <30 HU (Hounsfield Unit) is definitely the most vulnerable. The risk of plaque complications increases significantly in relation to the degree of stenosis. However, it should be considered at the epidemiological level (and therefore in terms of clinical impact on the patient), that being the plaques with a grade of stenosis <50% the most frequent, the absolute number of events is very high even in this situation (Fig. 7). Identifying this risk condition would allow establishing an optimal medical therapy and a more targeted warranty period than just considering the risk factors, which may not even be present.

To obtain the highest benefit from hybrid imaging and a risk stratification (Table 1) as complete as possible, it is crucial to have a precise characterization of the individual patient and even more important the definition of the belonging cluster. A two-step approach might be warranted (Fig. 8). The first objective is to assess the pre-test probability and in this regard the variables to be used include risk factors, symptoms, current and previous therapies, geometry parameters, and ventricular function, including contractile reserve and possible dyssynchrony. The second step is determining a reliable post-test probability, taking into account an exercise electrocardiogram, associated cardiac and vascular diseases and recent or previous myocardial infarction. Regarding this last aspect, if present, it would be necessary to acquire resid-

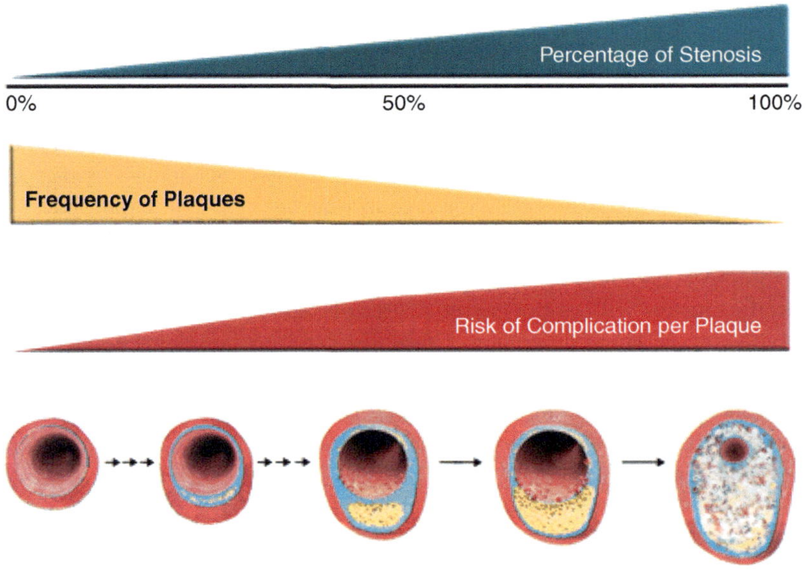

Fig. 7 From vulnerable plaque to vulnerable patient (Naghavi et al.—Circulation 2003)

Table 1 Patel et al. JACC 2017—AUC for coronary revascularization in patients with SHID

Noninvasive Risk Stratification
High risk (>3% annual death or MI)
1. Severe resting LV dysfunction (LVEF <35%) not readily explained by noncoronary causes
2. Resting perfusion abnormalities ≥10% of the myocardium in patients without prior history or evidence of MI
3. Stress ECG findings including ≥2 mm of ST-segment depression at low workload or persisting into recovery, exercise-induced ST-segment elevation, or exercise-induced VT/VF
4. Severe stress-induced LV dysfunction (peak exercise LVEF <45% or drop in LVEF with stress ≥10%)
5. Stress-induced perfusion abnormalities encumbering ≥10% myocardium or stress segmental scores indicating multiple vascular territories with abnormalities
6. Stress-induced LV dilation
7. Inducible wall motion abnormality (involving >2 segments or 2 coronary beds)
8. Wall motion abnormality developing at low dose of dobutamine (≤10 mg/kg/min) or at a low heart rate (<120 beats/min)
9. CAC score >400 Agatston units
10. Multivessel obstructive CAD (≥70% stenosis) or left main stenosis (≥50% stenosis) on CCTA
Intermediate risk (1% to 3% annual death or MI)
1. Mild/moderate resting LV dysfunction (LVEF 35% to 49%) not readily explained by noncoronary causes
2. Resting perfusion abnormalities in 5% to 9.9% of the myocardium in patients without a history or prior evidence of MI
3. ≥1 mm of ST-segment depression occurring with exertional symptoms
4. Stress-induced perfusion abnormalities encumbering 5% to 9.9% of the myocardium or stress segmental scores (in multiple segments) indicating 1 vascular territory with abnormalities but without LV dilation
5. Small wall motion abnormality involving 1 to 2 segments and only 1 coronary bed
6. CAC score 100 to 399 Agatston units
7. One vessel CAD with ≥70% stenosis or moderate CAD stenosis (50% to 69% stenosis) in ≥2 arteries on CCTA
Low risk (<1% annual death or MI)
1. Low-risk treadmill score (score ≥5) or no new ST segment changes or exercise-induced chest pain symptoms; when achieving maximal levels of exercise
2. Normal or small myocardial perfusion defect at rest or with stress encumbering <5% of the myocardium*
3. Normal stress or no change of limited resting wall motion abnormalities during stress
4. CAC score <100 Agaston units
5. No coronary stenosis >50% on CCTA

*Although the published data are limited; patients with these findings will probably not be at low risk in the presence of either a high-risk treadmill score or severe resting LV dysfunction (LVEF <35%).
Reproduced from Fihn et al. (3).

CAC indicates coronary artery calcium; CAD, coronary artery disease; CCTA, coronary computed tomography angiography; LV, left ventricular; LVEF, left ventricular ejection fraction; and MI, myocardial infarction.

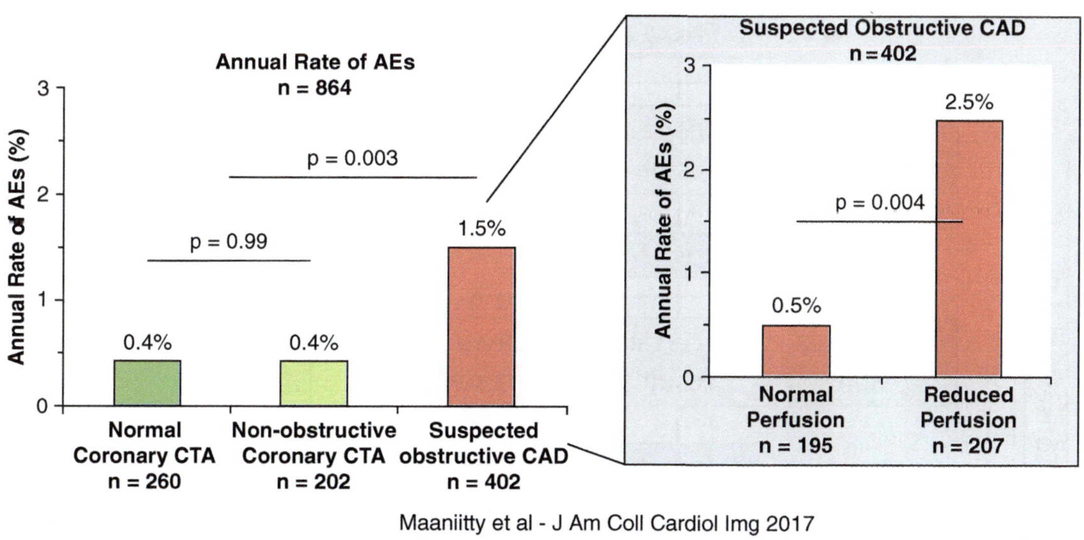

Fig. 8 CT followed by selective PET (Maaniitty et al.—J Am Coll Cardiol Img 2017)

ual viability parameters to be associated with the myocardial regions downstream of the detected stenosis. Even better, when possible, is the regional association of adrenergic imaging with vitality and stenosis, due to the possible presence of a dysinnervation or denervation.

Conclusions

Hybrid anatomical-functional imaging is an ideal combination as the advantages of one exam mutually overcome the limits of the other exam. When coronary artery disease is present, the role of functional examination is important for the modest positive predictive value of CT, a fact already received by the guidelines for which it is necessary to document the presence of myocardial ischemia and viability downstream of a stenosis for a correct indication to myocardial revascularization therapy. When functional data is normal, the role of CT is decisive in identifying the possible presence of coronary heart disease that would require specific medical therapy and/or an increase of monitoring frequency (Figs. 9 and 10).

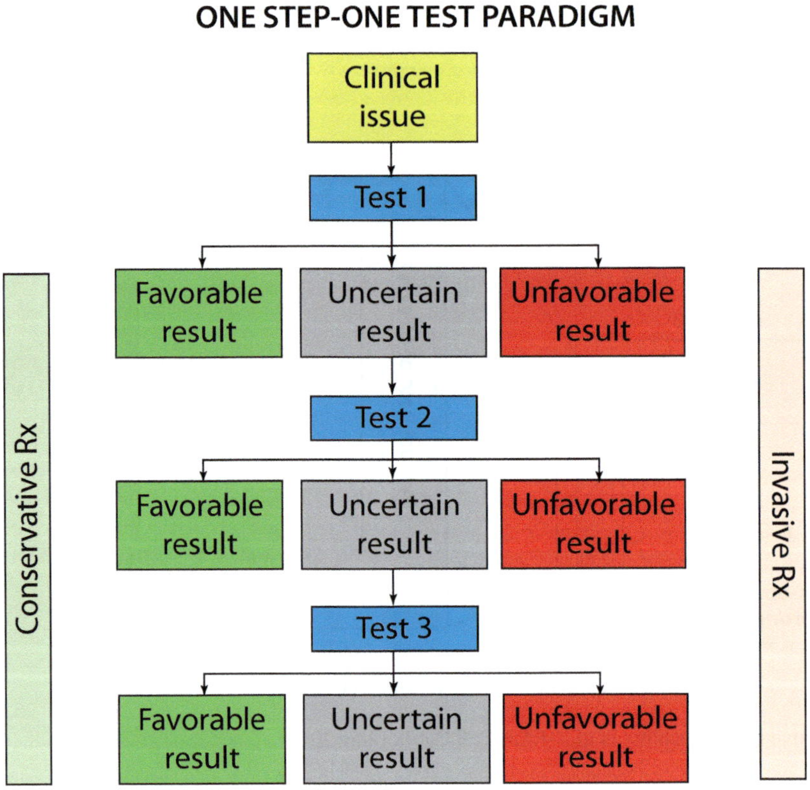

Fig. 9 Traditional diagnostic paradigm (Nudi et al.—J Nucl Cardiol 2019)

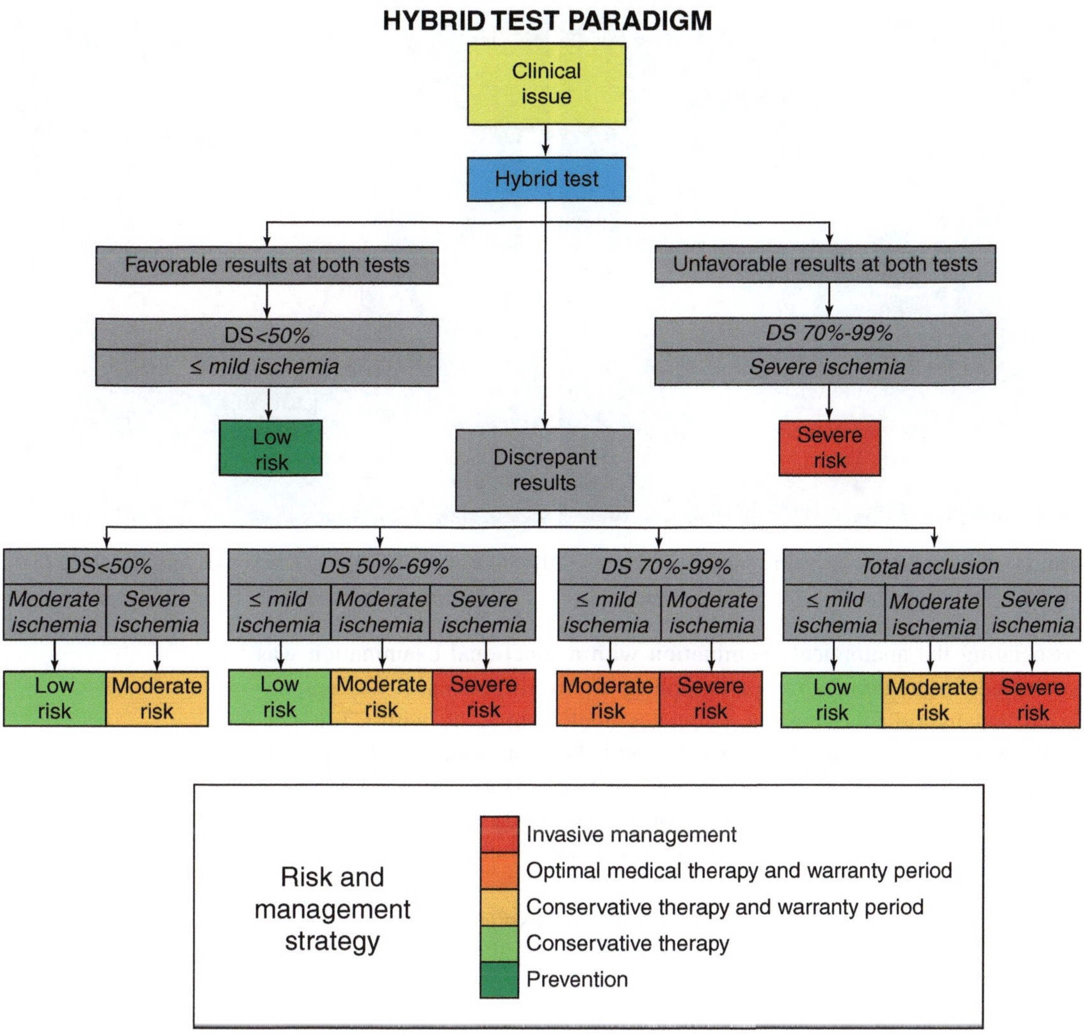

Fig. 10 Hybrid cardiac imaging diagnostic paradigm (Nudi et al.—J Nucl Cardiol 2019)

The possibility of recognizing the patient with normal coronary arteries but with alterations of the functional data is potentially interesting too. The result of this examination completes the cluster enriching it with key details for choosing the proper clinical path.

The gold standard for assessing the extent of the benefit, once straight coronary angiographic stenosis, is evolving towards a more comprehensive clinical evaluation that takes into consideration in particular major events, unexpected soft events, and quality of life.

In the recent recommendations on noninvasive imaging in coronary syndromes by the European Association of Cardiovascular Imaging and the American Society of Echocardiography, in collaboration with the American Society of Nuclear Cardiology, Society of Cardiovascular Computed Tomography, and Society for Cardiovascular Magnetic Resonance (Fig. 11), the role of diagnostic tests used in isolation, as a single examination, or by

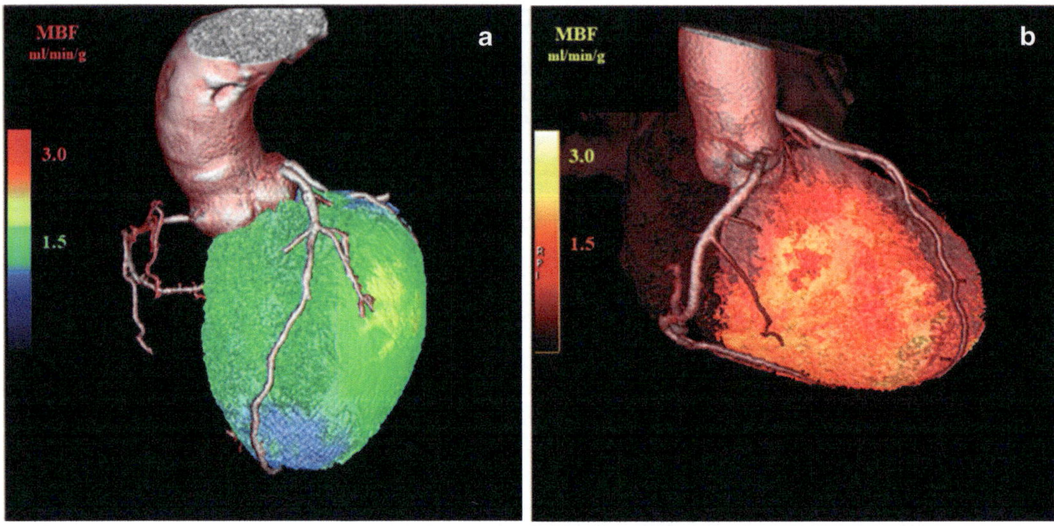

Fig. 11 Non-invasive imaging in coronary syndromes (Edvardsen et al., Eur Heart J Cardiovasc Imaging. 2022 Jan)

associating the anatomical examination with a functional examination was evaluated. In the concluding paragraph on future directions, it was emphasized that hybrid imaging that associates nuclear imaging with CT is currently the exam with the highest value and the best prospects. In the near future the study of stenosis and ischemia, CT or NMR imaging of coronary plaque morphology and nuclear imaging of metabolic or inflammatory processes may be added, perhaps with the prospect of integrating the tests and generating a single comprehensive report.

The chapters of the volume will outline and explain many of the cited aspects.

Service of Hybrid Cardio Imaging
Madonna della Fiducia Clinic,
Rome, Italy

Francesco Nudi

Part I

Specialists' Perspectives to Hybrid Cardiac Imaging

1 Hybrid Cardiac Imaging for the Clinical Cardiologist

Samia Massalha and Ora Israel

1.1 Coronary Artery Disease

Coronary artery disease (CAD) is the leading cause of death in developed countries. An estimated 20.1 million Americans above the age of 20 have CAD. Approximately every second american will have an acute myocardial infarction (AMI) with an estimated 605,000 new and 200,000 recurrent events each year [1]. As such the diagnosis, risk stratification, and adequate management of CAD is crucial.

Noninvasive testing for the presence or absence of CAD has been the focus of research over the last decades. The CCTA technology has evolved to high-resolution, multi-slice detector dual-source technology. CCTA can identify and differentiate high-risk vulnerable plaques versus low-risk plaques according to features such as their shape, the presence or absence of a "napkin ring," of positive remodeling, or spotty calcification. There has been also fast development and improvement in both hardware and software in the field of nuclear cardiology aiming to identify hemodynamically significant CAD.

While CCTA is superior with its negative predictive value (NPV) that exceeds 99% [2], it has limitations in the presence of severe coronary calcification or previously known severe CAD, whether post stenting or post coronary artery bypass grafting (CABG). These limitations arise due to artifacts attributed to metal and calcification such as beam hardening and partial volume effect in addition to blooming artifacts. While the major goal of evaluating patients after CABG with CCTA is to evaluate the patency of grafts, many reports will end up only mentioning a severe disease in the native coronary arteries.

Cardiac MRI and CT perfusion tests are not used routinely, being performed mostly in large academic centers for research purposes. The most widely used myocardial perfusion imaging tests are SPECT and PET. These technologies are based on the relative regional differences in radiotracer uptake determined by the coronary flow to that specific territory. As compared to SPECT, PET adds information to our understanding of physiological and pathophysiological cardiovascular conditions. Beyond its ability to assess for ischemia PET surpasses SPECT with its diagnostic accuracy in detecting hemodynamically significant obstructive CAD. The factors

Dr. Samia Massalha has no conflict of interest. Dr. Ora Israel is a consultant for General Electric Healthcare.

S. Massalha (✉)
Department of Nuclear Medicine, Haifa, Israel

Department of Non-invasive Cardiology, Rambam Health Care Campus, Haifa, Israel
e-mail: S_massalha@rambam.health.gov.il

O. Israel
Rappaport School of Medicine, Technion—Israel Institute of Technology, Haifa, Israel
e-mail: O_israel@rambam.health.gov.il

F. Nudi et al. (eds.), *Hybrid Cardiac Imaging for Clinical Decision-Making*,
https://doi.org/10.1007/978-3-030-99391-7_1

responsible for the better performance of PET are its higher spatial resolution and the better extraction fraction of PET radiotracers. In addition, PET has the ability to quantify the absolute myocardial perfusion rather than relative, as well as the coronary flow reserve. While SPECT quantitation of myocardial flow reserve (MFR) is a new tool mainly used at present for research, it might be available for clinical use in the near future. Additional strength of PET is its ability to visualize and quantify disease processes such as inflammation, innervation, and metabolism at molecular levels.

The above mentioned cardiac imaging modalities have common features and can provide similar information. However, they also vary in some complementary features. If two modalities are combined, the clinical evaluation will benefit from additional information provided by this new tool with incremental value in the assessment of different entities.

Myocardial perfusion imaging (MPI) including single-photon emission computed tomography (SPECT) and positron emission tomography (PET), and computed tomography (CT) are well-established noninvasive modalities for the investigation, prognostication, and management of patients with known or suspected CAD. These technologies provide both anatomical—degree of stenosis, plaque characterization, and quantification, as well as functional information regarding the hemodynamic significance of a presumed atherosclerotic plaque. Using these imaging techniques in a multimodality, hybrid mode, SPECT/CT and PET/CT results in high diagnostic accuracy and robust prognostic stratification.

Hybrid SPECT/CT and PET/CT technologies use attenuation correction (AC) algorithms from the CT component for post-processing to improve the image quality and diagnostic accuracy. Not all annihilated photons or positrons are detected by the SPECT or PET respectively since they are absorbed by different tissues in the body thus leading to attenuation. This process differs, of course, according to the tissue density. If attenuation is not corrected during post-processing it can cause significant artifacts leading to misdiagnosis. The use of a low dose CT scan can correct such attenuation, furthermore improving the diagnostic accuracy of CAD, mainly by a significant improvement in specificity, which increases from 73% in non-AC studies to 81% with AC [3].

The CT component performed for AC can also provide measurements of calcium scoring (CAS) as an add-on to the cardiac SPECT and PET perfusion studies. CAS increases the certainty of the CAD diagnosis. A high CAS in cases with normal MPI has been reported to shift management of the patient to a preventive medicine path since it is highly predictive of risk [4]. CAS provides an index of the plaque burden and as such the presence of subclinical atherosclerosis and will thus help identify asymptomatic individuals at high risk for the development of CAD [5]. This can encourage patients to adopt a healthier lifestyle and the clinicians to prescribe statins for primary prevention. In patients with equivocal MPI studies, the use of CAS can help by providing a final report with more clarity and certainty. A CAS of zero increases the certainty of differentiating between a potentially artifactual finding versus a true perfusion defect. On the other hand, in cases with near normal MPI in the presence of severe coronary artery calcifications, the report should discuss potential underestimation of the amount of perfusion defects and the presence of multivessel disease, especially when combined with other features of the MPI such as the decrease of the left ventricular ejection fraction (LVEF) at stress as compared to rest, and/or the development of regional wall motion at stress.

A low dose CT component of cardiac SPECT/CT or PET/CT also carries great importance for the detection of chest pain due to etiologies other than CAD. CT performed for AC can detect incidental findings (Fig. 1.1a–d).

In its early stages, hybrid imaging was limited by the increased exposure to ionizing radiation. However, the advancement of cardiac imaging technologies, both at the level of hardware and software, adapting newer scanning protocols when performing CCTA, such as prospective acquisition and a high pitch mode, in addition to the introduction of iterative reconstruction for

a

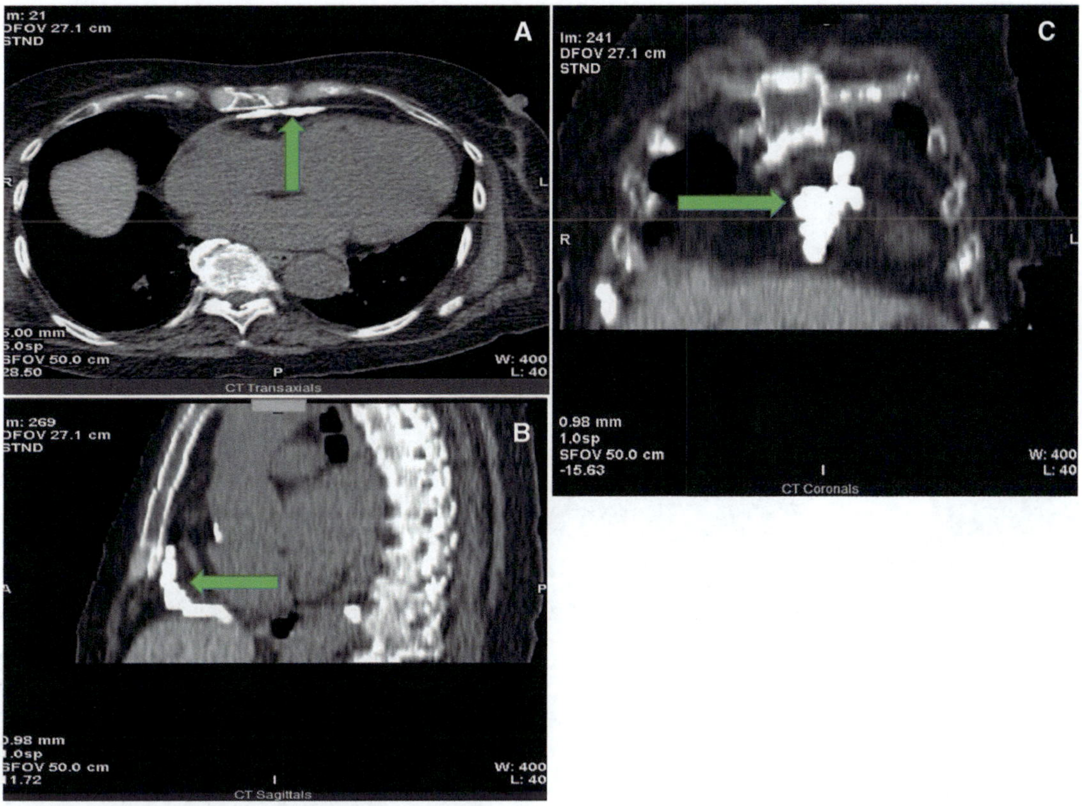

Fig. 1.1 (**a**) A 68-year-old female patient with diabetes, hypertension, and hyperlipidemia was admitted to the hospital due to recurrent chest pain and shortness of breath. A SPECT MPI was ordered and performed to rule out ischemia. The perfusion scan was normal however on the CT portion of the study that is performed for attenuation correction a significant pericardial calcification was noted and represents recurrent pericarditis. (A) Trans-axial view of CT at the level of the heart showing a four chamber view with pericardial calcifications close to the RV free wall. (B) Coronal view of the CT showing severe pericardial calcification close to the apex. (C) Sagittal view of the CT showing the same severe calcification. (**b**) A 57-year-old male patient referred for investigation of chest pain and an electrocardiographically positive exercise test. A, B, and C show a trans-axial, sagittal, and coronal views of the low dose attenuation correction CT portion of the SPECT perfusion study. The images show a significantly dilated esophagus. Further testing revealed achalasia. The myocardial perfusion study was negative for ischemia. (**c**) A 63-year-old male patient admitted to the hospital due to shortness of breath and mild elevation of troponin levels. Referred to rule out myocardial ischemia. SPECT perfusion study was negative for ischemia; however, the attenuation correction CT showed a severely dilated main pulmonary artery, further investigation with an echocardiogram revealed severe pulmonary hypertension. (**d**) A 63-year-old female patient with multiple risk factors including cigarette smoking was referred for investigation for chest pain and shortness of breath. A, B, and C are Trans-axial, coronal, and sagittal views of the lung from the CT for attenuation correction of the MPI. The arrow is pointed to an incidental finding of a mass in the right upper lung. Further evaluation was recommended and the referring physician was contacted and informed of the finding. D Trans-axial view of a high-resolution CT, the arrow points to the same finding. Biopsy from this mass revealed an adenocarcinoma of the lung

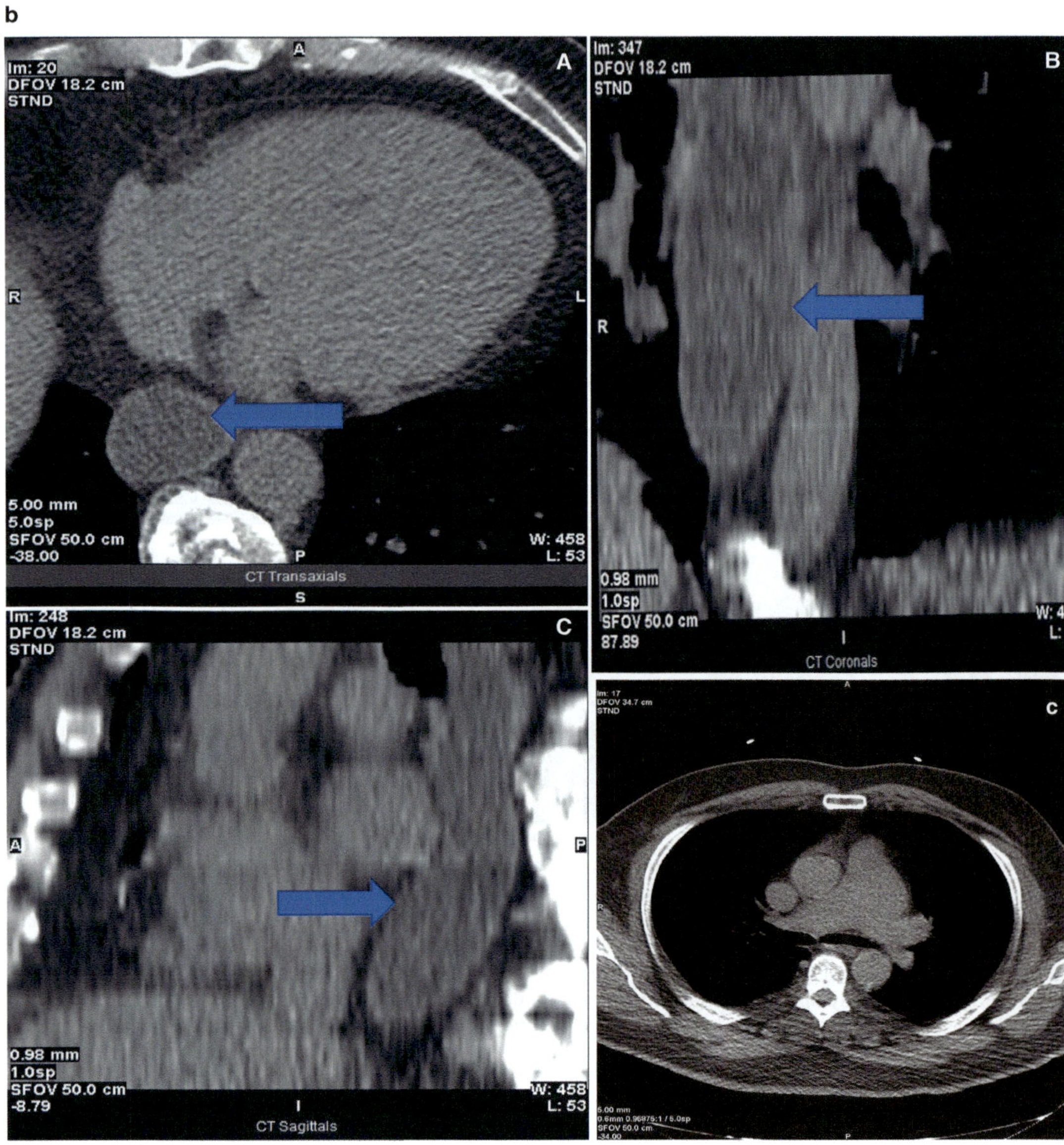

Fig. 1.1 (continued)

d

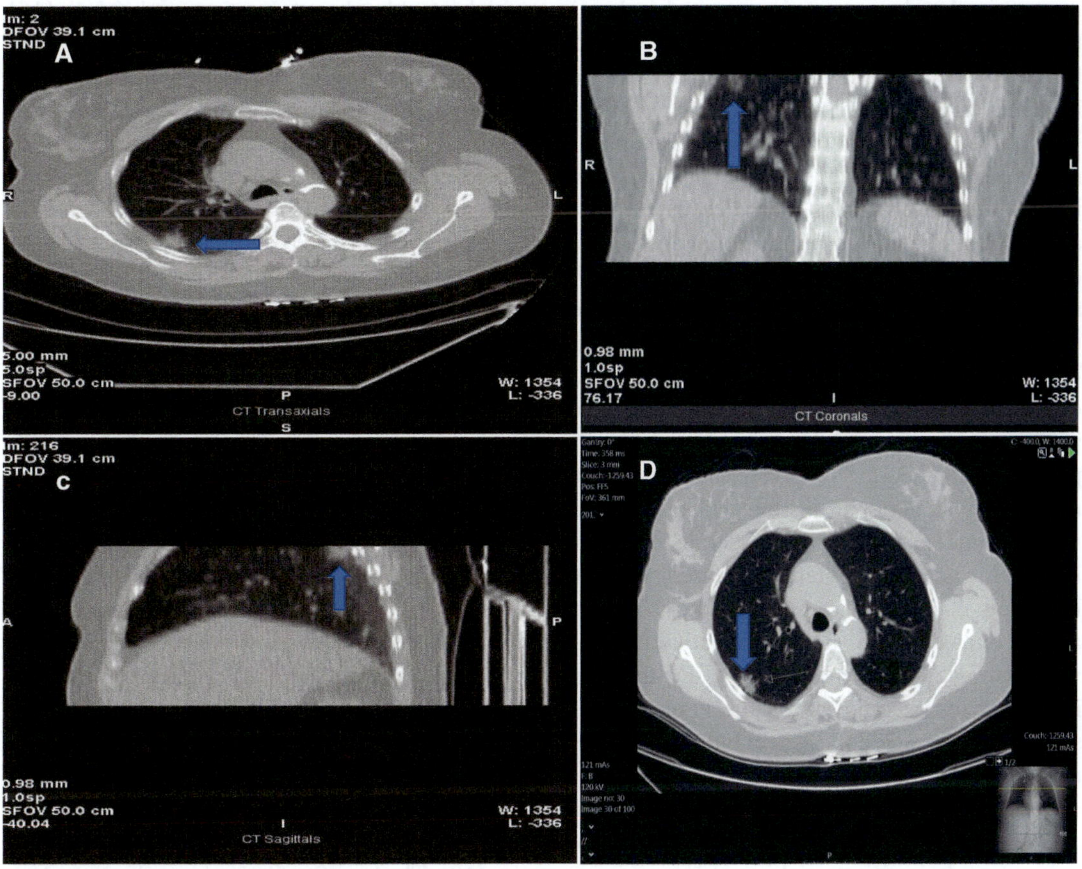

Fig. 1.1 (continued)

post-processing of data, have led to a significant decrease in patients exposure to ionizing radiation.

The use of hybrid imaging should be directed towards compensating for the stand-alone modality's weak points. The additional value of using hybrid SPECT/CCTA was investigated when the gold standard was not only invasive coronary angiography but also the fractional flow reserve (FFR) value and revealed an improved diagnostic performance when compared to each modality alone. The positive predictive value (PPV) of SPECT, 85%, and CCTA, 77%, significantly rose to 96% for the SPECT/CCTA analysis. In addition, the NPV of SPECT, 89%, improved to 95% with SPECT/CCTA [6]. Hybrid analysis of SPECT/CCTA and PET/CCTA is performed using an optimized alignment tool, allowing projection of the MPS image on the left ventricular epicardial surface obtained from the CCTA, allowing a panoramic view of the coronary artery tree projected onto the left ventricular myocardial perfusion territories.

The main objectives of therapies for stable ischemic heart disease are to alleviate symptoms, achieved via improvement of myocardial blood flow (MBF) and/or reduction in myocardial oxygen demand, in addition to prolonging life. Both optimal medical therapy (OMT) and revascularization approaches are clearly effective in relieving symptoms. Until recently, management of CAD was largely dictated by symptoms and by the presence or absence of obstructive disease detected by an anatomical imaging modality. Over the last two decades, multiple large randomized clinical trials compared optimal medical therapy versus revascularization for the treatment of CAD. None of the studies showed long-term benefit of revascularization over optimal medical therapy in the absence of documented ischemia by functional testing [7–9]. The randomized FAME trial has highlighted the pivotal role of ischemia-targeted revascularization in patients with stable CAD. This study showed that optimal medical therapy in patients with no hemodynamically significant stenosis measured by FFR had an excellent outcome, whereas percutaneous coronary angioplasty (PCI) driven by a positive FFR and optimal medical therapy decreased the rate of urgent revascularization [10]. Furthermore, the ISCHEMIA trial results clearly showed the lack of any superiority in choosing initial revascularization versus optimal medical therapy in the presence of moderate or severe ischemia documented by functional testing [11]. However, symptomatic patients with moderate or severe ischemia who were treated with earlier revascularization had greater improvement in their angina-related health status than patients treated with optimal medical therapy [12]. It is therefore important to not only assess the hemodynamic significance of a stenotic vessel but also to determine the degree of significance.

Documenting myocardial ischemia for management of CAD is already implemented in current revascularization guidelines [13].

The latest results from the ISCHEMIA trial will influence the next updated revascularization guidelines. These data emphasize the importance of interrogating both morphology and function in patients with stable CAD in order to offer the most appropriate treatment strategy hence the incorporation of ischemia evaluation in the current guidelines for revascularization [13]. Although the hemodynamic significance of certain stenosis can be measured by FFR during invasive angiography, this parameter should be also available using noninvasive imaging techniques such as PET/CT and SPECT/CT thus reducing complications and costs. One should keep in mind that FFR was validated by MFR derived from cardiac PET [14]. Cardiac CTA-derived FFR was recently developed using artificial intelligence and algorithms to calculate fluid hemodynamics. This technique is still expensive and time-consuming, especially the need to send the CCTA to a specialized center for processing, which could take at least around 24 h [15]. Treatment driven by functional measurements of coronary stenoses, such as FFR, have been shown to improve outcomes compared to anatomy-guided therapy and medical therapy [16]. However, in high-risk lesions, such as a significant stenosis of the left main or the proximal left anterior descending (LAD) coronary artery, a population excluded from enrolment in the ISCHEMIA trial, both functional and anatomical information are necessary, and this is where hybrid cardiac imaging plays an important role.

Hybrid cardiac imaging increases the diagnostic accuracy when compared to stand-alone technologies and has also an incremental prognostic value [17, 18]. Through spatial co-registration of anatomical and functional information, hybrid imaging may not only improve the diagnostic accuracy of noninvasive CAD assessment but also provide vessel-specific functional information to allow targeted revascularization strategies. This is of great importance especially while there is a disagreement between the severity of the disease, anatomically demonstrated by coronary angiography, and its hemodynamic significance represented by myocardial perfusion abnormalities [19]. The benefit of hybrid imaging was demonstrated in the large multicenter EVINCI study that showed that hybrid imaging prevents errors of standardized left ventricular segments in predicting hemodynamically significant coronary lesions due to the large variability in coronary anatomy. It also proved the reproducibility and feasibility of the co-registration of a three-dimensional CCTA and MPI [20].

Hybrid imaging is of great value in cases with multivessel CAD for planning the treatment of the individual patient, tailoring the revascularization procedure to the hemodynamically significant disease. Luminal stenosis does not necessarily predict the timing or the location of an acute coronary syndrome. Angiography alone lacks the ability to evaluate the functional significance of both 50–75% and 75–90% stenosis [19, 21].

Coronary artery anatomy varies considerably among individuals and may disagree with standardized vascular territories in up to 72% of patients referred to MPI. This is why the standard assumption of the vascular territory of a perfusion defect may be inaccurate [20, 22]. This applies particularly to the inferior and inferolateral walls, territories which traditionally show the largest variability in coronary anatomy. The incremental value of hybrid cardiac imaging resides in the accurate spatial co-localization of myocardial perfusion defects and subtending coronary arteries.

Cardiac PET/MRI has been in use since 2010, either through sequential acquisition or using integrated scanner platforms. Cardiac MRI on its own can provide quantification of cardiac chamber size, global and regional function, and tissue characterization using different sequences, T1, T2, T2*, in order to evaluate for the presence of scar, edema, sedimentation of substrate such as in hemochromatosis and other pathologies. PET/MRI can also detect cardiovascular disease with the advantage of no additional radiation exposure as compared to PET/CT. It can assess anatomy, function, the presence of scars related to previous MI or inflammation, such as myocarditis, and cardiomyopathies of different etiologies. PET/MRI can also provide information about the presence of edema in the acute phase of diseases. Currently, MRI angiography has limitations in the diagnosis of CAD beyond the proximal and mid-segments due to the small vessel caliber. Future advancements using fusion of PET and MR data sets may overcome these hurdles of MR coronary angiography [23].

In the subacute period after MI, the size of the infarct is of major importance for the prediction of outcome. PET/MRI enables the differential diagnosis between myocardial edema, microvascular obstruction, and intra-myocardial hemorrhage, the indicators for reperfusion injury and the infarct size being demonstrated by both late Gadolinium (Gd) enhancement and reduced 18F-fluoro-deoxyglucose (FDG) uptake. The incremental value of PET/MRI was demonstrated in a series of patients in whom segments of the myocardium showing wall motion abnormalities, decreased FDG uptake but no Gd enhancement had only partial improvement after revascularization [24]. Differentiating between reversible and nonreversible myocardial dysfunction determines left ventricular recovery post revascularization.

The main limitation of cardiac PET/MRI studies is the long scanning time of more than an hour. Since both MRI and PET provide some overlapping diagnostic parameters such as perfusion and viability, work in progress aims towards shorter study protocols by potentially reducing the redundancy of duplicate information extracted from both technologies.

Experimental animal studies in rats have explored the potential role of PET/CT in the diagnosis of arterial thrombus stability, which in turn is very important to determine management [25]. Furthermore, the future holds promise for a central role for hybrid cardiac PET/MRI and PET/CT for the diagnosis of arterial plaque, thrombus stabilization, and arterial inflammation, and for the evaluation of plaque vulnerability [26–28].

1.2 Heart Failure

The incidence of heart failure (HF) is high, with more than 800,000 new cases a year being reported in the US. The prevalence of HF could exceed eight million adult cases by the year 2030. By that time projections suggest that there will be a 127% increase in the cost of management of patients with HF, reaching 69.8 billion US$ [1]. Mortality rates attributed to HF after hospitalization at 30-days, 1-year, and 5-years are 10.4%, 22%, and 42.3%, respectively [29]. Evaluating patients with HF with reduced ejection fraction (HFrEF) begins with the assessment of the etiology, whether it is of ischemic or non-ischemic cause, considering that mortality rates of ischemic heart failure reach 80% and 70% for medically managed and surgically treated patients, respectively. Even though mortality rates seem lower among surgically treated patients, early mortality rates, in the first 30 days after surgery, are as high as 8%. Thus, there is a need for careful and thorough evaluation of these patients, including the diagnosis and differentiation between a scar and viable myocardium.

Despite the advancement in treatment strategies for ischemic heart disease, CAD is still the most common cause of HF. The role of revascularization and its benefit in the management of patients with ischemic HF (IHF) with moderate and severe reduction of left ventricular systolic function (LVF), below 35%, has been debated for many years, namely since the emergence of the terms "hibernation," "stunning," and "viability" more than three decades ago. The use of viability imaging relies on the notion that recovery of the LVF compromised due to CAD can be achieved by coronary revascularization. Chronic impairment of myocardial perfusion results in contractile dysfunction, a state referred to as hibernation. Rahimtoola suggested this condition could be treated by revascularization leading to functional recovery [30].

There are two types of viable dysfunctional myocardium, stunned and hibernating myocardium. While stunning occurs when the myocardium is challenged with short episodes of ischemia resulting in dysfunctional segments that do not deteriorate to an MI, hibernation is the result of reduced resting perfusion due to reduction in blood flow following repetitive ischemia with retained glucose metabolic activity. Contractility reduction occurs in both types; however, stunning might recover spontaneously, while on the contrary, hibernation must be treated with revascularization in order to prevent deterioration into a nonviable dysfunctional scar. When evaluating the myocardial viability, the scar-to-viable tissue ratio will eventually determine whether functional recovery of the myocardium is likely to occur if suitable revascularization is performed.

The literature is very rich with research demonstrating the benefit of revascularization when noninvasive imaging showed evidence of viable myocardium, both in terms of guiding therapy, improving survival and LVF recovery [31–36]. Assessment of viability is recommended by cardiology and cardiac imaging societies prior to decisions on management strategies [13]. On the other hand, the viability sub-study of the STICH trial (surgical treatment for ischemic heart failure) showed a significant association between the presence of viable myocardium and outcome by univariate but not multivariate analysis [37]. This sub-study was non- randomized, and as such this might have led to some selection bias. Furthermore, only a small percentage, 19%, of patients were treated with CABG while deemed to have negative tests for myocardial viability, and this again may affect the power of the study. The other limitation of the STICH trial was the use of a rather less sensitive modality to assess viability, SPECT rather than PET, in addition to stress echo. Finally, there was no recommendation for management following testing for viability, all patients had surgery and they were not managed as per the results of the viability tests.

Among several diagnostic techniques available for the evaluation of viable myocardium, SPECT using ^{201}Thallium chloride (Tl) or ^{99m}Technetium Sestamibi (Tc-MIBI) can assess cell membrane integrity and mitochondrial function.

Tl is a monovalent cationic radionuclide analog of potassium. The uptake of Tl into cardiac myocytes relies on both coronary flow and integrity of cell membrane and depends mainly on the presence of the functioning Na+/K+ATP-ase pump. In the presence of impaired flow, the speed of uptake is reduced significantly and the final radiotracer concentration is lower. Following the intracellular uptake there is an exchange between the myocytes and the blood pool, a process called redistribution, usually completed within 3–4 h, but may take up to 24 h. Reinjection of Tl can be used to enhance the contrast between regions of normal and abnormal uptake. Tl-MPI is a highly sensitive test for the detection of viable myocardium, in agreement with cardiac FDG imaging results [38].

FDG-PET/CT is so far considered the gold standard for the detection of viable myocardium. While it has the highest sensitivity for the prediction of LVF recovery after revascularization when compared to other imaging modalities, tests such as cardiac MR and stress echo, are more specific than FDG-PET/CT [39, 40]. The hallmark of viable myocardium is the metabolic adaptation made by chronically ischemic cardiomyocytes to optimize energy production in response to poor perfusion. Thus, in the presence of chronic ischemia, cardiomyocytes will shift their primary energy substrate from free fatty acid (FFA) to glucose. This process can be detected using FDG imaging. Preserved FDG uptake in a dysfunctional segment indicates a hibernating myocardium while the lack of uptake in a dysfunctional segment is indicative of nonviable tissue or scar. FDG uptake in more than 50% of the wall thickness of a dysfunctional LV segment, when compared to normally contracting remote segments, defines viable myocardium that will likely improve after revascularization of the supplying vessel [39].

In recent years contrast-enhanced cardiac MR (CMR) has been used for the detection of myocardial scar and its extend. Owing to its high-resolution, MR provides both anatomically and functionally valuable information. The presence of less than 50% transmurality of late Gd enhancement of the ventricular wall at a certain segment, when compared to remote non-dysfunctional segment, is considered a marker of viable myocardium. Integrating CMR with late Gd acquisition together with FDG-PET/CT provides information on high-resolution anatomy owing to the high spatial resolution of MR and myocardial metabolism all together. FDG-PET/CT adds sensitivity while it detects even small amounts of viable myocardium and MR measures the extend of scar since it relies on the inert molecule of Gd that measures the amount of the extracellular matrix scar. Therefore, the use of hybrid PET/MR appears potentially attractive for increasing the diagnostic accuracy, combining the high specificity of MR with the high sensitivity of PET.

The failing heart has increased sympathetic activity that leads to progressive remodeling of the myocardium that eventually leads to further reduction in LVF. Patients with IHF are at increased risk of fatal ventricular arrhythmias and sudden cardiac death [41]. Disruption of the balance and inhomogeneity of the left ventricular sympathetic innervation contributes to the development of arrhythmia.

Hybrid PET/CT and SPECT/CT imaging play an important role in identifying these patients. PET/CT using the radiotracer ^{11}C-meta-hydroxyephedrine (C-HED) could identify patients with ischemic cardiomyopathy with moderately to severely reduced LVF with an EF of below, or up to 35%, who are at high risk for a sudden cardiac arrest [42]. The risk of sudden cardiac arrhythmia was related to the innervated myocardium, independent of all other parameters such as the size of an MI, the presence or absence of viable myocardium, or the degree of LVF reduction. These results can help identify candidates that should receive an intracardiac cardioversion device (ICD) for primary prevention.

Imaging the sympathetic innervation of the heart can be also performed with SPECT/CT using the radiotracer ^{123}I-meta-iodobenzylguanidine (MIBG). This radiotracer enables the scintigraphic evaluation of the presynaptic sympathetic nerve endings and assessment of the cardiac innervation status. Several studies have demonstrated an association between the reduction of MIBG uptake and the development of malignant arrhythmia, worse outcome, frequent rehospitalization due to exacerbated HF symptoms and cardiac mortality [43, 44].

Hybrid imaging also plays a role in the assessment of the right ventricular function in the presence of pulmonary hypertension, a progressive disease that leads to an increase in pulmonary vascular resistance and can eventually cause right HF. So far CMR or three-dimensional echocardiography are the best modalities for assessing right ventricular function. CMR can measure right ventricular EF as well as other parameters such as cardiac output. An increase in pulmonary arterial pressure is associated with increased right ventricular FDG uptake, which indicates pressure overload and correlates with the progression of disease and unfavorable outcome [45]. When RV dysfunction is measured by the CMR component of the study it seems to correlate with increased FDG uptake in the right ventricle. Therefore, the integrated PET/MR design can provide both functional, hemodynamic, as well as metabolic information about the right heart [46].

1.3 Hybrid Imaging for Valvular Diseases

Valvular heart disease (VHD) is found in 1 out of 2 older adults, the most common pathology in the developed world being aortic valve stenosis, especially in light of the increase in life expectancy [47]. Assessment of the severity of the stenosis is crucial for patient management, which is straightforward in clearly graded stenosis. However, some cases are in the gray zone and determining the degree of stenosis can be very challenging.

While Doppler echocardiography is the primary imaging modality used in the assessment of VHD, it has some limitations. Approximately 40% of patients with aortic valve stenosis show a discrepancy between the severity of stenosis measured by pressure gradients across the valve, and the calculated aortic valve area. This condition is referred to as the low gradient aortic valve stenosis, further divided into subtypes: (1) classical low flow low gradient aortic valve stenosis with reduced LVF; (2) normal flow low gradient aortic valve stenosis; (3) paradoxical low flow low gradient aortic valve stenosis, usually in small LV cavity size resulting in low left ventricular stroke volume [48]. It is important to differentiate true severe aortic valve stenosis from pseudo-severe stenosis in the abovementioned cases, prior to making decisions on the further treatment strategy.

Hybrid imaging has been implemented to accurately assess the severity of stenosis. Multidetector CT may be used to measure the amount of calcification on the aortic valve. The degree of aortic valve calcification using the Agatston method can predict the hemodynamic significance and the rate of disease progression. Recent guidelines implemented the use of valvular calcium score in the assessment of stenosis severity and defining the treatment strategy. It is considered a criteria that increase the likelihood of severe aortic valve stenosis [49]. In addition, recent developments in nuclear cardiology can be used in the diagnosis of significant valvular stenosis. Aortic valve calcification has been established as an inflammatory process characterized by the accumulation and infiltration of lipid, macrophages, and T-lymphocytes. FDG uptake correlates with macrophage concentrations in calcified and atherosclerotic lesions. By assessment of the presence or absence of fibrosis, hybrid imaging can determine whether cardiac changes associated with afterload alteration, mainly in the case of aortic valve stenosis, are reversible or irreversible. FDG-PET can assess disease activity while anatomical information of either CT or MRI is necessary for both perfusion and viability. PET/CT imaging identifies anatomically and quantifies structures metabolically, including measurement of valve calcification (Fig. 1.2).

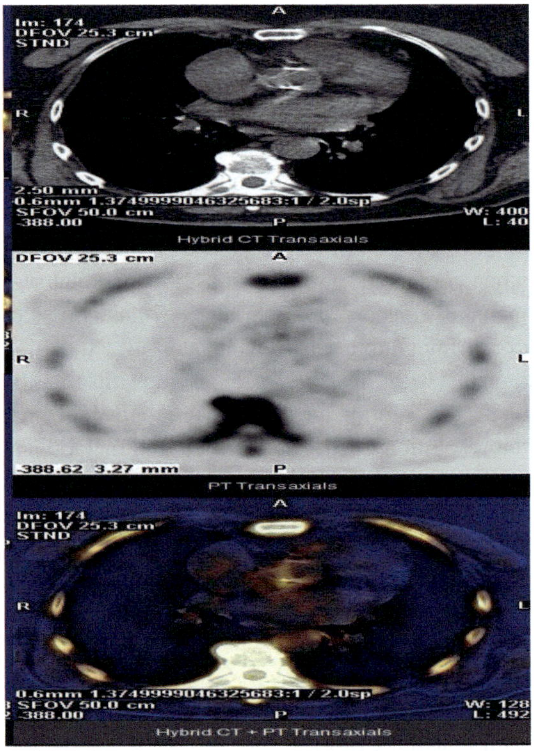

Fig. 1.2 In a 74-year-old female patient with syncope, an echocardiogram showed severe aortic valve stenosis, PET scan with sodium fluoride showed increased tracer uptake at the level of the aortic valve (maximal SUV = 3.2 mSv). The patient had a bioprosthesis implanted by trans-apical approach due to porcelain aorta. NAF-PET trans-axial images show severe aortic valve calcification seen in the Hybrid CT portion of the study (upper image). Increased radiotracer uptake at the level of the aortic valve by PET images (middle) and the bottom image—the hybrid CT and PET shows increased uptake as well

There are two main PET tracers used for this purpose. FDG, the glucose analog, enters the cells via glucose transport proteins and is then partially metabolized by the glycolytic metabolic pathway. After it passes the first hexokinase step, FDG-6-phosphate cannot be metabolized any further and is therefore trapped inside cells with high metabolic requirements including inflamed and high division capacity tissue ^{18}F-Sodium fluoride (NaF) is another PET tracer which directly incorporates into exposed bone crystal, hydroxyapatite, by an exchange with hydroxyl groups, leading to the detection of areas of novel calcification and calcium remodeling. In the clinical routine, NaF is used in the detection of primary osteoblastic tumors or bone metastases. Uptake of NaF can be used as a marker of calcification in atherosclerotic plaques [50].

The assessment of disease progression by these metabolic markers of disease activity in the case of aortic valve stenosis is promising. The early inflammation, detected by FDG uptake, plays an important role in valve calcification and its progression [51]. It enables the assessment of the hemodynamic significance of valve stenosis, it can also predict the risk of disease progression and prognosis [52, 53].

1.4 Cardiac Sarcoidosis

Sarcoidosis is a multisystem disease histologically characterized by non-necrotizing granulomatous inflammation affecting multiple organs. It involves mainly the lymph nodes and lungs but can also affect the heart. The disease occurs mostly at the age of 25–60 years, with the highest prevalence in women aged 25–44 years, around 100 cases over a population of 100,000 [54]. While being spread worldwide, it is more common in Northern Europe and among African Americans, particularly women. Among lethal cases, 50% of deaths occur in patients with cardiac sarcoidosis (CS), and therefore its early diagnosis is mandatory. The unknown etiology of the disease together with the lack of sensitive and specific diagnostic tests makes the diagnosis of CS challenging and involves a long and complex workup, based in part on the exclusion of other pathologies, and may include invasive procedures.

While autopsy studies supported by cardiac Gd-based MR have found cardiac involvement in 20–50% of cases of sarcoidosis (in US and Japanese statistics, respectively), clinical manifestations are likely to be found in only around 5–10% of patients. Undiagnosed CS was the cause of sudden cardiac death in as many as 14% of cases [55]. In up to 35% of patients below the age of 60, presenting with ventricular tachycardia (VT) or complete atrioventricular block, the underlying etiology is undiagnosed SC [56]. Furthermore, another study showed that biopsies documented the presence of undiagnosed CS in up to 3.5% of patients receiving a left ventricular assist device because of HF with reduced EF [57].

The clinical presentation of CS varies from conduction heart block due to invasion of the conduction system, HF, and ventricular tachycardia attributed to scarring leading to sudden cardiac death. Most patients with clinically manifest CS have less expression of extracardiac manifestation and have a worse outcome [55]. This makes the diagnosis of isolated CS even more challenging if currently available diagnostic criteria are applied. These criteria include endomyocardial biopsy with a sensitivity of 30% (due to the patchy nature of the disease) and require the presence of extracardiac involvement. The advancement of imaging technologies has led to the factitious impression of increase in the incidence of CS [58]. Two sets of diagnostic criteria are available, published by the Japanese Ministry of Health and Welfare (JMHW) in 2006, and the more recent Heart Rhythm Society consensus [59]. There are two pathways for diagnosis of CS: (1) histology obtained from myocardial tissue, with a sensitivity of only 19–30% [60]; (2) clinical diagnosis based on invasive and noninvasive studies. The probability of CS in patients with histological evidence of extracardiac sarcoidosis, after other causes of cardiac manifestations have been excluded, is based on the presence of at least one of the following:

- Steroid +/− immunosuppressant responsive cardiomyopathy or heart block
- Unexplained reduced LVEF (<40%)
- Unexplained sustained (spontaneous or induced) VT
- Mobitz type II second degree or third degree heart block
- Patchy uptake on cardiac PET (in a pattern consistent with CS)
- Late Gd enhancement on CMR (in a pattern consistent with CS)
- Positive ^{67}Ga uptake (in a pattern consistent with CS)

FDG helps differentiate between normal and inflamed tissue based on its higher metabolic rates and resulting greater glucose utilization. FDG-PET/CT has a high sensitivity of 82–100% for the diagnosis of CS with a specificity of 39–91% [60]. The pattern of FDG uptake is either focal or focal-on-diffuse uptake. FDG-PET/CT imaging in CS has been suggested for the management of patients with CS (Figs. 1.3 and 1.4). For FDG imaging of myocardial inflammation, it is important to understand that the healthy myocardium utilizes both glucose and free fatty acids, depending on the patient's nutrition and fasting status. To achieve high contrast between inflammatory infiltrates and normal myocardium, it is necessary to suppress myocardial glucose metabolism, this can be obtained by different protocols including prolonged fasting, high-fat low carbohydrate diet, fatty acid loading, and unfractionated heparin loading.

A strict suppression of physiological glucose uptake in myocytes by appropriate protocol is crucial to obtain an accurate scan (Fig. 1.3). Understanding the importance of patient prepara-

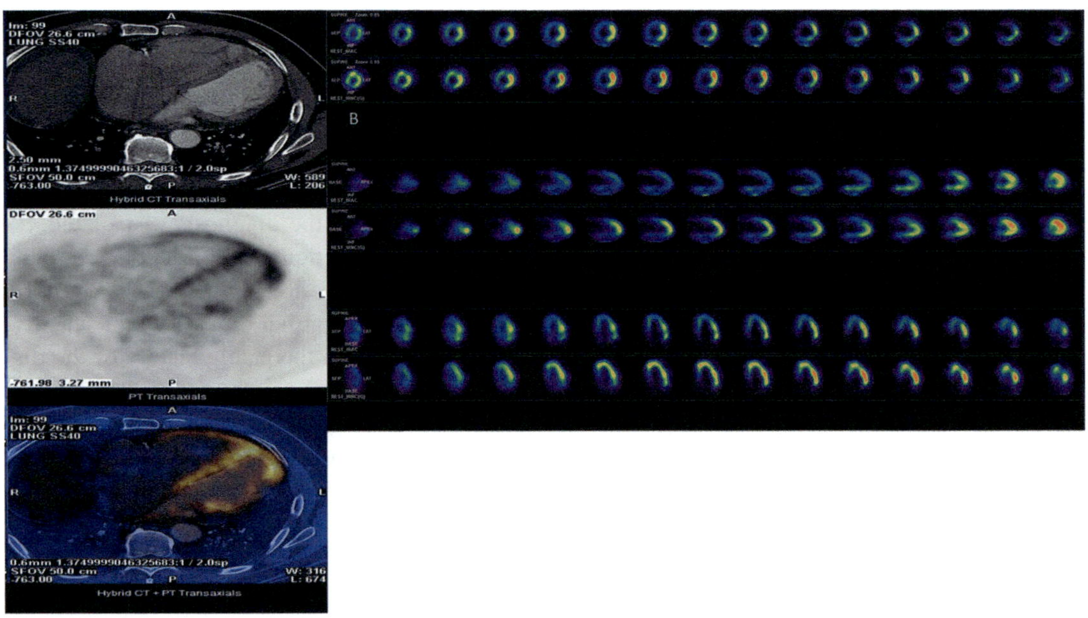

Fig. 1.3 A 58-year-old male patient with a main complaint of weakness and shortness of breath, on presentation his ECG showed complete atrioventricular block, lab work showed increases NT-PRO-BNP and troponin, echocardiography showed severely enlarged right ventricle and right atrium, severely reduced left and right ventricular systolic function and severe pulmonary hypertension. FDG-PET/CT (A) showed increased FDG uptake in the septum, apex of the left ventricle, basal lateral wall, and the RV free wall. A SPECT MPI scan (B) upper row non-attenuation correction and bottom row is the corrected images) showed reduced radiotracer uptake in the septum, apex, and basal inferolateral wall. These mismatched areas represents areas suspected of cardiac sarcoidosis. Echocardiography-guided myocardial biopsy showed interstitial aggregates of histiocytes (positive for CD68), associated with giant cells and small T-lymphocytes (positive for CD3), consistent with granulomas. Few scattered T-lymphocytes and histiocytes were seen, between the myocyte fibers. The findings were consistent with cardiac sarcoidosis

tion by the referring clinical cardiologist is of paramount importance in order to give the patient detailed preparation instructions.

FDG imaging provides information about the metabolic state of the myocardium and detects the presence of active granuloumatous disease when adequately performed and when the physiological uptake of glucose by myocytes is suppressed. The advantage of FDG imaging is in the early, active stages of the disease, when immunosuppressive therapy can make a difference in risk stratification and outcome. Higher FDG activity measured as standardized uptake values (SUV), mainly in basal segments, is associated with an increased risk for cardiac events, such as arrhythmias, VT, atrioventricular block, and HF [61].

Combination of both ^{82}Rubidium (Rb) or ^{13}N-ammonia (N)-PET/CT or SPECT MPI using ^{99m}Tc-based radiotracers with FDG allows toe difference between the different stages of the disease as well as between uptake due to inadequate dietary preparation and true findings related to the inflammatory process (Fig. 1.4). FDG-PET/CT is of value not only in the diagnosis and risk stratification of CS but also in the follow up of the disease and to monitor disease response to immunosuppressive treatment (Fig. 1.4). Patients with CS are treated with high-dose steroids, and then tapering down or continuation of these doses, or switching to other medications, will depend on the degree of response to treatment.

Based on FDG-PET/CT patterns the likelihood and stage of CS are classified as follows:

- Normal: normal perfusion, absence of cardiac FDG uptake.
- Early stage: mild perfusion defect, increased FDG uptake.
- Progressive myocardial impairment stage: severe perfusion defects, increased FDG uptake.
- Fibrosis stage: severe perfusion defect, minimal or no FDG uptake.

Gd-based contrast media used for MRI are inert and do not cross the cell membrane. In the presence of a scar in the post inflammatory state,

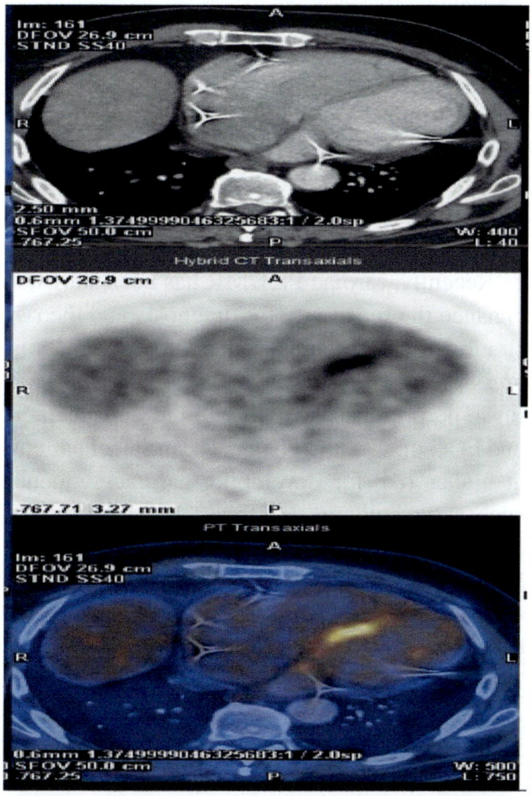

Fig. 1.4 Trans-axial FDG-PET/CT scan images from the same patient in Fig. 1.3 after 3 months of treatment with steroids. No FDG uptake is noticed in the right ventricular free wall, left ventricular apex, or basal lateral wall

Gd leaks into the interstitial space where it is temporarily trapped. After a time interval, Gd-enhanced areas will show slow washout of the contrast. CMR can detect even small areas of myocardial necrosis and/or fibrosis at areas of late Gd enhancement and with T1 mapping which is specific for fibrosis. In addition, CMR can detect regional and global dysfunction, assess for myocardial edema by T2 maps, as well as hyperemia and pericardial effusion. However, CMR has its own limitations beyond the presence of intracardiac defibrillation devices and pacemakers in this patient population, especially in patients with diffuse inflammatory disease such as chronic myocarditis. Furthermore, although the sensitivity of CMR for diagnosis of CS reaches 95% [62], due to the dynamic nature of the disease and the shifting between active inflammation and advanced fibrosis and scar, CMR might be less sensitive during the early, inflammatory stages of the disease.

These are the cases that would benefit most from the specific characteristics of MR combined with the high sensitivity and outstanding quantification capabilities of FDG-PET which hybrid imaging can offer.

Recently, cardiac PET/MR has been shown to enhance the sensitivity for diagnosis and the risk stratification of patients with CS. It can define areas of active disease versus fibrosis and scarring. The presence of both late Gd enhancement and FDG uptake on PET/CMR can select patients at higher risk for developing cardiac sequellae such as arrhythmia, HF, heart block, and SCD [63]. Some case reports describing the use of PET/MRI for detection of myocarditis showed overlapping of late Gd enhancement and decreased FDG uptake in the sub-epicardium. Although CMR is sufficient for diagnosis, this emphasizes the values of FDG-PET in identifying cardiac inflammation.

Non-FDG tracers targeting other inflammatory factors such as chemokines that cause some cellular changes in the myocardium are promising in cardiac PET/MRI in the future [64].

1.5 Infiltrative Diseases

1.5.1 Cardiac Amyloidosis

Amyloidosis is a group of diseases with similar pathogenesis of deposition of misfolded, insoluble fibrillary protein inside the extracellular matrix resulting in the loss of the normal tissue architecture. When involving the heart, amyloidosis is characterized by a progressive increase in wall thickness and stiffness. This leads to restrictive cardiomyopathy and progressive diastolic dysfunction that eventually deteriorates to systolic HF. If diagnosis is delayed or if left untreated, cardiac amyloidosis (CA) is associated with high morbidity and significant mortality. The diagnosis of CA is far from straightforward, especially since it can occur with no evidence of systemic disease [65]. There is also a long list of differential diagnoses of increased left ventricular wall thickness, including hypertensive disease, aortic valve stenosis, hypertrophic cardiomyopathy, left ventricular non-compaction, and Anderson–Fabry disease.

Different subtypes of CA have been described, depending on the deposited protein. These subtypes have different pathophysiological substrates and may vary significantly in their course of disease, prognosis, and therapeutic options [66, 67]. There are three major subtypes. (1) Acquired monoclonal immunoglobulin light chain amyloidosis (AL); these immunoglobulins are produced by clonal plasma cells in the bone marrow. Cardiac involvement is common and reaches up to 75%. It is a rapidly progressive disease if left untreated, with a median survival of less than 6 months. Therapy improves survival to 5–10 years [68]. (2) Wild type transthyretin-related CA (ATTRwt), the systemic senile amyloidosis, mainly affects elderly men. Cardiac involvement is the predominant clinical presentation. (3) Hereditary, mutant type transthyretin-related (ATTRm) caused by a protein is synthesized by the liver by dozens of mutations.

AL is relatively rare, up to 40.5/1,000,000 cases. The other two subtypes have a high prevalence and might reach up to 6% of the elderly patients with HF. The CA subtypes have a different clinical course, require a different treatment approach, and have therefore also different prognosis [69, 70].

Clinical presentation can vary significantly from asymptomatic patients to symptoms including shortness of breath, orthopnea, paroxysmal nocturnal dyspnea, palpitations, effort intolerance, dizziness, or fatigue. In the absence of a clear etiology such as ischemic heart disease or valvular problems, an increased wall thickness of more than 12 mm and diastolic dysfunction should definitely raise the suspicion of an infiltrative disease especially in the presence of multistructure involvement such as valves, muscle, ventricles, and atrial involvement. Clinical cardiologists should be familiar with the diagnostic algorithms, as well as with the indications, contraindications, and limitations of imaging modalities used in the diagnosis of CA.

The gold standard for the diagnosis of CA is endomyocardial biopsy, which is highly sensitive (100%). However, it is impractical as a screening test, and cannot assess the disease burden or be used as a follow-up tool to determine response to therapy. Different imaging modalities may facilitate early diagnosis such as CMR, radionuclide imaging with bone-avid radiotracers, and echocardiography. Current diagnostic approaches include at least one of these diagnostic modalities [67].

Echocardiography and CMR are excellent tools for the diagnosis of CA but have only limited diagnostic utility in the early phases of the disease. Furthermore, they cannot distinguish between the different types of CA. Molecular imaging with PET and SPECT plays a critical role in the diagnosis and the differentiation between the different subtypes of CA. Tc-labeled phosphonates agents used for bone scintigraphy bind strongly to ATTR amyloid and weakly or not at all to AA and AL amyloid. They can differentiate ATTR amyloidosis from patients without cardiac involvement in the disease (Fig. 1.5), and also can distinguish ATTR from AL-CA and other causes that lead to increased left ventricular wall thickness. Some reports demonstrated that NaF-PET/CT may be a potential tool to also differentiate between subtypes of CA [71].

In the absence of endomyocardial biopsy-proven disease, CA can be diagnosed using a combination of extracardiac biopsy, Tc-PYP/DPD/HMDP scintigraphy, myocardial uptake of targeted PET amyloid tracers, and echocardiographic and CMR findings [72].

ATTR amyloidosis and aortic valve stenosis may coexist in patients older than 75 years of age. In these cases, CA may mimic severe aortic valve stenosis in patients with actual moderate disease, a potential cause for misdiagnosis. In

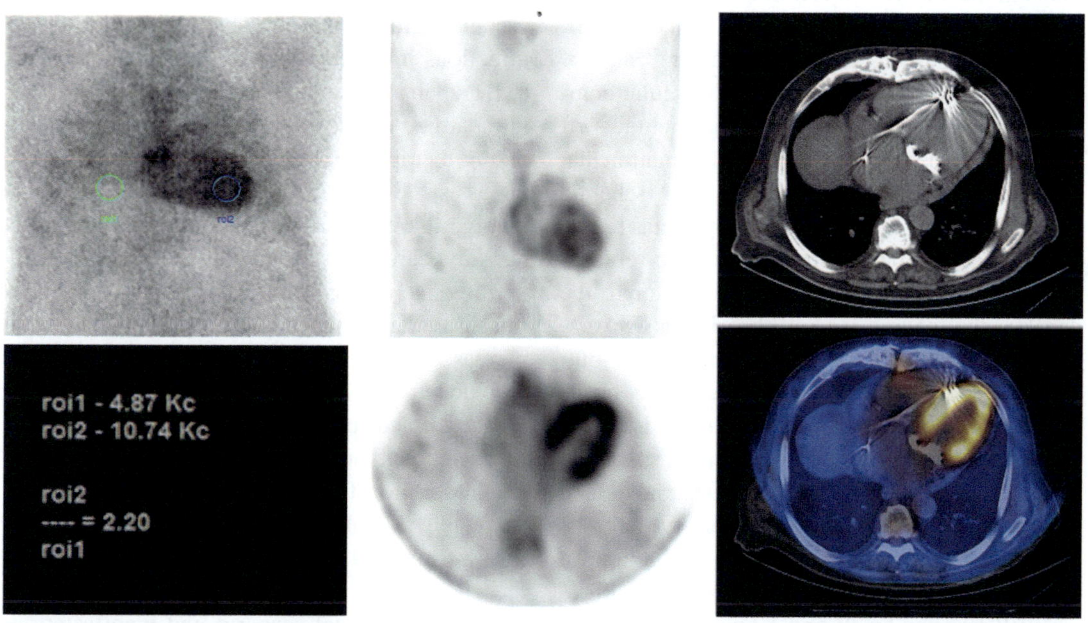

Fig. 1.5 Images from a ^{99m}Tc-PYP study of a 76-year-old patient referred due to worsening heart failure and concentric thickening of the left ventricle walls in ECHO. On the left is the static anterior image of the chest acquired 1 h after injection of ^{99m}Tc-PYP, displaying increased uptake in the myocardium compared to skeletal uptake, consistent with a visual score of 3. On the bottom left is the uptake ratio calculation between the heart and contralateral chest, equaling 2.2—consistent with ATTR and suggesting poor prognosis. On the right: SPECT/CT performed immediately following the static image, from left and clockwise: Maximal intensity projection (MIP) and axial slices of CT, fused SPECT/CT and SPECT, displaying the uptake is located in the myocardial wall and not in the blood pool, and the diffuse involvement of all walls of the left ventricle. The diagnosis of ATTR-CA was confirmed by endocardial biopsy in this patient. (Adapted with permission from Dr. Michal Weiler-Sagie, the Department of Nuclear Medicine, Rambam Healthcare Campus)

addition, CA can be a disease modifier that causes a more severe phenotype with worse HF, arrhythmia, and poorer prognosis. In this case diagnosis and the differentiation between hypertrophy attributed to severe aortic valve stenosis or that caused by cardiac amyloidosis is important to determine management and medical therapy in the presence of emerging therapies. Therefore, there is an increase in the use of bone scintigraphy in this group of patients.

1.5.2 Anderson–Fabry Disease

Anderson–Fabry disease (ADF) is an x-linked disorder that carries a grief prognosis if left untreated. A mutation in the gene coding for the lysosomal enzyme Alpha Galactosidase A leads to the accumulation of substrates, namely Globotriaosylceramide (GB3). This accumulation, found in the majority of cell lines is the reason for multiple organ involvement including the heart, kidneys, and nervous system. The leading cause of death in patients with AFD is cardiovascular complications. Cardiac manifestations include left ventricular hypertrophy, chronic inflammation that eventually leads to myocardial fibrosis, ischemic heart disease, dysfunction, and arrhythmias [73].

AFD is treatable by specific enzyme replacement and therefore early diagnosis, prior to the development of myocardial fibrosis, an irreversible condition, is of significance for better outcome. Besides measurement of enzyme levels when the disease is suspected, imaging is useful in the diagnosis or, at least, in the initial suspicion of AFD. CMR is of value in the diagnosis and follow up of the disease. It can identify the presence of inflammation and later in the course of the disease the replacement of myocytes by fibrosis, well-targeted by T1 and T2 native sequences, and low T1 mapping values together with late Gd enhancement once fibrosis develops. While there is no single imaging modality that can reliably rule in or rule out AFD, hybrid imaging offers a potential one-stop-shop for the diagnosis of AFD. PET/MRI has an additional value in differentiating between patients in the early stages of the disease who have mainly inflammation versus patients that already developed a scar. While FDG imaging facilitates detecting the presence of inflammation, late Gd enhancement corresponds to the presence of fibrotic scar tissue [74]. Additional information obtained from MR is related to parameters of the LV including hypertrophy and myocardial mass, mainly in patients who can develop myocardial fibrosis either prior to, or without hypertrophy. It is important to remember that low T1 maps are unique to AFD and can differentiate it from other diseases with left ventricular hypertrophy. CMR showing low T1 maps that represent the storage of GB3, in the absence of left ventricular hypertrophy, detects earlier systolic and diastolic dysfunction in patients with AFD.

1.5.3 Infection and Inflammation

Cardiac infections are mainly endocardial and can involve both native and prosthetic valves, vascular grafts, mainly aortic, in addition to infections involving cardiac implantable devices (CID) such as pacemakers (PM), devices used for intracardiac cardioversion (ICD), for resynchronizing therapies (CRT, CRTD) and left ventricular assist devices (LVAD). Infections may also involve the myocardium such as myocarditis or peri-myocarditis.

Infective endocarditis (IE) has high mortality rates if undiagnosed and untreated, in addition to increased rates of serious complications for those who do survive. So far diagnostic criteria depend on the clinical presentation, which at times can be unclear and not suggestive for the diagnosis of IE. In addition to clinical presentation and high suspicion, the diagnosis of IE is based on laboratory workup and imaging procedures, some being incorporated in the revised Duke criteria that include the clinical scenario and manifestations (septic emboli, new valvular dysfunction), blood workup including positive blood culture, and positive findings by echocardiogram. The primary imaging modality used in the diagnosis, prognostication and follow up during and after treatment of IE is transthoracic or transesophageal echocardiography, depending on the structure involved (i.e., tricuspid valve involvement versus left side valves, respectively).

In recent years, the diagnosis of IE also incorporates the use of other imaging modalities including CCTA, CMR, and FDG-PET/CT [75]. CCTA is used in the detection of complications of endocarditis such as abscesses, pseudoaneurysm formation, or fistulas. For this indication, CCTA has similar accuracy to transesophageal echo [76]. The latest European Society of Cardiology guidelines for the diagnosis and management of IE recommend the use of radiolabeled leukocyte scintigraphy and FDG-PET/CT in patients with CIDs and suspected endocarditis when echocardiography is negative [77]. The detection of abnormal activity by FDG-PET/CT or radiolabeled leukocytes SPECT/CT is defined as a major criterion according to these guidelines.

FDG-PET/CT has an incremental value both locally, at the site of the device/prosthetic valve where echocardiography is less sensitive due to artifacts and shadowing caused by the metal component of the device (Fig. 1.6), as well as for the diagnosis of remote foci of the disease, in detection of septic emboli to the lungs, spleen, and other organs. In patients with cardiac devices such as PM, the diagnosis of device infection is of extreme importance since the diagnosis will likely lead to the removal of the PM electrode, considered a high-risk procedure. Patients with back pain complaints should be suspected to have septic emboli in the spine. While CT or MR can be performed to confirm the diagnosis, whole-body FDG-PET/CT is an excellent alternative to provide more information on site and for remote seeding and septic emboli. FDG-PET/CT should be performed in patients with positive culture for S. Bovis or S. Gallolyticus, this condition is potentially associated with colorectal cancer. However, negative FDG-PET for gastrointestinal pathology does not rule out the diagnosis [78].

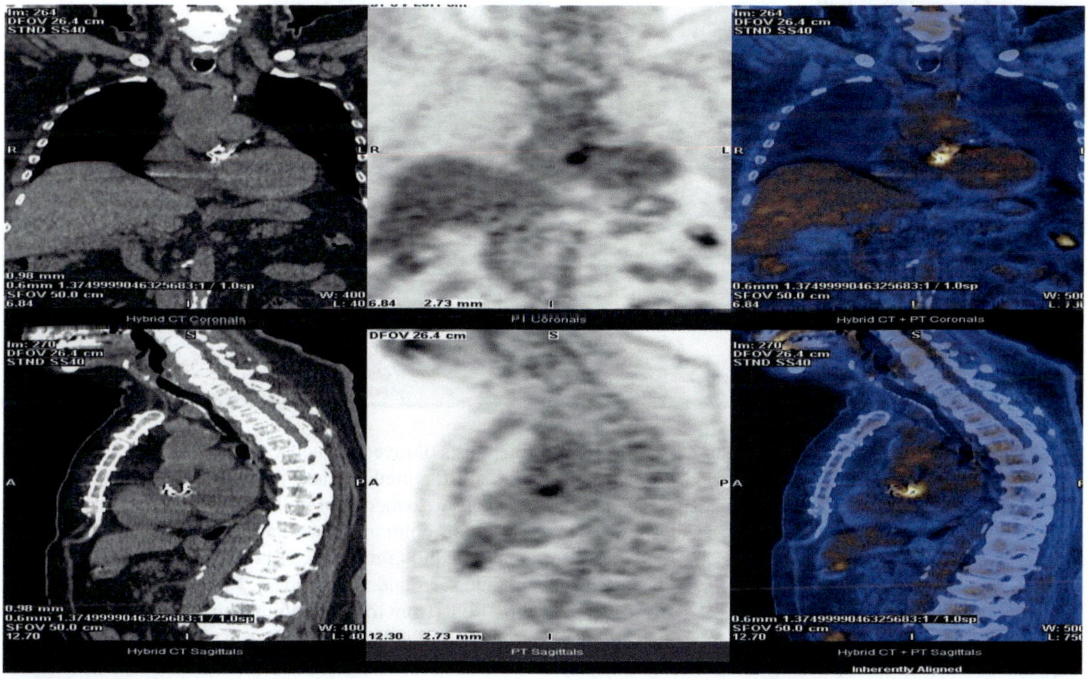

Fig. 1.6 An 82-year-old female patient post aortic valve replacement to a bioprosthesis (C.E 19) due to severe stenosis. Ten years later she presents with fever, blood cultures were positive for Enterococcus. Transthoracic echocardiogram was negative for vegetations however it demonstrated a moderately severe peri-prosthetic regurgitation originating from the posterior cusp. An FDG/PET showed increased focal tracer uptake in the posterior aspect of the bioprosthesis in the aortic position. This figure shows the CT, planar images, and SPECT images from left to right in both AP and sagittal views from in the upper and lower rows, respectively. Maximal SUV = 5.5 mSv

The use of hybrid FDG-PET/CTA in the management of patients suspected of IE lies in its ability to identify a large number of pathologies, in particular, in patients with complex anatomy after surgery or in patients with congenital disease (i.e., pulmonic valve that is hard to image by echocardiography, especially after surgical intervention). FDG-PET/CT also plays an important role in the diagnosis of vascular infections along the vascular tree such as infected aneurysms or pseudoaneurysms (Fig. 1.7a and b).

The fact that FDG is taken up by inflammatory processes makes it also an excellent agent for the diagnosis of noninfectious inflammation such as vasculitis. Large vessel vasculitis is a devastating disease, its diagnosis can be challenging and carries a grave prognosis if left untreated. Large vessel vasculitis can be diagnosed by ultrasonography for assessment of patency of vessels, MRI for thickening of vessel walls, or vascular wall biopsy. In some patients, all these diagnostic tools can be negative. In cases with a high clinical suspicion an FDG-

a

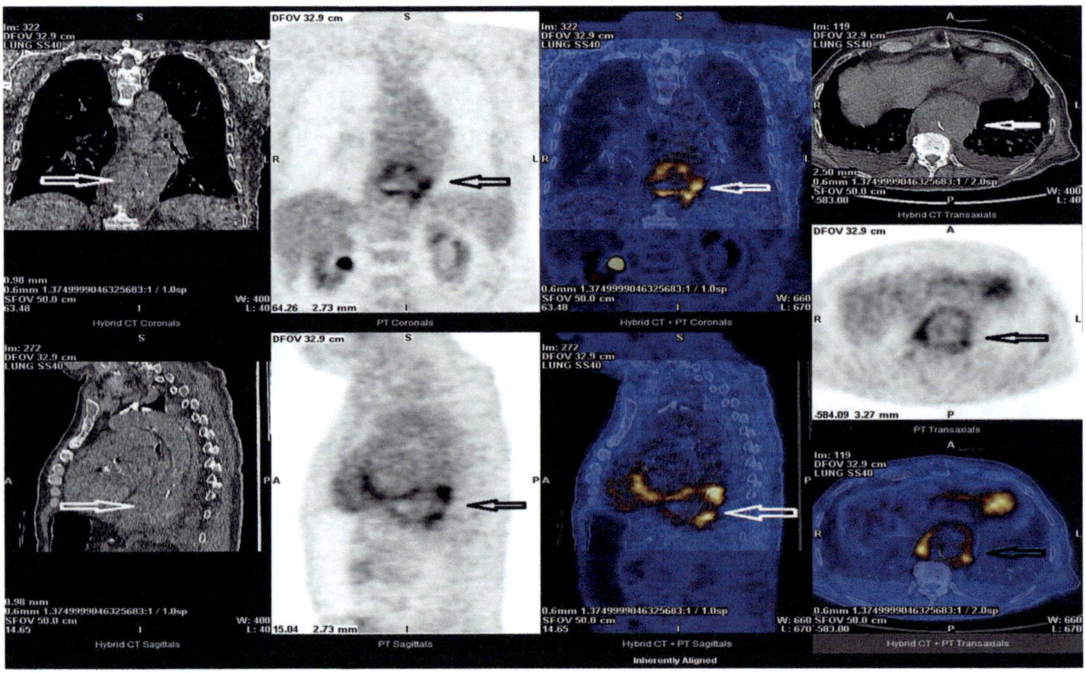

Fig. 1.7 (**a**) A 78-year-old male patient, known to have hypertension, hyperlipidemia, chronic kidney disease (due to severe bilateral renal artery stenosis) and monoclonal gammopathy of unknown significance. Admitted to the hospital for investigation of fever and Methicillin-sensitive Staphylococcus Aureus (MSSA) bacteremia, initial workup including a transthoracic echocardiogram that was negative. Later on he developed dyspnea and paroxysmal nocturnal orthopnea, general weakness, and abdominal pain. FDG/PET CT study showed pathological FDG uptake surrounding a structure measuring 6.8 cm around the descending thoracic aorta above the diaphragm, the CT portion of the study showed dilated aorta at the site of uptake and bilateral pleural effusion. Chest CTA showed descending thoracic aorta aneurysm at the level of D10–11, measuring 4.5 × 5.0 × 5.5 cm, this aneurysm is surrounded by a hypodense finding with density of fluid with a wall that is enhanced with contrast. This finding by the CTA was concluded as in keeping with the diagnosis of mycotic aneurysm surrounded by an inflamed fluid, differential diagnosis includes thrombosis surrounding a pseudoaneurysm with secondary infection. The far right end column shows trans-axial hybrid CT showing the descending thoracic aorta with a mild atherosclerotic plaque surrounded by a mass, PET, and fused hybrid CT and PET (from top to bottom, respectively). The top three images on the left show coronal views of the hybrid CT, PET, and hybrid CT and PET from left to right respectively, the finding is pointed out with an arrow. The bottom three images from the left show sagittal views of the hybrid CT, PET, and hybrid CT fused with PET from left to right, respectively. (**b**) CHEST CTA. (A) Sagital view shows the descending aorta, the aortic aneurysm, and the surrounding inflamed tissue. (B) Trans-axial view showing the descending thoracic aorta, aortic aneurysm, and the surrounding infectious inflammation and the pleural effusion. (C) Volume rendering showing the Aorta and the aortic aneurysm-arrows

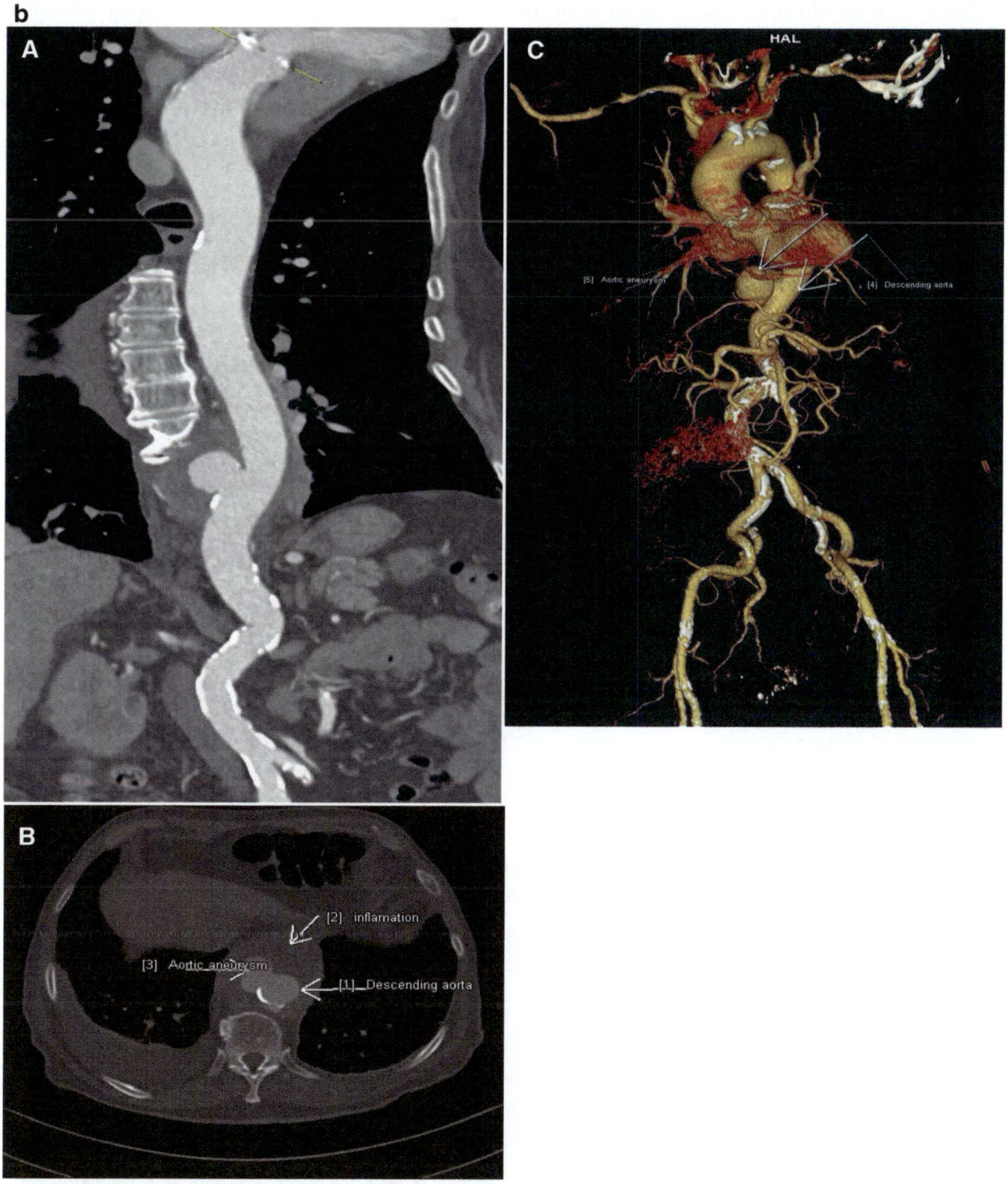

Fig. 1.7 (continued)

PET/CT study should be the diagnostic modality of choice to rule out or confirm the diagnosis and has been recommended for diagnosis and follow up of vasculitis by the EANM and ASNC [79]. FDG-PET/CT has a unique feature of whole-body scanning which is responsible for its good diagnostic accuracy. FDG-PET/CT also plays an important role in patients' follow up and monitoring treatment efficacy in large vessel vasculitis (Fig. 1.8a and b) [80].

a

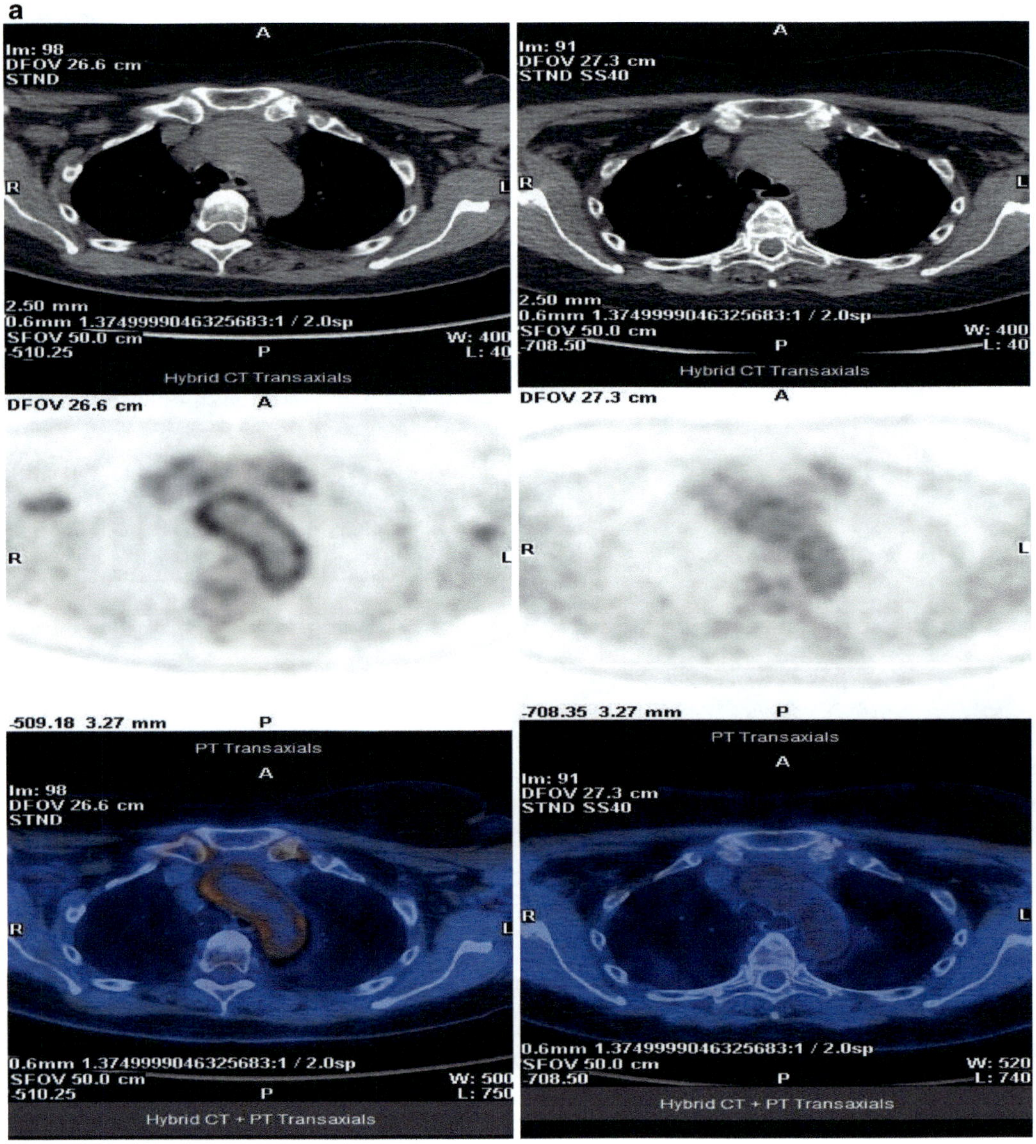

Fig. 1.8 (**a**) A 54-year-old female patient admitted to the hospital for investigation of severe headache and numbness in her left arm. CT angiogram showed stenosis of her left brachial artery. FDG-PET scan showed increased diffuse pathological nonhomogenous FDG uptake in the large vessels of the neck, Chest, and abdomen. She was diagnosed with Takayasu. The left panel of this figure from top to bottom demonstrates a trans-axial hybrid CT view at the level of the aortic arch followed at the middle left by a same view same level PET scan and at the bottom a fusion of the hybrid CT and PET scan, the corresponding images on the right are same view same level images posttreatment with steroids. (**b**) Same patient as in Fig. 1.8a. Left column top to bottom shows a hybrid CT scan in a tran-axial view at the cervical level followed by a PET scan showing increased FDG uptake in the right and left carotid arteries. The bottom image shows fusion of the hybrid CT and PET. The right column shows corresponding images from the same patient after treatment with steroids

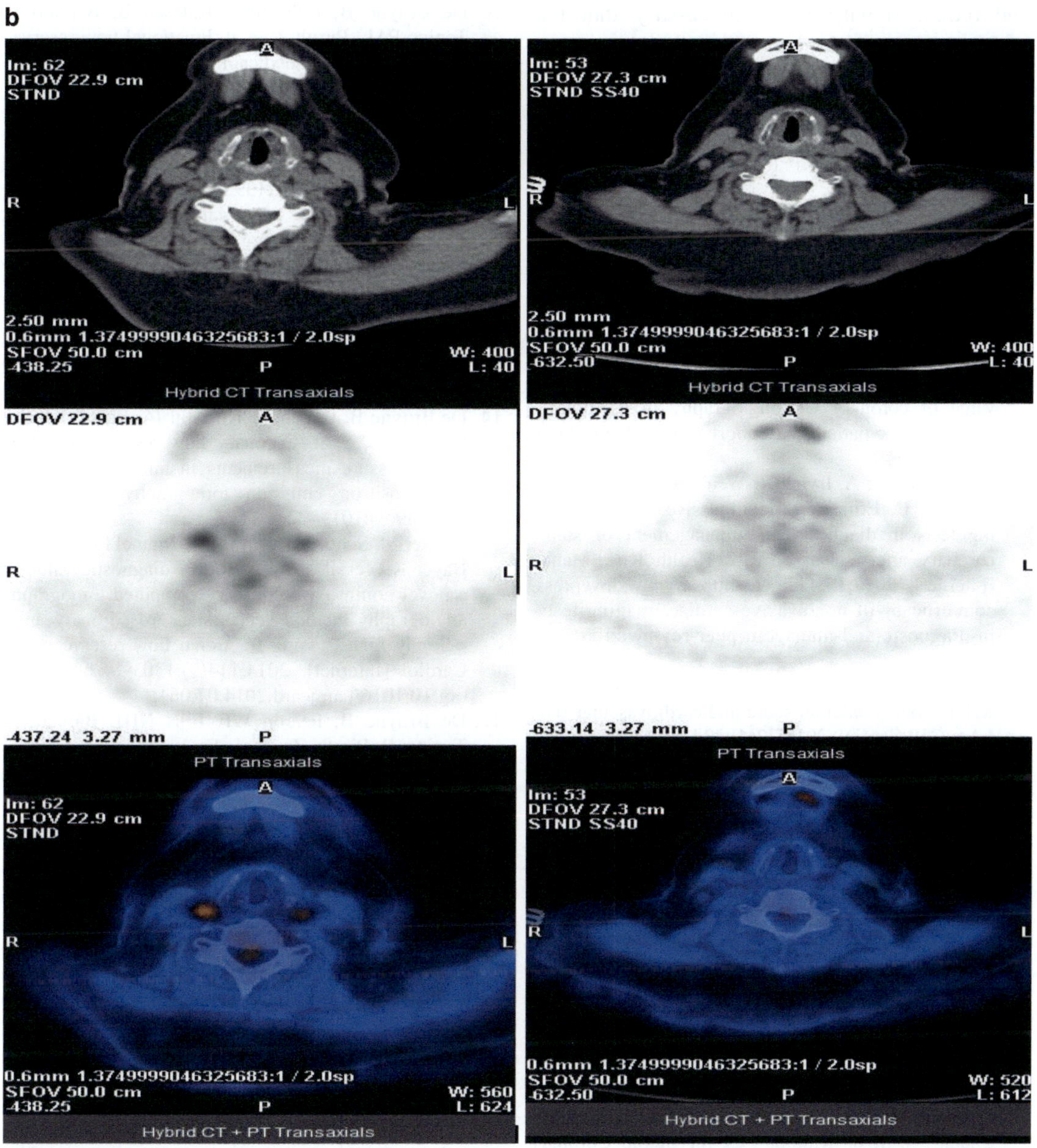

Fig. 1.8 (continued)

1.6 Summary

The major advancement in the available noninvasive diagnostic tools especially in the era of artificial intelligence that enables the combination of the different imaging modalities requires that clinical cardiologists have a full grasp and understanding of the different tools that are available in their armamentarium. It is of great importance to understand what each modality can offer, and what the indications and contraindications for their use are. This will result in more accurate and earlier diagnoses, increase the cost effectiveness of patient management, reduce ionizing radiation exposure of both patients and staff when an imaging modality is used appropriately, and reduce downstream unnecessary that has both major psychological effects on the patient and financial burden on the medical system.

References

1. Virani SS, Alonso A, Aparicio HJ, Benjamin EJ, Bittencourt MS, Callaway CW, et al. Heart disease and stroke statistics—2021 update: a report from the American Heart Association. Circulation. 2021;143(8):e254–743.
2. Plank F, Friedrich G, Dichtl W, Klauser A, Jaschke W, Franz WM, et al. The diagnostic and prognostic value of coronary CT angiography in asymptomatic high-risk patients: a cohort study. Open Heart. 2014;1(1):1–9.
3. Mordi I, Badar A, Irving R, Weir-McCall J, Houston G, Lang C. Efficacy of noninvasive cardiac imaging tests in diagnosis and management of stable coronary artery disease. Vasc Health Risk Manag [Internet]. 2017;13:427–37. https://www.dovepress.com/efficacy-of-noninvasive-cardiac-imaging-tests-in-diagnosis-and-managem-peer-reviewed-article-VHRM.
4. Greenland P, Blaha MJ, Budoff MJ, Erbel R, Watson KE. Coronary calcium score and cardiovascular risk. J Am Coll Cardiol. 2018;72(4):434–47.
5. Schenker MP, Dorbala S, Hong ECT, Rybicki FJ, Hachamovitch R, Kwong RY, et al. Interrelation of coronary calcification, myocardial ischemia, and outcomes in patients with intermediate likelihood of coronary artery disease: a combined positron emission tomography/computed tomography study. Circulation. 2008;117(13):1693–700.
6. Schaap J, Kauling RM, Matthijs Boekholdt S, Nieman K, Bob Meijboom W, Post MC, et al. Incremental diagnostic accuracy of hybrid SPECT/CT coronary angiography in a population with an intermediate to high pre-test likelihood of coronary artery disease. Eur Heart J Cardiovasc Imaging. 2013;14(7):642–9.
7. Boden WE, O'Rourke RA, Teo KK, et al. for the COURAGE Trial Research Group*. Optimal Medical Therapy with or without PCI for Stable Coronary Disease. NEJM, 2007;56(15):1503–15.
8. Raymond E, Pisano E, Gatsonis C, Boineau R, Domanski M, Troutman C, et al. New England Journal. SCD-Heft. Heart Fail. 2011;364(6):225–37.
9. Hachamovitch R, Hayes SW, Friedman JD, Cohen I, Berman DS. Comparison of the short-term survival benefit associated with revascularization compared with medical therapy in patients with no prior coronary artery disease undergoing stress myocardial perfusion single photon emission computed tomography. Circulation. 2003;107(23):2900–6.
10. De Bruyne B, Pijls NHJ, Kalesan B, Barbato E, Tonino PAL, Piroth Z, et al. Fractional flow reserve–guided PCI versus medical therapy in stable coronary disease. N Engl J Med. 2012;367(11):991–1001.
11. Maron DJ, Hochman JS, Reynolds HR, Bangalore S, O'Brien SM, Boden WE, et al. Initial invasive or conservative strategy for stable coronary disease. N Engl J Med. 2020;382:1395–407.
12. Spertus JA, Jones PG, Maron DJ, O'Brien SM, Reynolds HR, Rosenberg Y, et al. Health-status outcomes with invasive or conservative care in coronary disease. N Engl J Med. 2020;382:1408–19.
13. Neumann FJ, Sousa-Uva M, Ahlsson A, Alfonso F, Banning AP, Benedetto U, et al. 2018 ESC/EACTS guidelines on myocardial revascularization. Eur Heart J. 2019;40(2):87–165.
14. De Bruyne B, Baudhuin T, Melin JA, Pijls NHJ, Sys SU, Bol A, et al. Coronary flow reserve calculated from pressure measurements in humans: validation with positron emission tomography. Circulation. 1994;89(3):1013–22.
15. Renker M, Schoepf UJ, Wang R, Meinel FG, Rier JD, Bayer RR, et al. Comparison of diagnostic value of a novel noninvasive coronary computed tomography angiography method versus standard coronary angiography for assessing fractional flow reserve. Am J Cardiol [Internet]. 2014;114(9):1303–8. https://doi.org/10.1016/j.amjcard.2014.07.064.
16. De Bruyne B, Fearon WF, Pijls NHJ, Barbato E, Tonino P, Piroth Z, et al. Fractional flow reserve–guided PCI for stable coronary artery disease. N Engl J Med. 2014;371(13):1208–17.
17. Biondi-Zoccai G, Versaci F, Iskandrian AE, Schillaci O, Nudi A, Frati G, et al. Umbrella review and multivariate meta-analysis of diagnostic test accuracy studies on hybrid non-invasive imaging for coronary artery disease. J Nucl Cardiol. 2020;27(5):1744–55.
18. Pazhenkottil AP, Nkoulou RN, Ghadri JR, Herzog BA, Buechel RR, Küest SM, et al. Prognostic value of cardiac hybrid imaging integrating single-photon emission computed tomography with coronary computed tomography angiography. Eur Heart J. 2011;32(12):1465–71.
19. Tonino PAL, Fearon WF, De Bruyne B, Oldroyd KG, Leesar MA, Ver Lee PN, et al. Angiographic versus functional severity of coronary artery stenoses in the FAME study. Fractional flow reserve versus angiography in multivessel evaluation. J Am Coll Cardiol [Internet]. 2010;55(25):2816–21. https://doi.org/10.1016/j.jacc.2009.11.096.
20. Liga R, Vontobel J, Rovai D, Marinelli M, Caselli C, Pietila M, et al. Multicentre multi-device hybrid imaging study of coronary artery disease: results from the EValuation of INtegrated Cardiac Imaging for the Detection and Characterization of Ischaemic Heart Disease (EVINCI) hybrid imaging population. Eur Heart J Cardiovasc Imaging. 2016;17(9):951–60.

21. Hoffmann U, Ferencik M, Udelson JE, Michael H, Truong QA, Patel MR, et al. HHS Public Access. 2018;135(24):2320–32.
22. Javadi MS, Lautamäki R, Merrill J, Voicu C, Epley W, McBride G, et al. Definition of vascular territories on myocardial perfusion images by integration with true coronary anatomy: a hybrid PET/CT analysis. J Nucl Med. 2010;51(2):198–203.
23. Robson PM, Dweck MR, Trivieri MG, Karakatsanis NA, Contreras J, Gidwani U, et al. HHS Public Access. 2018;10:1103–12.
24. Grothoff M, Elpert C, Hoffmann J, Zachrau J, Lehmkuhl L, De Waha S, et al. Right ventricular injury in ST-elevation myocardial infarction risk stratification by visualization of wall motion, edema, and delayed-enhancement cardiac magnetic resonance. Circ Cardiovasc Imaging. 2012;5(1):60–8.
25. Aziz K, Berger K, Claycombe K, Huang R, Patel R, Abela GS. Noninvasive detection and localization of vulnerable plaque and arterial thrombosis with computed tomography angiography/positron emission tomography. Circulation. 2008;117(16):2061–70.
26. Gorog DA, Fayad ZA, Fuster V. Arterial thrombus stability: does it matter and can we detect it? J Am Coll Cardiol. 2017;70(16):2036–47.
27. Kang MK, Kim CJ, Choo EH, Han EJ, Hwang BH, Kim JJ, et al. Anti-inflammatory effect of statin is continuously working throughout use: a prospective three time point 18F-FDG PET/CT imaging study. Int J Cardiovasc Imaging [Internet]. 2019;35(9):1745–53. https://doi.org/10.1007/s10554-019-01584-y.
28. Sriranjan RS, Tarkin JM, Evans NR, Le EPV, Chowdhury MM, Rudd JHF. Atherosclerosis imaging using PET: insights and applications. Br J Pharmacol. 2021;178:2186–203.
29. Abbafati C, Machado DB, Cislaghi B, Salman OM, Karanikolos M, McKee M, et al. Global burden of 369 diseases and injuries in 204 countries and territories, 1990–2019: a systematic analysis for the global burden of disease study 2019. Lancet. 2020;396(10258):1204–22.
30. Rahimtoola SH. Myocardial hibernation: clinical manifestations and importance. Dialogues Cardiovasc Med. 1997;2(2):59–75.
31. Beanlands RSB, Nichol G, Huszti E, Humen D, Racine N, Freeman M, et al. F-18-Fluorodeoxyglucose positron emission tomography imaging-assisted management of patients with severe left ventricular dysfunction and suspected coronary disease. A randomized, controlled trial (PARR-2). J Am Coll Cardiol. 2007;50(20):2002–12.
32. Ghosh N, Rimoldi OE, Beanlands RSB, Camici PG. Assessment of myocardial ischaemia and viability: role of positron emission tomography. Eur Heart J. 2010;31(24):2984–95.
33. Abraham A, Nichol G, Williams KA, Guo A, de Kemp RA, Garrard L, et al. 18F-FDG PET imaging of myocardial viability in an experienced center with access to 18F-FDG and integration with clinical management teams: the Ottawa-FIVE substudy of the PARR 2 trial. J Nucl Med [Internet]. 2010;51(4):567–74. http://jnm.snmjournals.org/cgi/doi/10.2967/jnumed.109.065938.
34. McArdle B, Shukla T, Nichol G, Dekemp RA, Bernick J, Guo A, et al. Long-term follow-up of outcomes with F-18-fluorodeoxyglucose positron emission tomography imaging-assisted management of patients with severe left ventricular dysfunction secondary to coronary disease. Circ Cardiovasc Imaging. 2016;9(9):1–8.
35. Ling LF, Marwick TH, Flores DR, Jaber WA, Brunken RC, Cerqueira MD, et al. Identification of therapeutic benefit from revascularization in patients with left ventricular systolic dysfunction inducible ischemia versus hibernating myocardium. Circ Cardiovasc Imaging. 2013;6(3):363–72.
36. Schinkel AFL, Bax JJ, Poldermans D, Elhendy A, Ferrari R, Rahimtoola SH. Hibernating myocardium: diagnosis and patient outcomes. Curr Probl Cardiol. 2007;32(7):375–410.
37. Bonow RO, Maurer G, Lee KL, Holly TA, Binkley PF, Desvigne-Nickens P, et al. Myocardial viability and survival in ischemic left ventricular dysfunction. N Engl J Med. 2011;364(17):1617–25.
38. Dilsizian V, Perrone-Filardi P, Arrighi JA, Bacharach SL, Quyyumi AA, Freedman NMT, et al. Concordance and discordance between stress-redistribution-reinjection and rest-redistribution thallium imaging for assessing viable myocardium: comparison with metabolic activity by positron emission tomography. Circulation. 1993;88(3):941–52.
39. Rischpler C, Langwieser N, Souvatzoglou M, Batrice A, Van Marwick S, Snajberk J, et al. PET/MRI early after myocardial infarction: evaluation of viability with late gadolinium enhancement transmurality vs. 18F-FDG uptake. Eur Heart J Cardiovasc Imaging. 2015;16(6):661–9.
40. Stuijfzand WJ, Raijmakers PG, Driessen RS, van Royen N, Nap A, van Rossum AC, et al. Value of hybrid imaging with PET/CT to guide percutaneous revascularization of chronic total coronary occlusion. Curr Cardiovasc Imaging Rep. 2015;8(7):1–14.
41. Leimbach WN, Wallin BG, Victor RG, Aylward PE, Sundlöf G, Mark AL. Direct evidence from intraneural recordings for increased central sympathetic outflow in patients with heart failure. Circulation. 1986;73(5):913–9.
42. Fallavollita JA, Heavey BM, Luisi AJ, Michalek SM, Baldwa S, Mashtare TL, et al. Regional myocardial sympathetic denervation predicts the risk of sudden cardiac arrest in ischemic cardiomyopathy. J Am Coll Cardiol. 2014;63(2):141–9.
43. Jacobson AF, Senior R, Cerqueira MD, Wong ND, Thomas GS, Lopez VA, et al. Myocardial iodine-123

meta-iodobenzylguanidine imaging and cardiac events in heart failure. Results of the prospective ADMIRE-HF (AdreView Myocardial Imaging for Risk Evaluation in Heart Failure) study. J Am Coll Cardiol. 2010;55(20):2212–21.
44. Tamaki S, Yamada T, Okuyama Y, Morita T, Sanada S, Tsukamoto Y, et al. Cardiac iodine-123 metaiodobenzylguanidine imaging predicts sudden cardiac death independently of left ventricular ejection fraction in patients with chronic heart failure and left ventricular systolic dysfunction. Results from a comparative study with Si. J Am Coll Cardiol. 2009;53(5):426–35.
45. Ohira H, de Kemp R, Pena E, Davies RA, Stewart DJ, Chandy G, et al. Shifts in myocardial fatty acid and glucose metabolism in pulmonary arterial hypertension: a potential mechanism for a maladaptive right ventricular response. Eur Heart J Cardiovasc Imaging. 2016;17(12):1424–31.
46. Kazimierczyk R, Szumowski P, Nekolla SG, Blaszczak P, Malek LA, Milosz-Wieczorek B, et al. Prognostic role of PET/MRI hybrid imaging in patients with pulmonary arterial hypertension. Heart. 2021;107(1):54–60.
47. D'Arcy JL, Coffey S, Loudon MA, Kennedy A, Pearson-Stuttard J, Birks J, et al. Large-scale community echocardiographic screening reveals a major burden of undiagnosed valvular heart disease in older people: the OxVALVE population cohort study. Eur Heart J. 2016;37(47):3515–22.
48. Clavel MA, Magne J, Pibarot P. Low-gradient aortic stenosis. Eur Heart J. 2016;37(34):2645–57.
49. Baumgartner H, Falk V, Bax JJ, De Bonis M, Hamm C, Holm PJ, et al. 2017 ESC/EACTS guidelines for the management of valvular heart disease. Eur Heart J. 2017;38:2739–2786p.
50. Derlin T, Wisotzki C, Richter U, Apostolova I, Bannas P, Weber C, et al. In vivo imaging of mineral deposition in carotid plaque using 18F-sodium fluoride PET/CT: correlation with atherogenic risk factors. J Nucl Med. 2011;52(3):362–8.
51. Abdelbaky A, Corsini E, Figueroa AL, Subramanian S, Fontanez S, Emami H, et al. Early aortic valve inflammation precedes calcification: a longitudinal FDG-PET/CT study. Atherosclerosis. 2015;238(2):165–72.
52. Dweck MR, Jones C, Joshi NV, Fletcher AM, Richardson H, White A, et al. Assessment of valvular calcification and inflammation by positron emission tomography in patients with aortic stenosis. Circulation. 2012;125(1):76–86.
53. Marincheva-Savcheva G, Subramanian S, Qadir S, Figueroa A, Truong Q, Vijayakumar J, et al. Imaging of the aortic valve using fluorodeoxyglucose positron emission tomography: increased valvular fluorodeoxyglucose uptake in aortic stenosis. J Am Coll Cardiol [Internet]. 2011;57(25):2507–15. https://doi.org/10.1016/j.jacc.2010.12.046.
54. Dumas O, Abramovitz L, Wiley AS, Cozier YC, Camargo CA. Epidemiology of sarcoidosis in a prospective cohort study of U.S. women. Ann Am Thorac Soc. 2016;13(1):67–71.
55. Ekström K, Lehtonen J, Nordenswan HK, Mäyränpää MI, Räisänen-Sokolowski A, Kandolin R, et al. Sudden death in cardiac sarcoidosis: an analysis of nationwide clinical and cause-of-death registries. Eur Heart J. 2019;40(37):3121–8.
56. Kandolin R, Lehtonen J, Kupari M. Cardiac sarcoidosis and giant cell myocarditis as causes of atrioventricular block in young and middle-aged adults. Circ Arrhythm Electrophysiol. 2011;4(3):303–9.
57. Segura AM, Radovancevic R, Demirozu ZT, Frazier OH, Buja LM. Granulomatous myocarditis in severe heart failure patients undergoing implantation of a left ventricular assist device. Cardiovasc Pathol [Internet]. 2014;23(1):17–20. https://doi.org/10.1016/j.carpath.2013.06.005.
58. Kandolin R, Lehtonen J, Airaksinen J, Vihinen T, Miettinen H, Ylitalo K, et al. Cardiac sarcoidosis: epidemiology, characteristics, and outcome over 25 years in a nationwide study. Circulation. 2015;131(7):624–32.
59. Birnie DH, Sauer WH, Bogun F, Cooper JM, Culver DA, Duvernoy CS, et al. HRS expert consensus statement on the diagnosis and management of arrhythmias associated with cardiac sarcoidosis. Heart Rhythm [Internet]. 2014;11(7):1304–23. https://doi.org/10.1016/j.hrthm.2014.03.043.
60. Ohira H, Tsujino I, Yoshinaga K. 18F-fluoro-2-deoxyglucose positron emission tomography in cardiac sarcoidosis. Eur J Nucl Med Mol Imaging. 2011;38(9):1773–83.
61. Flores RJ, Flaherty KR, Jin Z, Bokhari S. The prognostic value of quantitating and localizing F-18 FDG uptake in cardiac sarcoidosis. J Nucl Cardiol [Internet]. 2020;27(6):2003–10. https://doi.org/10.1007/s12350-018-01504-y.
62. Kandolin R, Lehtonen J, Graner M, Schildt J, Salmenkivi K, Kivistö SM, et al. Diagnosing isolated cardiac sarcoidosis. J Intern Med. 2011;270(5):461–8.
63. Wicks EC, Menezes LJ, Barnes A, Mohiddin SA, Sekhri N, Porter JC, et al. Diagnostic accuracy and prognostic value of simultaneous hybrid 18 F-fluorodeoxyglucose positron emission tomography/magnetic resonance imaging in cardiac sarcoidosis. Eur Heart J Cardiovasc Imaging. 2018;19(7):757–67.
64. Ardehali H, Howard DL, Hariri A, Qasim A, Hare JM, Baughman KL, et al. A positive endomyocardial biopsy result for sarcoid is associated with poor prognosis in patients with initially unexplained cardiomyopathy. Am Heart J. 2005;150(3):459–63.
65. Arbustini E, Verga L, Concardi M, Palladini G, Obici L, Merlini G. Electron and immuno-electron microscopy of abdominal fat identifies and char-

acterizes amyloid fibrils in suspected cardiac amyloidosis. Amyloid Int J Exp Clin Invest [Internet]. 2002;9(2):108–14.
66. Rapezzi C, Merlini G, Quarta CC, Riva L, Longhi S, Leone O, et al. Systemic cardiac amyloidoses: disease profiles and clinical courses of the 3 main types. Circulation. 2009;120(13):1203–12.
67. Gillmore JD, Maurer MS, Falk RH, Merlini G, Damy T, Dispenzieri A, et al. Nonbiopsy diagnosis of cardiac transthyretin amyloidosis. Circulation. 2016;133(24):2404–12.
68. Zhang KW, Stockerl-Goldstein KE, Lenihan DJ. Emerging therapeutics for the treatment of light chain and transthyretin amyloidosis. JACC Basic Transl Sci [Internet]. 2019;4(3):438–48. https://doi.org/10.1016/j.jacbts.2019.02.002.
69. Quock TP, Yan T, Chang E, Guthrie S, Broder MS. Epidemiology of AL amyloidosis: a real-world study using US claims data. Blood Adv. 2018;2(10):1046–53.
70. González-López E, Gallego-Delgado M, Guzzo-Merello G, De Haro-Del Moral FJ, Cobo-Marcos M, Robles C, et al. Wild-type transthyretin amyloidosis as a cause of heart failure with preserved ejection fraction. Eur Heart J. 2015;36(38):2585–94.
71. Van Der Gucht A, Galat A, Rosso J, Guellich A, Garot J, Bodez D, et al. [18F]-NaF PET/CT imaging in cardiac amyloidosis. J Nucl Cardiol. 2016;23(4):846–9.
72. Dorbala S, Ando Y, Bokhari S, Dispenzieri A, Falk RH, Ferrari VA, et al. ASNC/AHA/ASE/EANM/HFSA/ISA/SCMR/SNMMI expert consensus recommendations for multimodality imaging in cardiac amyloidosis: part 2 of 2—Diagnostic criteria and appropriate utilization. J Nucl Cardiol [Internet]. 2019. https://doi.org/10.1007/s12350-019-01761-5.
73. Baig S, Edward NC, Kotecha D, Liu B, Nordin S, Kozor R, et al. Ventricular arrhythmia and sudden cardiac death in Fabry disease: a systematic review of risk factors in clinical practice. Europace. 2018;20:f153–61.
74. Nappi C, Altiero M, Imbriaco M, Nicolai E, Giudice CA, Aiello M, et al. First experience of simultaneous PET/MRI for the early detection of cardiac involvement in patients with Anderson-Fabry disease. Eur J Nucl Med Mol Imaging. 2015;42:1025–31.
75. Horgan SJ, Mediratta A, Gillam LD. Cardiovascular imaging in infective endocarditis: a multimodality approach. Circ Cardiovasc Imaging. 2020;13(7):1–11.
76. Feuchtner GM, Stolzmann P, Dichtl W, Schertler T, Bonatti J, Scheffel H, et al. Multislice computed tomography in infective endocarditis. Comparison with transesophageal echocardiography and intraoperative findings. J Am Coll Cardiol. 2009;53(5):436–44.
77. Medicine N, Grazia M, France JC, Del F, El G, Anna P, et al. 2015 ESC guidelines for the management of infective endocarditis the task force for the management of infective endocarditis of the European Society of Cardiology (ESC) endorsed by: European Association for Cardio-Thoracic Surgery. Eur Heart J 2015;36:3075–3123p.
78. Pizzi MN, Roque A, Fernández-Hidalgo N, Cuéllar-Calabria H, Ferreira-González I, Gonzàlez-Alujas MT, et al. Improving the diagnosis of infective endocarditis in prosthetic valves and intracardiac devices with F-fluordeoxyglucose positron emission tomography/computed tomography angiography: initial results at an infective endocarditis referral center. Circulation. 2015;132:1113–26.
79. Slart RHJA, Slart RHJA, Glaudemans AWJM, Chareonthaitawee P, Treglia G, Besson FL, et al. FDG-PET/CT(A) imaging in large vessel vasculitis and polymyalgia rheumatica: joint procedural recommendation of the EANM, SNMMI, and the PET Interest Group (PIG), and endorsed by the ASNC. Eur J Nucl Med Mol Imaging. 2018;45(7):1250–69.
80. Lee YH, Choi SJ, Ji JD, Song GG. Diagnostische Genauigkeit der 18F-FDG PET bzw. PET/CT für Vaskulitiden großer Gefäße: Eine Metaanalyse. Z Rheumatol. 2016;75(9):924–31.

Hybrid Cardiac Imaging for the Cardiologist with Expertise in Echocardiography

2

Eugenio Picano and Paul Leeson

2.1 Introduction

Echocardiography remains the cornerstone of medical imaging in cardiology for its undisputed advantages of widespread diffusion, portability, versatility, safety, and radiation-free nature, with no need for iodine and gadolinium-based contrast agents [1–3]. Echocardiography also has key advantages for economic and environmental sustainability, with a lack of ionizing radiation significantly reducing the downstream cancer risk induction [4] and a low environmental footprint, estimated to be 100-times less than a cardiac magnetic resonance [5].

Still, echocardiography faces limitations because of its operator-dependence, which results in greater subjectivity of interpretation. In addition, in recent years the tremendous versatility of the technique has resulted in a huge increase in the information that can be extracted from ultrasound imaging, which can be difficult for the cardiologists to handle and interpret. They now, receive information on anatomy, function, flow, cardiac structure, coronary supply, and lung appearances, with different techniques such as M-mode, two-dimensional (2D), color-, continuous wave-, pulsed-, and tissue-Doppler, contrast, three-dimensional (3D), and deformation (strain) imaging [6, 7]. Artificial intelligence (AI) and hybrid imaging approaches may provide a solution to simplify the handling of this wealth of this imaging information (Fig. 2.1) with four main aims [8]: (1) to make objective what is currently done by the "naked eye" (for instance regional wall motion analysis) or by "hand measurements" (for instance ejection fraction from left ventricular end-diastolic and end-systolic volumes); (2) to detect what is undetectable by "natural" intelligence (for instance, myocardial fibrosis with conventional gray level analysis of 2D image texture); (3) to combine in a single image information coming from different imaging sources: for instance, fluoroscopy and trans-esophageal echocardiography (TEE) in hybrid imaging during transcatheter mitral valve repair; (4) to mine big data with techniques such as network analysis to identify interconnected variables and thereby optimize risk stratification for individual patients.

AI is an umbrella term that has expanded in use to encompass different approaches, which

No conflict of interest declared by the authors. Paul Leeson is a founder and shareholder of Ultromics Ltd. an AI imaging company.

E. Picano (✉)
Biomedicine Department, Institute of Clinical Physiology, National Council Research, Pisa, Italy
e-mail: picano@ifc.cnr.it

P. Leeson
Cardiovascular Clinical Research Facility, RDM Division of Cardiovascular Medicine, University of Oxford, Oxford, UK
e-mail: paul.leeson@cardiov.ox.ac.uk

F. Nudi et al. (eds.), *Hybrid Cardiac Imaging for Clinical Decision-Making*,
https://doi.org/10.1007/978-3-030-99391-7_2

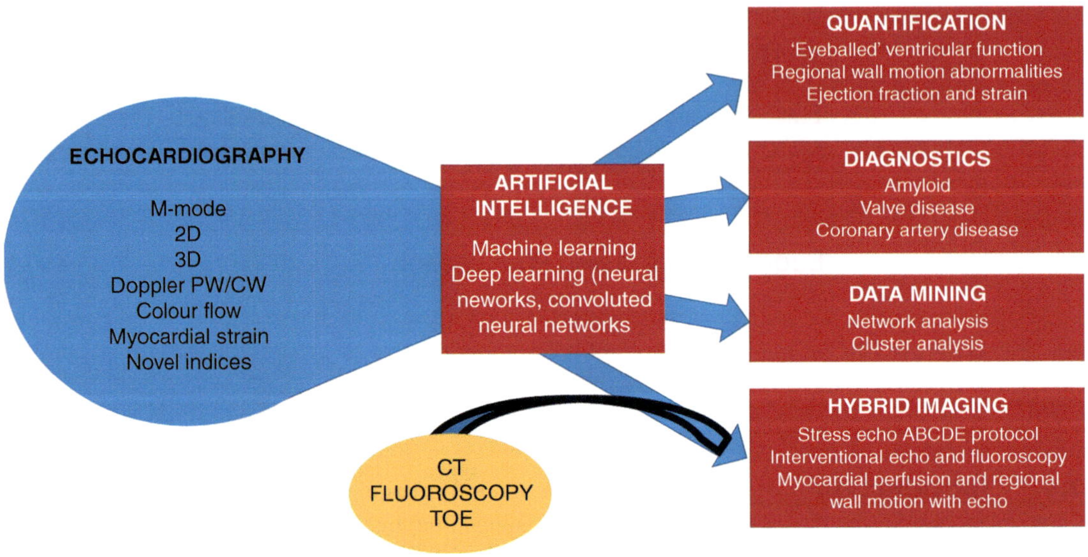

Fig. 2.1 Artificial Intelligence and hybrid imaging for echocardiography. Diagram to illustrate the potential applications of AI to large-scale echocardiography data sets and clinical practice

have evolved as the methodology has developed: **machine learning** describes the ability of machines to learn for themselves using big datasets with minimal supervision; **deep learning** is a type of machine learning that makes decisions based on networks of decision nodes that mimic the human brain neural network and, more specifically, the human retinal neural connections; **convolutional neural networks** are a specific type of deep learning neural network that has multiple interconnected layers of nodes [9] that have proved particularly effective for learning about image structure. For instance, a convolutional neural network can be developed to recognize an image by dividing the image into separate features, which are then considered by the different layers of the network, from deepest to more superficial. The lowest layer might recognize simple features such as edges. The next layer would recognize combinations of simple features such as edges and circles or gray levels. Each level provides increasing levels of complexity and definition allowing some conclusion about the likely nature of the image. The features of the top layer are then typically used in a multinomial logistic regression model to generate a classification of the image based on a probabilistic output. Once a process, or "algorithm," has been developed using AI to process images, whether simply to recognize the image, or make quantifiable conclusions from the image, the next critical step is to test the "algorithm" to ensure it continues to accurately make predictions when faced with new data [10].

2.2 From Eyeballing to Quantification

Some of the first applications of AI within echocardiography have been to make operator-independent what is currently done "by hands" and "by eyes." Recognition of a correct echocardiographic view [11, 12] or calculation of left ventricular ejection fraction have now been effectively performed with AI [13, 14]. AI-based approaches can even overcome technical challenges such as the identification of borders in poor quality images, which limit other automated approaches. "*A computer that has never seen an image before can now take an echocardiogram, look at 2 views and, without any user input or need to contour the ventricle, estimate what it thinks is the ejection fraction with astonishing precision*" [15]. Traditionally, ejection fraction interpretation at point of care has been conducted through visual estimation, but variation in clinician experience across point-of-care settings has raised concerns about accuracy. AI software that uses advanced pattern recognition algorithms to imitate the way the human eye identifies borders and motion should remove this variability between operators.

Another example of AI replacing or corroborating naked eye diagnosis is regional wall motion abnormalities at rest and during stress. A deep learning approach has the same accuracy as experienced readers in identifying regional wall motion abnormalities and has now been applied both in resting conditions [16] and during stress [17].

As AI-based approaches are further developed, traditionally complex, time-consuming, and technically demanding measurements performed by eye or hand should start to be undertaken in automated and highly reproducible ways. These approaches should be able to encompass assessment of right ventricular size and function [18], automatic quantification of mitral regurgitation [19], measurements of mitral valve [20], aortic root [21], or left ventricular filling pressures [22].

2.3 Exposing Information Missed by the Eye

AI methods may also allow extraction of information missed by the "eye." For years videodensitometric features of the 2D image have been used to identify myocardial fibrosis as increased gray levels and reduced cyclic variation from systole to diastole [23, 24]. This approach has never been implemented clinically due to sources of error such as nonlinearity between displayed signal and received signal, possibility of artifacts, anisotropy of myocardial walls showing different reflectivity features in different projections. Now a cardiac ultrasonic fingerprinting approach has shown potential to identify myocardial fibrosis, consistent with findings from the gold standard of delayed gadolinium enhancement. This method combines information on gray levels, global longitudinal strain, left ventricular volumes, and clinical risk factors [25].

A similar approach can be applied to the detection of complex carotid plaque morphology. Ultrasound has the clear potential to identify a lipid core separated from fibrotic and calcified plaque components. Therefore the texture and morphological features of a complex, rupture-prone plaque may be identifiable with image processing and generate greater insights about clinical plaque stability than can be achieved just by relying on plaque geometry and stenosis [26, 27]. By undertaking this analysis with machine learning, the approach should allow identification of vulnerable plaques in a solid, operator-independent manner [28] that might further expand the potential of a comprehensive risk stratification based on the integration of resting carotid scan and stress echo.

2.4 Hybrid Imaging

Echocardiography is generally used as a stand-alone technique, independently of other imaging techniques. A different approach is hybrid imaging, a multimodal approach using information derived from different techniques, usually complementary in nature (e.g., anatomical and functional) rather than overlapping (anatomical and anatomical) [29] Hybridization implies the simultaneous interpretation of obtained scans for critical on-line decision-making (for instance in echocardiography-fluoroscopy fusion) but may also imply a simultaneous interpretation of different sets of images obtained independently and combined off-line for purposes of interpretation for instance to match an anatomic disease (most typically a coronary atherosclerotic plaque) with a functional defect (usually a stress-induced perfusion defect or a regional wall motion abnormality. However, no application in cardiology has reached the clinical acceptance of hybrid imaging with PET-CT in oncology.

The main application of real-time fusion imaging in echocardiography is the combination with fluoroscopy in percutaneous structural heart interventions to increase procedural success. The method is based on the localization of the TEE probe into the fluoroscopic space, allowing to detect the position and orientation of the TEE probe from fluoroscopic data [30].

The commercially available fusion systems can reduce procedural time and fluoroscopic time due to better and faster understanding of the combination of soft tissue anatomy and catheter devices, resulting in less need for X-ray during the procedure [30]. Typically, interventional cardiologists are more familiar with fluoroscopic than ultrasound images. Information from TEE images is therefore transposed onto the fluoroscopic images. Fusion imaging facilitates improved understanding of anatomical structures and the spatial relation between the X-ray and ultrasound images, improves communication between imaging and interventional cardiologists, ability of the interventionalist to manipulate the 3D-TEE images, and improved confidence when positioning the interventional device and guiding interventional procedures [31]. The benefits and weaknesses of echocardiography-fluoroscopy fusion are summarized in Table 2.1.

Table 2.1 Hybrid imaging with echocardiography-fluoroscopy fusion during percutaneous interventions

Strengths	Weaknesses
Same visual perspective	Same vendor for X-ray and TEE
Better team communication	Proprietary software needed
Improved visual guidance	Extra-cost of hardware
More efficient navigation	3D echo probe required
Less radiation for patients	Not feasible for children <20 kg
Less radiation for doctors	Intracardiac US not supported
Harmonization of images	Poor image quality impairs fusion
Lower procedural time	Dedicated learning curve required

Many procedures have been combined with fusion imaging with obvious benefits. Congenital and structural heart disease interventions benefit most from fusion imaging, and include transseptal catheterization, atrial septal defect closure, ventricular septal defect closure, stenting of pulmonary vein stenosis (either congenital or iatrogenic caused by atrial fibrillation ablation), Mitraclip, paravalvular leak closure, and left atrial appendage occlusion among others [32]. In principle, any intervention that requires image guidance using ultrasound modalities and x-rays may benefit from fusion technology [33]. Each one poses special opportunities and challenges. For instance, transcatheter mitral valve repair guidance can be performed with either Mitraclip or Cardioband systems (Fig. 2.2). According to the pioneering experience of Faletra, Agricola et al., in this specific application fusion imaging is especially helpful in: (a) guiding the search of transseptal puncture site; (b) navigating in the left atrium (to avoid impinging on the lateral wall or left lateral ridge); (c) assessing superior-inferior clip trajectory; and (d) localizing the origin of regurgitant jet on fluoroscopy. On the other hand, not all authors reported a reduction in radiation exposure with this specific application, and the handling of a huge amount of visual data can be distractive ("fusion or confusion?") for the interventional cardiologist, who may be reluctant to adopt this technique in absence of convincing evidences and large scale evidences, not available as yet [34].

Another less mature field of application of fusion imaging is coronary artery disease. The combination of coronary computed tomography angiography and strain maps of deformation imaging obtained with 3D echocardiography can show match or mismatch between anatomic coronary stenosis and longitudinal strain maps, allowing direct visualization of each coronary artery and myocardial longitudinal in its territory [35]. This approach can be derived from deformation maps at rest or—more conveniently—with strain maps during stress, and hybrid fusion software are available allowing anatomical matching between 3D strain stress data sets superimposed on 3D coronary computed tomog-

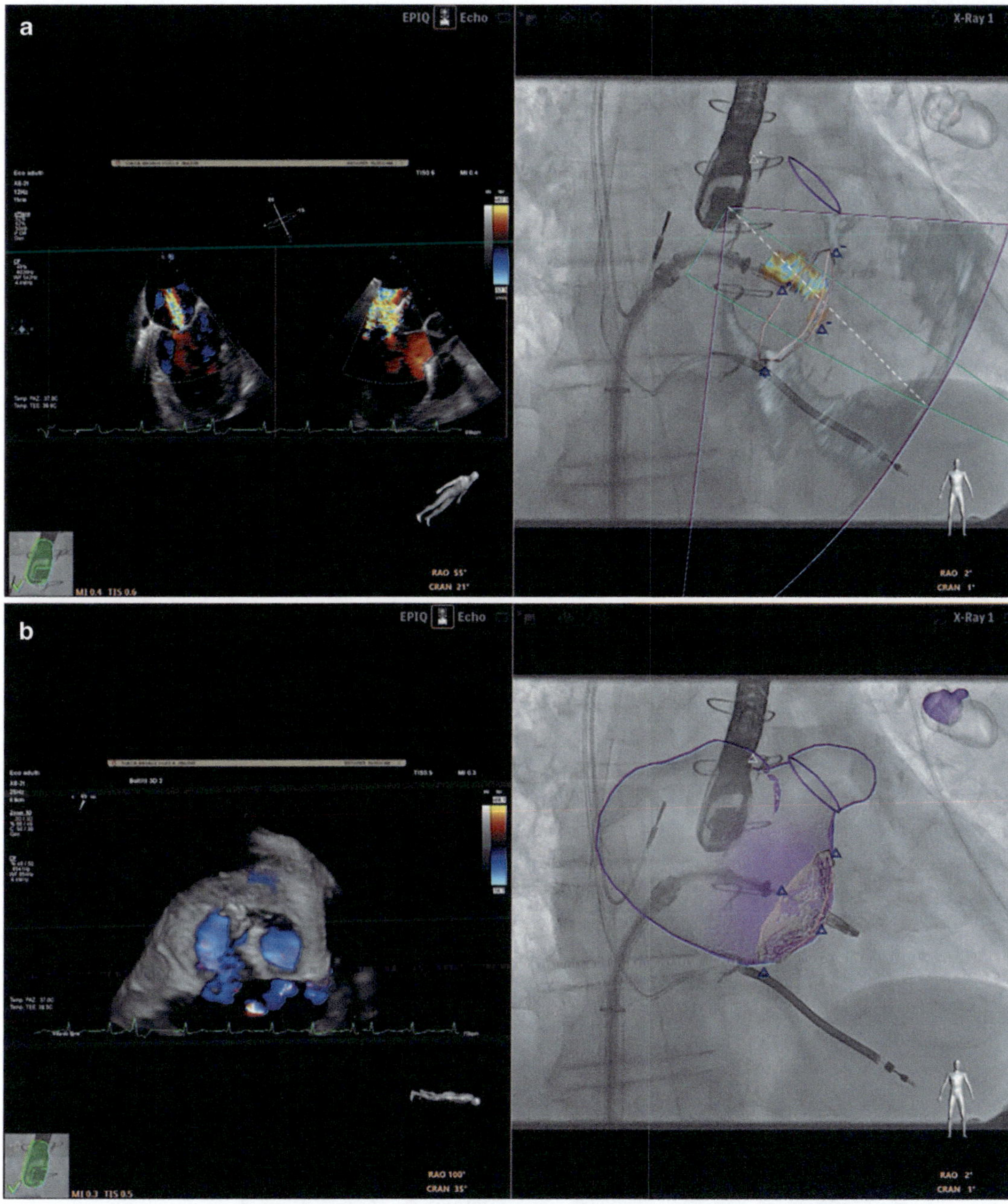

Fig. 2.2 Fusion imaging with Heart Model during MitraClip procedure. (**a**) Color Doppler and mitral valve model superimposed to Right Anterior Oblique and Caudal fluoroscopic projection. (**b**) After Clip release. (By courtesy of Professor Eustachio Agricola, Vita-Salute University, San Raffaele Hospital, Milan, Italy)

raphy datasets. These packages allow a spectacular comprehensive anatomic and functional representation of coronary anatomy and regional stress myocardial function at the same time [36].

2.5 Data Handling: Network Analysis

Increasingly it is being realized that regional wall motion analysis on its own is insufficient for accurate diagnosis and risk stratification of a patient with suspected or known coronary artery disease and/or heart failure. However, a rational approach that can combine the enormous amount of information available on individual patients to provide optimal risk prediction has been lacking. Network analysis is ideally suited to mine big data and could be used to identify key variables and optimize risk stratification. For instance, in coronary artery disease multiple clusters of information can be collected during stress echo that may be of benefit for diagnosis [36, 37]. Five key parameters, in particular, have been defined that converge conceptually, logistically, and methodologically in the ABCDE protocol of stress echo (Fig. 2.3). These capture the many vulnerabilities of the patient above and beyond critical coronary artery stenosis: epicardial coronary artery stenosis, pulmonary congestion, and interstitial pulmonary edema (B-lines), global myocardial function, coronary small vessels, and cardiac autonomic nervous system imbalance. The five steps of the ABCDE protocol are: (1) step A: regional wall motion abnormalities by 2D (possibly enriched and strengthened by quantitative assessment or regional and global longitudinal strain); (2) step B: B-lines by lung ultrasound (with the 4-site simplified scan of third intercostal space) assessing the shape of lung water and pulmonary congestion [38, 39]; (3) step C: left ventricular contractile reserve assessed as the

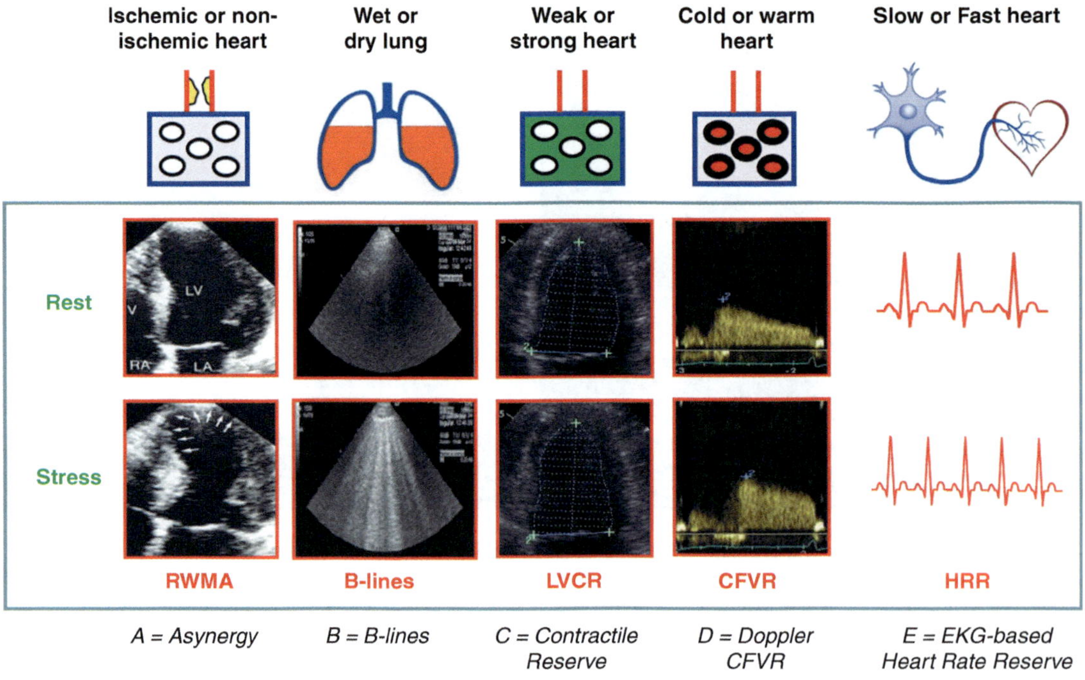

Fig. 2.3 The targets of integrated ABCDE stress echo. The five pathophysiological targets of ABCDE-SE: epicardial coronary artery stenosis (with RWMA); lung water (with B-lines); myocardial function (with left ventricular end-systolic area); small vessels (with coronary flow velocity reserve); cardiac autonomic balance (with heart rate reserve). (Modified and adapted from Picano E, 2018 [36] http://creativecommons.org/licenses/by/4.0/. From Picano E et al. [36], http://creativecommons.org/licenses/by/4.0/)

stress/rest ratio of force (systolic arterial pressure by cuff sphygmomanometer/end-systolic volume from 2D) or more simply as left ventricular cavity dilation during stress [40, 41]; (4) step D: Doppler-based assessment of coronary flow velocity reserve in left anterior descending coronary with pulsed-wave Doppler; (5) step E: imaging-independent EKG-based assessment of heart rate reserve (peak/rest heart rate) [42, 43]. The same transducer is used for both the cardiac and ultrasound scan. The cutoff values are stress-independent for A, B, and D, but stress-specific for C and E, since vasodilators are a weaker inotropic and chronotropic stress than exercise and dobutamine. The abnormal cutoff value for contractile reserve is based on receiver-operating characteristics validation for outcome measures and is lower for vasodilators (≤1.1) compared to exercise or dobutamine stress (≤2.0). The abnormal cutoff value for chronotropic reserve is lower for vasodilators (heart rate reserve ≤1.22) compared to exercise or dobutamine stress (≤1.80). Chronotropic incompetence is associated with a worse prognosis independently of induced ischemia with all forms of physical and pharmacological stress. The combination of these 5 ABCDE parameters in a single test allows a more comprehensive risk stratification than regional wall motion abnormalities alone. Each cluster of rest and stress imaging data is combined with clinical, electrocardiographic, and other imaging data to identify specific phenotypes (with prevalent regional ischemia, increased myocardial stiffness and pulmonary congestion, global left ventricular hyper- or hypo-contractile dysfunction and myocardial fibrosis, microcirculatory disease, autonomic dysfunction). Each specific phenotype requires a targeted approach, which can be neutral or even detrimental for other forms of diseases sharing the same symptoms and the same morphology and function at rest.

2.6 Conclusion

AI-echocardiography describes the application of the overlapping fields of machine learning, deep learning, and network analysis to echocardiography image processing and analysis. The technologies are also ideally suited for analyzing hybrid imaging data and have the potential to dramatically simplify the lives of cardiologists and echocardiographers. AI will shift the cardiologist's time from tedious training, analysis, and archiving to integration and innovation. AI will close the gap between experts and beginners potentially allowing unsupervised diagnosis. Echocardiography and stress echo generates an immense amount of digital data that can be combined with traditional risk factors, clinical presentation, other imaging techniques, and laboratory biomarkers. Making sense of this landslide of data is a challenge even for the best cardiologist but AI provides a potential key for interpretation and data mining. The methods could uncover complex clinical relationships that redefine disease and previously unseen clinically relevant information hidden within ultrasound images [44]. The trend for the use of data mining will allow extraction of data currently buried in the image and make them readily available for clinical use. Echocardiography could become not only the first-line cardiology imaging test but, increasingly, the only and final test required by cardiologists to reach a diagnosis and management plan [45]. For individual centers and echocardiography labs increased precision and reproducibility derived from AI means volumes of activity will no longer be necessary to guarantee accuracy of measures [46, 47]. With AI-echocardiography and AI-stress echo we are witnessing a new exciting era that will rapidly change the daily life of our laboratories, allowing integration, quantification, and operator-independence, so that echocardiography can be established as the definitive, quantitative, unsupervised, and objective imaging test.

References

1. Knuuti J, Wijns W, Saraste CD, Barbato E, Funck-Brentano C, Prescott E, Storey RF, Deaton C, Cuisset T, Agewall S, Dickstein K, Edvardsen T, Escaned J, Gersh BJ, Svitil P, Gilard M, Hasdai D, Hatala R, Mahfoud F, Masip J, Muneretto C, Valgimigli M,

Achenbach S, Bax JJ, ESC Scientific Document Group. ESC guidelines for the diagnosis and management of chronic coronary syndromes. Eur Heart J. 2019;2020(41):407–77. https://doi.org/10.1093/eurheartj/ehz425.
2. Picano E, Vañó E, Rehani MM, Cuocolo A, Mont L, Bodi V, Bar O, Maccia C, Pierard L, Sicari R, Plein S, Mahrholdt H, Lancellotti P, Knuuti J, Heidbuchel H, Di Mario C, Badano LP. The appropriate and justified use of medical radiation in cardiovascular imaging: a position document of the ESC associations of cardiovascular imaging, percutaneous cardiovascular interventions and electrophysiology. Eur Heart J. 2014;35:665–72.
3. Lancellotti P, Pellikka PA, Budts W, Chaudry F, Donal E, Dulgheru R, Edvarsen T, Garbi M, Ha JW, Kane G, Kreeger J, Mertens L, Pibarot P, Picano E, Ryan T, Tsutsui J, Varga A. Recommendations for the clinical use of stress echocardiography in non-ischemic heart disease: joint document of the European Association of Cardiovascular Imaging and the American Society of Echocardiography. Eur Heart J Cardiovasc Imaging. 2016;17:1191–22.
4. Pellikka PA, Arruda-Olson A, Chaudhry FA, Chen MH, Marshall JE, Porter TR, Sawada SG. Guidelines for performance, interpretation, and application of stress echocardiography in ischemic heart disease: from the American Society of Echocardiography. J Am Soc Echocardiogr. 2020;33:1–41.e8.
5. Picano E. Sustainability of medical imaging. BMJ. 2004;328:578–80. https://doi.org/10.1136/bmj.328.7439.578.
6. Marwick TH, Buonocore J. Environmental impact of cardiac imaging tests for the diagnosis of coronary artery disease. Heart. 2011;97:1128–31. https://doi.org/10.1136/hrt.2011.227884.
7. Picano E, Pellikka PA. Stress echo applications beyond coronary artery disease. Eur Heart J. 2014;35:1033–40. https://doi.org/10.1093/eurheartj/eht350.
8. Garcia-Fernandez MA. Artificial intelligence in echocardiography. The future is here. Argentinian J Cardiol. 2019;87:469–72.
9. Alsharqi M, Upton R, Mumith A, Leeson P. Artificial intelligence: a new clinical support tool for stress echocardiography. Expert Rev Med Devices. 2018;15:513–5. https://doi.org/10.1080/17434440.2018.1497482.
10. Dey D, Slomka PJ, Leeson P, Comaniciu D, Shrestha S, Sengupta PP, Marwick TH. Artificial intelligence in cardiovascular imaging: JACC state-of-the-art review. J Am Coll Cardiol. 2019;73:1317–35. https://doi.org/10.1016/j.jacc.2018.12.054.
11. Khamis H, Zurakhov G, Azar V, Raz A, Friedman Z, Adam D. Automatic apical view classification of echocardiograms using a discriminative learning dictionary. Med Image Anal. 2017;36:15–21. https://doi.org/10.1016/j.media.2016.10.007.
12. Madani A, Arnaout R, Mofrad M, Arnaout R. Fast and accurate view classification of echocardiograms using deep learning. NPJ Digit Med. 2018;1:6. https://doi.org/10.1038/s41746-017-0013-1.
13. Narula S, Shameer K, Salem Omar AM, Dudley JT, Sengupta PP. Machine-learning algorithms to automate morphological and functional assessments in 2D echocardiography. J Am Coll Cardiol. 2016;68:2287–95. https://doi.org/10.1016/j.jacc.2016.08.062.
14. Asch FM, Poilvert N, Abraham T, Jankowski M, Cleve J, Adams M, Romano N, Hong H, Mor-Avi V, Martin RP, Lang RM. Automated echocardiographic quantification of left ventricular ejection fraction without volume measurements using a machine learning algorithm mimicking a human expert. Circ Cardiovasc Imaging. 2019;12:e009303. https://doi.org/10.1161/CIRCIMAGING.119.009303.
15. Leeson P, Fletcher AJ. Combining artificial intelligence with human insight to automate echocardiography. Circ Cardiovasc Imaging. 2019;12:e009727. https://doi.org/10.1161/CIRCIMAGING.119.009727.
16. Kusunose K, Abe T, Haga A, Fukuda D, Yamada H, Harada M, Sata M. A deep learning approach for assessment of regional wall motion abnormality from echocardiographic images. JACC Cardiovasc Imaging. 2020;13(2 Pt 1):374–81. https://doi.org/10.1016/j.jcmg.2019.02.024.
17. Alsharqi M, Woodward WJ, Mumith JA, Markham DC, Upton R, Leeson P. Artificial intelligence and echocardiography. Echo Res Pract. 2018;5:R115–25. https://doi.org/10.1530/ERP-18-0056.
18. Genovese D, Rashedi N, Weinert L, Narang A, Addetia K, Patel AR, Prater D, Goncalves A, Mor-Avi V, Martin RP, Lang RM. Machine learning-based three-dimensional echocardiographic quantification of right ventricular size and function: validation against cardiac magnetic resonance. J Am Soc Echocardiogr. 2019;32(8):969–77. https://doi.org/10.1016/j.echo.2019.04.001.
19. Moghaddasi H, Nourian S. Automatic assessment of mitral regurgitation severity based on extensive textural features on 2D echocardiography videos. Comput Biol Med. 2016;73:47–55. https://doi.org/10.1016/j.compbiomed.2016.03.026.
20. Jeganathan J, Knio Z, Amador Y, Hai T, Khamooshian A, Matyal R, Khabbaz KR, Mahmood F. Artificial intelligence in mitral valve analysis. Ann Card Anaesth. 2017;20:129–34. https://doi.org/10.4103/aca.ACA_243_16.
21. Wojnarski CM, Roselli EE, Idrees JJ, Zhu Y, Carnes TA, Lowry AM, Collier PH, Griffin B, Ehrlinger J, Blackstone EH, Svensson LG, Lytle BW. Machine-learning phenotypic classification of bicuspid aortopathy. J Thorac Cardiovasc Surg. 2018;155:461–469.e4. https://doi.org/10.1016/j.jtcvs.2017.08.123.
22. Salem Omar AM, Shameer K, Narula S, Abdel Rahman MA, Rifaie O, Narula J, Dudley JT, Sengupta PP. Artificial intelligence-based assessment of left ventricular filling pressures from 2-dimensional cardiac ultrasound images. JACC Cardiovasc Imaging. 2018;11:509–10. https://doi.org/10.1016/j.jcmg.2017.05.003.

23. Picano E, Pelosi G, Marzilli M, Lattanzi F, Benassi A, Landini L, L'Abbate A. In vivo quantitative ultrasonic evaluation of myocardial fibrosis in humans. Circulation. 1990;81:58–64. https://doi.org/10.1161/01.cir.81.1.58.
24. Picano E, Faletra F, Marini C, Paterni M, Danzi GB, Lombardi M, Campolo L, Gigli G, Landini L, Pezzano A. Increased echodensity of transiently asynergic myocardium in humans: a novel echocardiographic sign of myocardial ischemia. J Am Coll Cardiol. 1993;21:199–207. https://doi.org/10.1016/0735-1097(93)90737-l.
25. Kagiyama N, Shrestha S, Cho SJ, Ashraf M, Khalil M, Hu L, Balla S, Casaclang-Verzosa G, Sengupta P. Cardiac ultrasonic fingerprinting: a radiomics approach for high-throughput feature phenotyping of dysfunctional myocardium. J Am Soc Echocardiogr. 2019, abstract YIA-1 JASE pgB3.
26. Picano E, Landini L, Distante A, Salvadori M, Lattanzi F, Masini M, L'Abbate A. Angle dependence of ultrasonic backscatter in arterial tissues: a study in vitro. Circulation. 1985;72:572–6. https://doi.org/10.1161/01.cir.72.3.572.
27. Urbani MP, Picano E, Parenti G, Mazzarisi A, Fiori L, Paterni M, Pelosi G, Landini L. In vivo radiofrequency-based ultrasonic tissue characterization of the atherosclerotic plaque. Stroke. 1993;24:1507–12. https://doi.org/10.1161/01.str.24.10.1507.
28. Lekadir K, Galimzianova A, Betriu A, Del Mar Vila M, Igual L, Rubin DL, Fernandez E, Radeva P, Napel S. A convolutional neural network for automatic characterization of plaque composition in carotid ultrasound. IEEE J Biomed Health Inform. 2017;21:48–55. https://doi.org/10.1109/JBHI.2016.2631401. Epub 2016 Nov 22. PMID: 27893402; PMCID: PMC5293622.
29. Juarez-Orozco LE, Martinez-Manzanera O, van der Zant FM, Knol RJJ, Knuuti J. Deep learning in quantitative PET myocardial perfusion imaging: a study on cardiovascular event prediction. JACC Cardiovasc Imaging. 2020;13(1 Pt 1):180–2. https://doi.org/10.1016/j.jcmg.2019.08.009.
30. Balzer J, Zeus T, Veulemans V, Kelm M. Hybrid imaging in the catheter laboratory: real-time fusion of echocardiography and fluoroscopy during percutaneous structural heart disease interventions. Interv Cardiol. 2016;11:59–64. https://doi.org/10.15420/icr.2016.11.1.59.
31. Jone PN, Haak A, Ross M, Wiktor DM, Gill E, Quaife RA, Messenger JC, Salcedo EE, Carroll JD. Congenital and structural heart disease interventions using echocardiography-fluoroscopy fusion imaging. J Am Soc Echocardiogr. 2019;32:1495–504. https://doi.org/10.1016/j.echo.2019.07.023.
32. Faletra FF, Biasco L, Pedrazzini G, Moccetti M, Pasotti E, Leo LA, Cautilli G, Moccetti T, Monaghan MJ. Echocardiographic-fluoroscopic fusion imaging in transseptal puncture: a new technology for an old procedure. J Am Soc Echocardiogr. 2017;30:886–95. https://doi.org/10.1016/j.echo.2017.05.001.
33. Faletra FF, Pozzoli A, Agricola E, Guidotti A, Biasco L, Leo LA, Taramasso M, Pasotti E, Kuwata S, Moccetti M, Tanner FC, Pedrazzini G, Nietlispach F, Moccetti T, Zuber M, Maisano F. Echocardiographic-fluoroscopic fusion imaging for transcatheter mitral valve repair guidance. Eur Heart J Cardiovasc Imaging. 2018;19:715–26. https://doi.org/10.1093/ehjci/jey067.
34. Maffessanti F, Patel AR, Patel MB, Walter JJ, Mediratta A, Medvedofsky D, Kachenoura N, Lang RM, Mor-Avi V. Non-invasive assessment of the haemodynamic significance of coronary stenosis using fusion of cardiac computed tomography and 3D echocardiography. Eur Heart J Cardiovasc Imaging. 2017;18:670–80. https://doi.org/10.1093/ehjci/jew147.
35. Pazhenkottil AP, Tanner FC, Buechel RR, Giannopoulos AA, Kaufmann PA, Zuber M. Cardiac hybrid imaging combining 3D-strain echocardiography with coronary computed tomography angiography. Eur Heart J. 2019;40(4):395–6. https://doi.org/10.1093/eurheartj/ehy700.
36. Picano E, Ciampi Q, Wierzbowska-Drabik K, Urluescu M-L, Morrone D, Carpeggiani C. The new clinical standard of integrated quadruple stress echocardiography with ABCD protocol. Cardiovasc Ultrasound. 2018;16:22. https://doi.org/10.1186/s12947-018-0141-z.
37. Ciampi Q, Zagatina A, Cortigiani L, Gaibazzi N, Daros CB, Zhuravskaya N, Wierzbowska-Drabik K, Kasprzak JD, de Castro JL, Pretto S, D'Andrea A, Djordjevic-Dikic A, Monte I, Simova I, Boshchenko A, Citro R, Amor M, Merlo PM, Dodi C, Rigo F, Gligorova S, Dekleva M, Severino S, Lattanzi F, Scali MC, Torres MA, Salustri A, Zanella H, Colonna P, Carpeggiani C, Picano E. Functional, coronary anatomic and prognostic correlates of coronary flow velocity reserve during stress echocardiography. J Am Coll Cardiol. 2019;74.2280–93.
38. Zagatina A, Zhuravskaya N, Shmatov D, Ciampi Q, Carpeggiani C, Picano E, Stress Echo 2020 Study Group of the Italian Society of Echocardiography, Cardiovascular Imaging. Exercise stress echocardiography with ABCDE protocol in unexplained dyspnoea. Int J Cardiovasc Imaging. 2020;36(5):823–31. https://doi.org/10.1007/s10554-020-01789-6.
39. Scali MC, Cortigiani L, Simionuc A, Gregori D, Marzilli M, Picano E. Exercise-induced B-lines identify worse functional and prognostic stage in heart failure patients with depressed left ventricular ejection fraction. Eur J Heart Fail. 2017;19(11):1468–78. https://doi.org/10.1002/ejhf.776. Epub 2017 Feb 15. PMID: 28198075.
40. Scali MC, Zagatina A, Ciampi Q, Cortigiani L, D'Andrea A, Djordjevic-Dikic A, Merlo PM, Lattanzi F, Simova I, Monte I, Dodi C, Kasprzak JD, Galderisi M, Boshchenko A, Rigo F, Varga A, Dekleva M, Re F, de Castro E Silva Pretto JL, Zhuravaskaya N, Stress Echo 2020 Study Group of the Italian Society of Cardiovascular Imaging. The functional mean-

ing of B-profile during stress lung ultrasound. JACC Cardiovasc Imaging. 12(5):928–30. https://doi.org/10.1016/j.jcmg.2018.10.017.
41. Cortigiani L, Huqi A, Ciampi Q, Bombardini T, Bovenzi FM, Picano E. Integration of wall motion, coronary flow velocity and left ventricular contractile reserve in a single test: prognostic value of vasodilator stress echocardiography in diabetic patients. J Am Soc Echocardiogr. 2018;31:692–701.
42. Chaowalit N, McCully RB, Callahan MJ, Mookadam F, Bailey KM, Pellikka PA. Outcomes after normal dobutamine stress echocardiography and predictors of adverse events: long-term follow-up of 3014 patients. Eur Heart J. 2006;27:3039–44.
43. Cortigiani L, Carpeggiani C, Landi P, Raciti M, Bovenzi F, Picano E. Blunted heart rate reserve as an imaging-independent prognostic predictor during dipyridamole-echocardiography test. Am J Cardiol. 2019;124:972–7.
44. Thrall JH. Trends and developments shaping the future of diagnostic medical imaging: 2015 annual oration in diagnostic radiology. Radiology. 2016;279:660–6. https://doi.org/10.1148/radiol.2016160293.
45. Picano E, Lattanzi F, Orlandini A, Marini C, L'Abbate A. Stress echocardiography and the human factor: the importance of being expert. J Am Coll Cardiol. 1991;17:666–9. https://doi.org/10.1016/s0735-1097(10)80182-2.
46. Varga A, Picano E, Dodi C, Barbieri A, Pratali L, Gaddi O. Madness and method in stress echo reading. Eur Heart J. 1999;20:1271–5. https://doi.org/10.1053/euhj.1999.1541.
47. Ciampi Q, Picano E, Paterni M, Daros CB, Simova I, de Castro E Silva Pretto JL, Scali MC, Gaibazzi N, Severino S, Djordjevic-Dikic A, Kasprzak JD, Zagatina A, Varga A, Lowenstein J, Merlo PM, Amor M, Celutkiene J, Perez JE, Di Salvo G, Galderisi M, Mori F, Costantino MF, Massa L, Dekleva M, Chaves DQ, Trambaiolo P, Citro R, Colonna P, Rigo F, Torres MAR, Monte I, Stankovic I, Neskovic A, Cortigiani L, Re F, Dodi C, D'Andrea A, Villari B, Arystan A, De Nes M, Carpeggiani C, Stress Echo 2020 Study Group of the Italian Society of Cardiovascular Echography. Quality control of regional wall motion analysis in stress echo 2020. Int J Cardiol. 2017;249:479–85.

Hybrid Cardiac Imaging for the Specialist with Expertise in Cardiac Magnetic Resonance

3

Jannike Nickander and Martin Ugander

3.1 Introduction

Correct medical treatment necessitates a correct diagnosis. Cardiac imaging aims to establish an accurate diagnosis without performing unnecessary invasive procedures, and there are several imaging modalities in clinical use today. Echocardiography, cardiac computed tomography (CCT), cardiac nuclear medicine imaging (NM), and cardiovascular magnetic resonance imaging (CMR) all convey valuable diagnostic information about the heart's anatomy and function. However, each technique has limitations ranging from radiation burden to a varying ability to perform myocardial tissue characterization. Consequently, hybrid imaging encompassing the combination of two or more imaging modalities is of interest. Hybrid imaging can incorporate anatomical and functional information from separate imaging modalities acquired in a single session—or through the fusion of independently acquired imaging modalities—to provide in-depth multimodality co-localized information about cardiac disease processes. The use of two or more techniques allows for the synergistic effect of combining the advantages of each technique, while simultaneously reducing the disadvantages of both. Hybrid imaging can thereby provide information on multiple aspects of structure, function, and metabolism that cannot always be obtained by a standalone imaging modality.

3.2 Brief Overview of Standalone Cardiac Imaging Modalities

Echocardiography, greatly simplified, generates images from ultrasound waves that are reflected in the heart and detected by a transducer. Echocardiography is particularly suitable for assessing left ventricular (LV) function [1], valve abnormalities, and pericardial effusion. While echocardiography is readily available and is the most common cardiac imaging, this imaging method has a limited ability to directly characterize myocardial tissue properties [2]. CCT has evolved into an important imaging method to evaluate coronary calcification [2], cardiac and coronary anatomy, and function [3]. The established method to quantify coronary calcification, the coronary artery calcium (CAC) score, can predict the likelihood of coronary events [4].

J. Nickander
Department of Clinical Physiology, Karolinska University Hospital, and Karolinska Institutet, Stockholm, Sweden
e-mail: jannike.nickander@ki.se

M. Ugander (✉)
Department of Clinical Physiology, Karolinska University Hospital, and Karolinska Institutet, Stockholm, Sweden

Kolling Institute, Royal North Shore Hospital, University of Sydney, Sydney, Australia

F. Nudi et al. (eds.), *Hybrid Cardiac Imaging for Clinical Decision-Making*,
https://doi.org/10.1007/978-3-030-99391-7_3

Coronary CT angiography (CTA) is another important cardiac CT technique. Coronary CTA has a very high specificity and negative predictive value (NPV). Coronary CTA has been shown to be an appropriate tool for use in intermediate risk patients who present with chest pain in the emergency room, to rule out acute coronary syndrome (ACS) [5, 6], and has become the gatekeeper to invasive angiography in the UK [7]. NM is an important tool for myocardial perfusion imaging (MPI) and myocardial viability assessment with the use of radiotracers in positron emission tomography (PET) and single-photon emission computed tomography (SPECT) [8]. SPECT MPI relies on the notion that a significant obstruction in a coronary artery will result in reduced blood flow in that particular perfusion territory relative to the remote myocardium, leading to a lower accumulation of perfusion-specific radiotracer in that particular territory. This will render a perfusion defect on SPECT scans, as the concentration of radiotracer is much higher in the remote myocardium compared to the ischemic region. The inherent diagnostic shortcoming of SPECT is that it relies on the quantification of relative difference in absolute myocardial perfusion, rendering difficulties making the diagnosis of multivessel disease or diffuse coronary microvascular disease (CMD). PET, by comparison, enables noninvasive quantification of absolute myocardial perfusion, which is also referred to myocardial blood flow (MBF). By calculating the ratio of the peak perfusion at maximal pharmacological vasodilatory stress to perfusion at rest, the coronary flow reserve (CFR) can be calculated. CFR is an important measure for evaluating the functional relevance of a coronary stenosis [9, 10]. PET thereby allows for both the detection of obstructive coronary artery disease (CAD) and diffuse CMD. The major drawback of PET, besides ionizing radiation, is the limited spatial resolution (1–3 mm) related to the physical limits inherent to the detection of positron decay and the resultant annihilated photons. Prior to the year 2000, PET was regarded as the reference standard for myocardial viability imaging. However, since the introduction of the CMR technique known as late gadolinium enhancement (LGE), which allows for detailed tissue characterization, LGE CMR has arguably become the modality of choice for viability imaging [11]. CMR has emerged as a robust imaging technique for a comprehensive set of states including cardiac anatomical morphology [12], tissue characterization with regards to both focal and diffuse myocardial fibrosis and edema [13–16], LV and right ventricular function [2, 17], myocardial wall thickness and viability [11, 18], myocardial perfusion assessed both visually and quantitatively [19–21], and blood flow across valves and in the great vessels [22]. Table 3.1 summarizes capabilities of the different standalone imaging modalities.

Table 3.1 Summary of typical standalone capability of different cardiac imaging modalities as used in clinical practice

	CCT	Ultrasound	CMR	Nuclear
Molecular	–	–	–	+++
Viability	+	+	+++	+++
Blood flow	–	+++	+++	+
Perfusion	+	+	+++	+++
Anatomy	+++	+++	+++	–
Spatial resolution	0.5–2.0 mm	0.5–5.0 mm	0.5–2.0 mm	0.5–5.0 mm
Temporal resolution	~80 ms	~10 ms	~30 ms	~60 ms
Penetration depth	No limit	mm-cm	No limit	No limit
Ionizing radiation	+	–	–	+

3.3 Hybrid Imaging

There is currently no clear definition of the term hybrid imaging, and it can be used to describe the simultaneously acquired images by a combined system, the co-registration of sequentially acquired images on separate systems, the merging of images acquired on separate systems at separate time points, or anything in between. This chapter aims to focus on the current knowledge on combined systems with MR however where combined systems are lacking, hybrid imaging applications in a broader sense will be described.

3.4 PET/MR Hybrid Imaging

Compared to other modalities, the ability to depict anatomy by PET is limited by a relatively lower both spatial and temporal resolution. In the 1990s, this led to extensive research efforts in image co-registration between PET and CT. These research efforts culminated in the success of combined PET/CT scanners in the early 2000s [23], after which the research focus turned to MR with its high soft tissue contrast, and the potential to reduce the radiation burden by replacing CT. The combination of MR and PET scanners posed several challenges. First, the static magnetic field of the MR scanner in combination with continuously changing gradient field and radiofrequency signals inhibits the photomultiplier tubes from working properly and interferes with the electronics in the PET detectors. The PET detector induces inhomogeneities in the magnetic field, causing eddy current effects and electromagnetic interference, which can seriously degrade the quality of the MR images. It was evident that a design where the elements of the two scanners were isolated from each other was needed. Several approaches have been reported including custom magnet architecture, field-cycled MR image acquisition [24], and redesigned PET photodetectors [25]. However, eventually two different designs were commercially available by 2010—an integrated system (Siemens Biograph mMR [26], GE Signa PET/MR) and separate scanners connected by a common patient table (Philips Ingenuity TF PET/MR [27], GE-PET/CT-MR).

3.4.1 PET/MR in Obstructive CAD

Coronary artery disease (CAD) is a dynamic process with the continuous accumulation of atherosclerotic lesions and functional disturbances in the coronary circulation, culminating in the foremost public health issue in Western societies. Traditionally, the anatomical luminal narrowing of coronary arteries identified during invasive angiography has visually been identified as obstructive and treated with percutaneous intervention. However, it has become apparent that myocardial ischemia is not exclusively an anatomical diagnosis, but a physiological one, where cardiac imaging has an important role to guide revascularization. As standalone cardiac imaging modalities SPECT, PET, and CMR all have a high sensitivity and specificity for detecting obstructive CAD, as well as reliable quantification of the extent of myocardial ischemia expressed as percent of the left ventricle [28]. CT with CCTA and CAC can identify atherosclerotic lesions and quantify calcification; however, cannot grade the functional relevance of an atherosclerotic lesion or quantify the extent of myocardial ischemia [29, 30]. MPI for the diagnostic work-up of CAD is well established, using both PET and CMR. PET MPI may be seen as the quantitative reference standard for myocardial blood flow and coronary flow reserve with the use of radiotracers (some of which have superior characteristics compared to gadolinium-based contrast agents) and spatial coverage of the left ventricle; however, CMR MPI has the advantages of being free from ionizing radiation and has a higher spatial resolution with the ability to reliably detect even subendocardial ischemia. PET and CMR show a good correlation for ischemia detection on a per slice and segment basis however CMR has been shown to underestimate coronary flow reserve due to overestimation of resting perfusion [31]. However, this may be mitigated by newly developed fully automated quantitative perfusion mapping [32], which has an excellent accuracy compared to PET [33]. This technique shows clinical promise as it accurately detects obstructive CAD [34] as determined by invasive fractional flow reserve (FFR) and CMD as determined by the invasive index of microcirculatory resistance (IMR) [35]. Synergistic effects of hybrid PET/MR include higher spatial resolution, where CMR can distinguish between endo- and epicardial perfusion. This is illustrated in a case where PET identified cavity dilation in a patient with hypertrophic cardiomyopathy, and CMR could demonstrate subendocardial ischemia [31]. Quantitative perfusion mapping by CMR has shown that CMD is common, and may be an early biomarker in hypertrophic cardiomyopathy [36]. One disadvantage of MR MPI is the lack of full spatial coverage of the left ventricle. The current clinical standard is to perform perfusion imaging in three short-axis slices. One key factor for therapy guidance is the extent of left ventricular ischemia [37], which may become inaccurate when only using three slices. Attempts to mitigate this using 3D first-pass perfusion CMR have been attempted [38]. However, this is not yet established in clinical routine. Currently, there is no support for a combined PET/MR approach to detect obstructive CAD beyond the standalone modalities [39]. However, CAD is a particularly interesting area for hybrid cardiac imaging. Hybrid techniques like PET/CT, SPECT/CT, and CT/MR are all of potential interest but will not be discussed further in this chapter. CT/MR for the diagnosis of obstructive CAD will be discussed in the CT/MR section.

3.4.2 PET/MR for Evaluating Myocardial Viability

Infarct size, viability, and area at risk are all major predictors for outcome after myocardial infarction and are paramount for further decision-making with regards to therapy in both acute and chronic disease. Repetitive ischemia or resting hypoperfusion may lead to a reduced left ventricular ejection fraction due to regional wall motion abnormalities or global hypokinesia. It is well known that the cardiomyocytes under this condition switch to glucose metabolism instead of free fatty acids. The regional wall motion abnormalities may be reversed if normal perfusion is reestablished [40], and this state is thus referred to as hibernating myocardium [41], and is associated with poor outcomes [42, 43]. There are several approaches to noninvasive image viability, including dobutamine stress echocardiography or CMR, and Thallium-201 SPECT, while the most commonly used techniques are ^{18}F-FDG PET and LGE CMR. ^{18}F-FDG PET is typically combined with a perfusion study to identify hibernating myocardium via the mismatch between increased glucose consumption and reduced perfusion, with good sensitivity and acceptable specificity [44]. Due to the high spatial resolution of CMR, LGE accurately displays the transmurality of myocardial infarction (an ischemic scar) and combined with wall motion abnormalities LGE can identify hibernating myocardium, that is likely to benefit from reperfusion, viable myocardium [11]. Hybrid PET/MR approaches have shown a moderate-to-good agreement between LGE and reduced ^{18}F-FDG uptake following an acute myocardial infarction [45–47]. Furthermore, CMR can differentiate between myocardial edema, microvascular obstruction, and intramyocardial hemorrhage, all of which carry prognostic information following an acute myocardial infarction [48–52]. It is important to be able to discriminate between reversible and irreversible myocardial dysfunction, since myocardial segments with reversible dysfunction will contribute to global left ventricular recovery if successfully revascularized. However, disagreement between PET and CMR has been observed. PET tends to underestimate infarct size, likely due to the lower spatial resolution compared to CMR, as well as the increased detection of small subendocardial infarctions by CMR. Furthermore, ^{18}F-FDG uptake has, compared to LGE, been shown to be a better predictor of functional recovery in regions with wall motion abnormalities after myocardial infarction [46]. However, this discrepancy may have been due to methodological differences since the definitions for reduced ^{18}F-FDG uptake and LGE were not exactly comparable. By comparison, cases with reduced ^{18}F-FDG uptake, no LGE, and wall motion abnormalities that do not recover over 6 months after acute infarction have been identified [53], and this highlights a future potential utility for hybrid cardiac PET/MR imaging in ischemic heart disease. Since PET and CMR can identify stunned or hibernating myocardium as standalone modalities [54, 55], PET/MR allows for more advanced diagnosis with regards to metabolism and molecular processes. In ischemic cardiomyopathy, LGE allows for precise assessment of scar transmurality, and simultaneous acquisition of perfusion with PET can aid the diagnosis. As LGE and perfusion provide

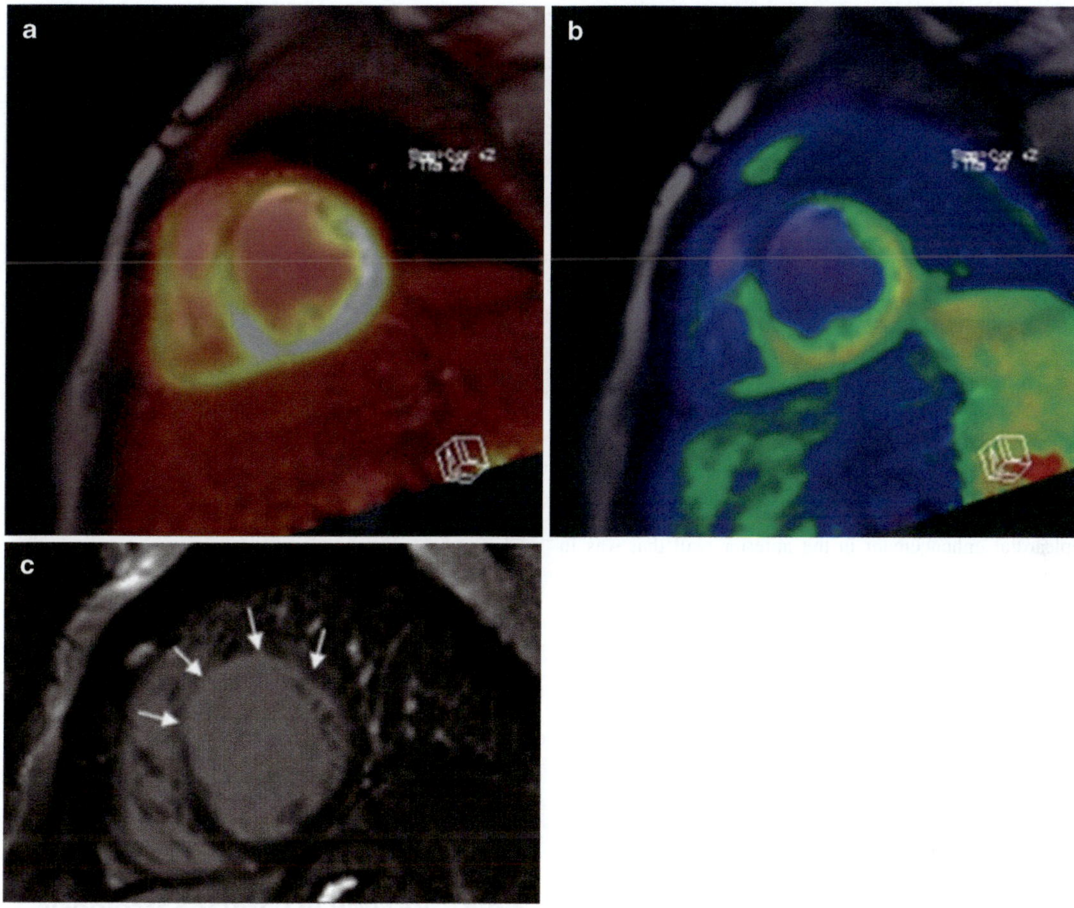

Fig. 3.1 Hybrid PET/MR of a patient with coronary artery disease. Cardiac PET/MR hybrid images showing missing 18F-FDG and 13N-NH3 uptakes in agreement with the presence of transmural late gadolinium enhancement (LGE) in the anteroseptal wall of the myocardium. (**a**) Image fusion of 18F-FDG PET and LGE CMR. (**b**) Image fusion of 13N-NH3 PET and LGE CMR. (**c**) Extent and transmurality of scar determined by CMR. (Reproduced from [39])

different information about the myocardium, the complementary value of the two techniques could improve both individual outcome prediction and risk assessment [39] however such studies remain to be performed (Fig. 3.1).

3.4.3 PET/MR in Nonischemic Heart Disease

CMR is an established cardiac imaging modality for clinical diagnosis and subsequent management of inflammatory heart disease. CMR allows for accurate detection of small areas of myocardial necrosis or fibrosis using LGE. Furthermore, CMR can identify myocardial edema with T2-weighted imaging, T1 and T2 mapping, as well as global and regional dysfunction and pericardial effusion. Taken together, the ability to detect or rule out these findings aid in the diagnosis of myocarditis. A combination of multiparametric mapping by CMR with metabolic characterization by ^{18}F-FDG PET has the potential to be a powerful imaging tool in cardiac inflammation. Furthermore, hybrid imaging could provide insights into pathophysiological mechanisms, for example, in Fabry disease, where PET/MR scans suggest that inflammation may be an important factor in disease progression [56, 57]. Another pathophysiological link may be

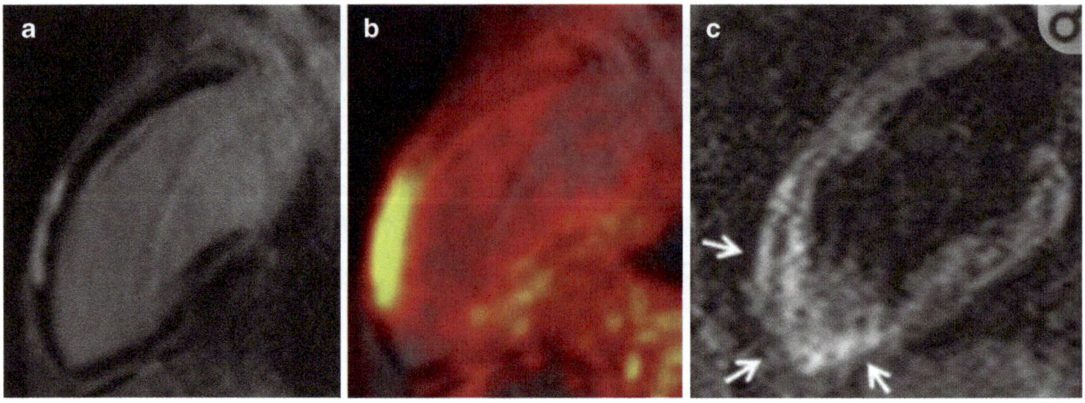

Fig. 3.2 Hybrid PET/MR of a patient with acute myocarditis. The images display 18F-FDG PET/MR in acute myocarditis. (**a**) Shows a late gadolinium enhancement image by CMR in long-axis view. There is a typical subepicardial enhancement in the anterior wall that was in excellent agreement with increased 18F-FDG uptake on fused images (**b**). (**c**) Shows a T2-weighted image, denoting edema (arrows) in the LV anterior wall. (Reproduced from [39])

CMD. Quantitative perfusion by CMR shows lower perfusion prior to developing traditional cardiac involvement in Fabry disease [58]. PET/MR may also identify characteristics of LGE in nonischemic disease, such as cardiac amyloidosis [59]. Hybrid PET/MR may allow for deeper characterization of subclinical or early disease states in nonischemic heart disease. The most important factor for ^{18}F-FDG PET in myocardial inflammation imaging is to properly suppress the myocardial glucose metabolism, in order to achieve high contrast between normal and inflamed myocardium. Different protocols including fasting, high-fat low-carbohydrate diet, fatty acid loading, and unfractionated heparin loading are utilized [60]. Of note, the suppression of myocardial glucose metabolism may fail in patients with diabetes and/or steroid/glucocorticoid treatment.

3.4.4 PET/MR in Acute Myocarditis

CMR alone is in many cases sufficient to diagnose acute myocarditis. However, the ability of PET to quantify inflammatory activity makes PET/MR of potential interest for disease monitoring in chronic myocarditis. Furthermore, PET/MR may improve diagnostic accuracy beyond differentiating between acute or chronic myocarditis by adding additional diagnostic information in cases with ambiguous CMR findings. The potential of PET/MR in myocarditis has been demonstrated in cases where intense ^{18}F-FDG uptake has closely matched the focal epicardial LGE, myocardial edema, and hyperemia in acute myocarditis [61, 62] (Fig. 3.2).

3.4.5 PET/MR in Cardiac Sarcoidosis

Cardiac involvement in sarcoidosis leads to focal nonischemic LGE findings, malignant arrhythmias, and heart failure, and is a strong predictor of poor outcomes. Therefore, early detection and differentiation between active and chronic disease, with subsequent treatment, improves morbidity and mortality. However, both accurate detection and disease monitoring remain a challenge. By comparison, invasive endomyocardial biopsy suffers from sampling error and may yield false-negative results. Both CMR and ^{18}F-FDG PET play important roles in the clinical work-up of cardiac sarcoidosis [63, 64], where expert consensus recommends ^{18}F-FDG PET [65, 66]. A hybrid approach with PET/MR, especially the combination of LGE with ^{18}F-FDG PET may have added benefit, as imaging of myocardial scarring guides electrode placement in ICD implantation [67]. Small studies and case reports have shown that hybrid PET/MR offers complementary information regarding pathophysiology, and incremental diagnostic information on injury pattern and disease activity [64, 68–72].

3.5 CT/MR Hybrid Imaging

CT, and in particular, coronary CTA is a noninvasive imaging technique that allows for direct visualization of CAD, accompanied by detailed cardiothoracic anatomy. Coronary CTA has a high both NPV and sensitivity, but a lower both PPV and specificity, and tends to overestimate the coronary stenosis grade compared to invasive angiography. Coronary CTA may therefore be considered a suboptimal indicator of flow-limiting CAD as false-positive rates may increase rates of cardiac catheterizations and unnecessary revascularization. CMR can also be used for direct visualization of the coronary circulation, however as of yet, not with the level of spatial resolution and detail as coronary CTA for detecting coronary stenosis [73]. Stress CMR may either be used to identify flow-limiting CAD by wall motion abnormalities or visualization of regional perfusion defects. A hybrid approach would allow for fusing the anatomical information with the functional perfusion data, which may overcome some of the limitations of coronary CTA, and thereby improve the diagnostic performance compared to the standalone imaging modalities. Currently, no clinical system for simultaneous CT/MR acquisition exists. Hybrid CT/MR imaging will be discussed in a broader sense, including complementary and comparative utilities.

3.5.1 CT/MR in Obstructive CAD

Coronary CTA and stress perfusion CMR are well-established noninvasive methods to detect obstructive CAD with good-to-excellent sensitivity and specificity compared to invasive angiography. In head-to-head comparisons of the respective methods, several studies reveal similar accuracies for detecting obstructive CAD [74], especially when adding CT stress-rest perfusion [75]. By comparison, CT delayed enhancement (CTDE) for detection of ischemic scar has been shown to not improve the accuracy of CT for detecting obstructive CAD, likely due to the moderate accuracy of CTDE compared to CMR LGE [76]. There is evidence that coronary CTA can replace invasive angiography in the diagnosis of obstructive CAD in combination with stress CMR [77]. Early studies of hybrid CT/MR diagnostic approaches suggested that there was no incremental improvement regardless of the parameter combination of the two imaging methods [78]. Later studies showed that combined use of coronary CTA and CMR improved both specificity and overall accuracy for detecting significant CAD while allowing identification of both cardiac and extracardiac findings [79]. Furthermore, fusion of coronary CTA and whole-heart perfusion CMR has been shown to refine the assessment of obstructive CAD, where hybrid CT/MR assessment led to reclassification of the relevance of the stenosis by CT in 17% of patients [80]. Most studies use invasive angiography as a golden standard. However, there is a growing body of evidence that diagnosis of CAD severity using invasive angiography is flawed, as angiographic appearance and severity do not necessarily reflect functional relevance. A recent meta-analysis of cardiac imaging methods for obstructive CAD using FFR as a reference standard revealed that CMR had the highest performance, and the anatomical methods, such as coronary CTA yielded lower specificity, even using the functional CT-derived FFR (FFR_{CT}) [81]. These results are supported by a recent single center study showing that coronary CTA, FFR_{CT}, and CMR have similar diagnostic accuracy compared to FFR from invasive angiography, where FFR_{CT} had the highest sensitivity, but CMR had the highest specificity [82]. Furthermore, a recent meta-analysis showed that hybrid coronary CTA and perfusion cardiac imaging improve diagnostic specificity for detecting obstructive CAD as compared to standalone coronary CTA [83].

3.5.2 CT/MR in Nonischemic Heart Disease

Given the relatively recent advancement in cardiac CT technology for the characterization of nonischemic heart disease, there are currently no studies on hybrid CT/MR approaches for diagnosing nonischemic heart disease. CT inherently lacks the level of tissue contrast that CMR provides, even though the technique offers high spatial and temporal resolution, rendering precise images of thoracic anatomy. Research efforts have been made into myocardial tissue characterization with CT, both with regards to delayed enhancement and extracellular volume (ECV) quantification. Several studies show that ECV quantification by CT is feasible and can differentiate between normal and diseased myocardium [84, 85], with good agreement compared to CMR ECV [86]. Small studies of CTDE show good agreement with CMR LGE and the possibility to differentiate between different etiologies [87, 88]. Limited experiences from using cardiac CT in a variety of different left ventricular myocardial diseases have been published and given today's state-of-the-art CT scanners, it has been shown that CT can quantify left ventricular volumes, measure myocardial wall thickness, quantify infarct size, and identify HCM, sarcoidosis, amyloidosis, non-compaction cardiomyopathy, and myocarditis. Taken together, this suggests that CT may be useful when echocardiography and CMR are not possible or suitable [89].

3.6 SPECT/MR Hybrid Imaging

Currently, no clinical system for simultaneous SPECT/MR acquisition exists. However, research efforts are being made both with regards to scanner prototypes [90], as well as contrast/isotopes agents [91]. However, one might argue that there is no need to fuse two functional imaging modalities, as opposed to a functional and anatomical modality (SPECT/CT, PET/CT). Therefore, the following section will focus on hybrid imaging using SPECT/MR in a broader sense, including complementary and comparative utilities.

3.6.1 SPECT/MR in Obstructive CAD

SPECT is a noninvasive imaging method that has been extensively validated, and is widely available and used clinically, with a high reported sensitivity of 87–89% [92], and an estimated specificity of 89% [93] for obstructive CAD. SPECT has also been shown to be a strong technique for guiding treatment [37]. The diagnostic limitations with SPECT include imaging difficulties in obesity, as well as in extensive multivessel disease or CMD. SPECT tends to underestimate the true ischemia extent in multivessel CAD [94], and obesity can lead to false-positive results. Stress CMR has a reported sensitivity of 90% and a specificity of 81% [95] for detecting obstructive CAD using qualitative or semi-quantitative approaches. Diagnostic limitations with CMR include so-called dark rim artifacts, but this may be mitigated by fully quantitative CMR approaches [32]. SPECT has been shown to underestimate left ventricular volumes and function compared to CMR [96], and CMR outperforms SPECT in head-to-head comparisons for detecting obstructive CAD [97, 98]. Notably, clinical studies on hybrid SPECT/MR for detecting obstructive CAD are currently lacking.

3.6.2 SPECT/MR in Acute Myocardial Ischemia

Final infarct size following acute myocardial infarction is determined by the size of the area at risk, reperfusion injury, and the duration of myocardial ischemia. Accurate imaging of area at risk is important, not only because it is linked to outcomes, but also because it is an important parameter for evaluating myocardial salvage in experimental/pharmaceutical studies. Previously, SPECT was regarded as the reference standard for imaging area at risk [99], but SPECT can be impractical in the acute setting. A hybrid approach to co-registration of SPECT and MR for quantifying myocardium at risk in experimental acute myocardial infarctions has been reported [100], and contrast-enhanced steady-state free precession (CE-SSFP) CMR has been validated both in vivo and ex vivo compared to SPECT [101]. CE-SSFP has also been validated in clinical patients [102], and CMR also allows for the quantification of salvage index, as LGE can be used to quantify infarct size, whereas SPECT cannot differentiate between myocardium at risk and infarct size.

3.6.3 SPECT/MR in Nonischemic Heart Disease

The role of SPECT in patients with nonischemic heart disease is unclear. A major advantage of SPECT regarding nonischemic diseases is the variety of radiotracers to detect different pathophysiological phenomena both regarding metabolism and neurotransmission. However, the use of different radiotracers allows for differences between hospitals with regard to the availability of tracers and local expertise. Abnormal myocardial perfusion in HCM and CMD detected by SPECT is linked to worse prognosis [103, 104]. Fascinating observations have been made with iodine-123-beta-methyl-iodophenylpentadecanoic acid (BIMPP, marker of fatty acid metabolism) and iodine-123-labeled metaiodobenzylguanidine (MIBG, tracker of presynaptic uptake of neurotransmitters) where BMIPP and MIBG uptake are reduced in HCM [105, 106]. CMR, with excellent spatial resolution, allows for a more extensive appreciation of the pattern and extent of hypertrophy compared to echocardiography, as well as reproducible quantification of left ventricular dimension, volume, and ejection fraction [107]. Only a few studies and case reports have studied the combination of SPECT and CMR showing associations between regional myocardial perfusion and regional hypertrophy [108], and as well as dyssynchrony on SPECT concordant with the extent of LGE [109].

3.6.4 SPECT/MR in Myocarditis

The sensitivity and specificity of SPECT are not adequate for the reliable diagnosis of myocarditis; however, case reports show identifiable perfusion defects using SPECT MPI in patients with myocarditis. CMR is well-established for both diagnosis and prognosis in patients with myocarditis [14]. Few case reports and small studies show discordant results of SPECT and CMR to detect chronic myocarditis [110], and contradicting results with concordant perfusion defects on SPECT with LGE on CMR have been reported [111] (Fig. 3.3). A hybrid approach of dual SPECT (BIMPP and ^{201}TlCL), ^{18}F-FDG-PET, and CMR in sarcoidosis revealed increased mismatch and defect scores in areas with LGE, suggesting that the combined approach can discriminate active inflammation and myocardial damage in sarcoidosis [112].

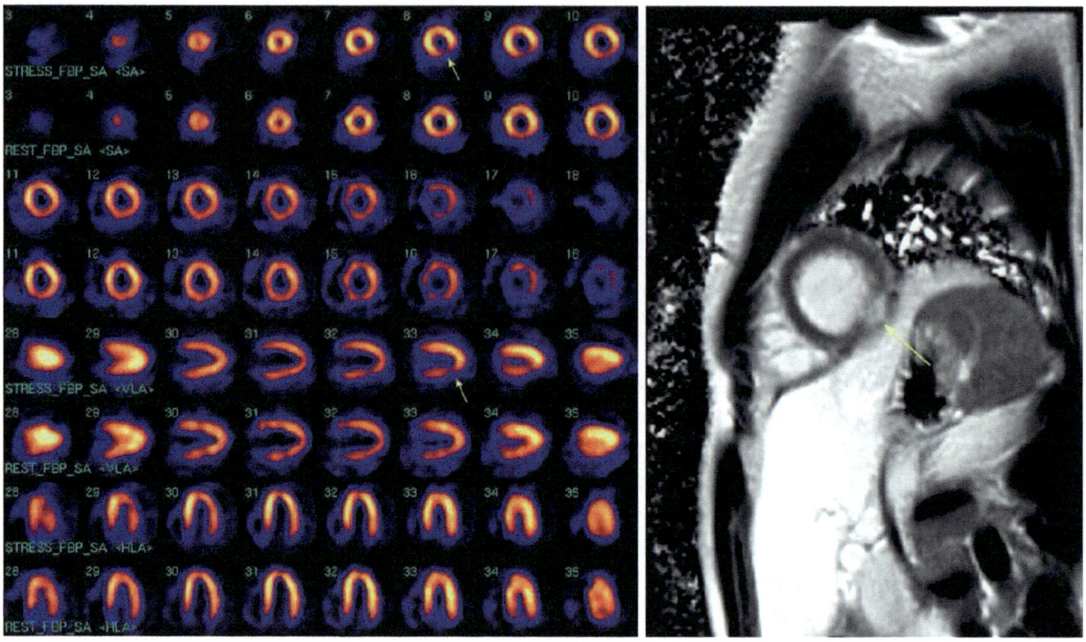

Fig. 3.3 A case of concordant perfusion defect on SPECT with LGE by CMR. SPECT myocardial perfusion images (Tc-99m sestamibi) at stress and rest are shown to the left. Arrows denote an area of reversible hypoperfusion in the inferolateral left ventricular wall. To the right, the late gadolinium enhancement image shows concordant LGE in the inferolateral wall (arrow). (Adapted from [111])

3.7 Ultrasound/MR Hybrid Imaging

Currently, no clinical system for simultaneous ultrasound/MR acquisition exists, and the literature on hybrid imaging is mostly related to valve and structural heart disease which is beyond the scope of this chapter.

References

1. Abraham TP, Dimaano VL, Liang HY. Role of tissue Doppler and strain echocardiography in current clinical practice. Circulation. 2007;116(22):2597–609.
2. Lam WC, Pennell DJ. Imaging of the heart: historical perspective and recent advances. Postgrad Med J. 2016;92(1084):99–104.
3. Cury RC, Nieman K, Shapiro MD, Butler J, Nomura CH, Ferencik M, et al. Comprehensive assessment of myocardial perfusion defects, regional wall motion, and left ventricular function by using 64-section multidetector CT. Radiology. 2008;248(2):466–75.
4. Detrano R, Guerci AD, Carr JJ, Bild DE, Burke G, Folsom AR, et al. Coronary calcium as a predictor of coronary events in four racial or ethnic groups. N Engl J Med. 2008;358(13):1336–45.
5. Litt HI, Gatsonis C, Snyder B, Singh H, Miller CD, Entrikin DW, et al. CT angiography for safe discharge of patients with possible acute coronary syndromes. N Engl J Med. 2012;366(15):1393–403.
6. Priest VL, Scuffham PA, Hachamovitch R, Marwick TH. Cost-effectiveness of coronary computed tomography and cardiac stress imaging in the emergency department: a decision analytic model comparing diagnostic strategies for chest pain in patients at low risk of acute coronary syndromes. JACC Cardiovasc Imaging. 2011;4(5):549–56.
7. SCOT-HEART Investigators. CT coronary angiography in patients with suspected angina due to coronary heart disease (SCOT-HEART): an open-label, parallel-group, multicentre trial. Lancet. 2015;385(9985):2383–91.
8. Ghosh N, Rimoldi OE, Beanlands RS, Camici PG. Assessment of myocardial ischaemia and viability: role of positron emission tomography. Eur Heart J. 2010;31(24):2984–95.
9. Di Carli M, Czernin J, Hoh CK, Gerbaudo VH, Brunken RC, Huang SC, et al. Relation among stenosis severity, myocardial blood flow, and flow reserve in patients with coronary artery disease. Circulation. 1995;91(7):1944–51.
10. Uren NG, Melin JA, De Bruyne B, Wijns W, Baudhuin T, Camici PG. Relation between myocar-

dial blood flow and the severity of coronary-artery stenosis. N Engl J Med. 1994;330(25):1782–8.
11. Kim RJ, Wu E, Rafael A, Chen EL, Parker MA, Simonetti O, et al. The use of contrast-enhanced magnetic resonance imaging to identify reversible myocardial dysfunction. N Engl J Med. 2000;343(20):1445–53.
12. Gupta A, Lee VS, Chung YC, Babb JS, Simonetti OP. Myocardial infarction: optimization of inversion times at delayed contrast-enhanced MR imaging. Radiology. 2004;233(3):921–6.
13. Hunold P, Schlosser T, Vogt FM, Eggebrecht H, Schmermund A, Bruder O, et al. Myocardial late enhancement in contrast-enhanced cardiac MRI: distinction between infarction scar and non-infarction-related disease. AJR Am J Roentgenol. 2005;184(5):1420–6.
14. Mahrholdt H, Wagner A, Judd RM, Sechtem U, Kim RJ. Delayed enhancement cardiovascular magnetic resonance assessment of non-ischaemic cardiomyopathies. Eur Heart J. 2005;26(15):1461–74.
15. Friedrich MG, Strohm O, Schulz-Menger J, Marciniak H, Luft FC, Dietz R. Contrast media-enhanced magnetic resonance imaging visualizes myocardial changes in the course of viral myocarditis. Circulation. 1998;97(18):1802–9.
16. Ferreira VM, Piechnik SK, Dall'Armellina E, Karamitsos TD, Francis JM, Choudhury RP, et al. Non-contrast T1-mapping detects acute myocardial edema with high diagnostic accuracy: a comparison to T2-weighted cardiovascular magnetic resonance. J Cardiovasc Magn Reson. 2012;14:42.
17. Schalla S, Nagel E, Lehmkuhl H, Klein C, Bornstedt A, Schnackenburg B, et al. Comparison of magnetic resonance real-time imaging of left ventricular function with conventional magnetic resonance imaging and echocardiography. Am J Cardiol. 2001;87(1):95–9.
18. Kim RJ, Fieno DS, Parrish TB, Harris K, Chen EL, Simonetti O, et al. Relationship of MRI delayed contrast enhancement to irreversible injury, infarct age, and contractile function. Circulation. 1999;100(19):1992–2002.
19. Lipton MJ, Bogaert J, Boxt LM, Reba RC. Imaging of ischemic heart disease. Eur Radiol. 2002;12(5):1061–80.
20. Mordini FE, Haddad T, Hsu LY, Kellman P, Lowrey TB, Aletras AH, et al. Diagnostic accuracy of stress perfusion CMR in comparison with quantitative coronary angiography: fully quantitative, semiquantitative, and qualitative assessment. JACC Cardiovasc Imaging. 2014;7(1):14–22.
21. McCommis KS, Goldstein TA, Zhang H, Misselwitz B, Gropler RJ, Zheng J. Quantification of myocardial blood volume during dipyridamole and doubtamine stress: a perfusion CMR study. J Cardiovasc Magn Reson. 2007;9(5):785–92.
22. Arheden H, Holmqvist C, Thilen U, Hanseus K, Bjorkhem G, Pahlm O, et al. Left-to-right cardiac shunts: comparison of measurements obtained with MR velocity mapping and with radionuclide angiography. Radiology. 1999;211(2):453–8.
23. Beyer T, Townsend DW, Brun T, Kinahan PE, Charron M, Roddy R, et al. A combined PET/CT scanner for clinical oncology. J Nucl Med. 2000;41(8):1369–79.
24. Gilbert KM, Scholl TJ, Handler WB, Alford JK, Chronik BA. Evaluation of a positron emission tomography (PET)-compatible field-cycled MRI (FCMRI) scanner. Magn Reson Med. 2009;62(4):1017–25.
25. Pichler BJ, Judenhofer MS, Catana C, Walton JH, Kneilling M, Nutt RE, et al. Performance test of an LSO-APD detector in a 7-T MRI scanner for simultaneous PET/MRI. J Nucl Med. 2006;47(4):639–47.
26. Delso G, Furst S, Jakoby B, Ladebeck R, Ganter C, Nekolla SG, et al. Performance measurements of the Siemens mMR integrated whole-body PET/MR scanner. J Nucl Med. 2011;52(12):1914–22.
27. Zaidi H, Ojha N, Morich M, Griesmer J, Hu Z, Maniawski P, et al. Design and performance evaluation of a whole-body ingenuity TF PET-MRI system. Phys Med Biol. 2011;56(10):3091–106.
28. Takx RA, Blomberg BA, El Aidi H, Habets J, de Jong PA, Nagel E, et al. Diagnostic accuracy of stress myocardial perfusion imaging compared to invasive coronary angiography with fractional flow reserve meta-analysis. Circ Cardiovasc Imaging. 2015;8(1):e002666.
29. Meijboom WB, Van Mieghem CA, van Pelt N, Weustink A, Pugliese F, Mollet NR, et al. Comprehensive assessment of coronary artery stenoses: computed tomography coronary angiography versus conventional coronary angiography and correlation with fractional flow reserve in patients with stable angina. J Am Coll Cardiol. 2008;52(8):636–43.
30. Misaka T, Sugitani Y, Asato N, Matsukubo Y, Uemura M, Ashikaga R, et al. Coronary artery to aortic luminal attenuation ratio in coronary CT angiography for the diagnosis of haemodynamically significant coronary artery stenosis. Br J Radiol. 2020;93(1105):20190003.
31. Kunze KP, Nekolla SG, Rischpler C, Zhang SH, Hayes C, Langwieser N, et al. Myocardial perfusion quantification using simultaneously acquired (13) NH3 -ammonia PET and dynamic contrast-enhanced MRI in patients at rest and stress. Magn Reson Med. 2018;80(6):2641–54.
32. Kellman P, Hansen MS, Nielles-Vallespin S, Nickander J, Themudo R, Ugander M, et al. Myocardial perfusion cardiovascular magnetic resonance: optimized dual sequence and reconstruction for quantification. J Cardiovasc Magn Reson. 2017;19(1):43.
33. Engblom H, Xue H, Akil S, Carlsson M, Hindorf C, Oddstig J, et al. Fully quantitative cardiovascular magnetic resonance myocardial perfusion ready

for clinical use: a comparison between cardiovascular magnetic resonance imaging and positron emission tomography. J Cardiovasc Magn Reson. 2017;19(1):78.
34. Knott KD, Camaioni C, Ramasamy A, Augusto JA, Bhuva AN, Xue H, et al. Quantitative myocardial perfusion in coronary artery disease: a perfusion mapping study. J Magn Reson Imaging. 2019;50(3):756–62.
35. Kotecha T, Martinez-Naharro A, Boldrini M, Knight D, Hawkins P, Kalra S, et al. Automated pixel-wise quantitative myocardial perfusion mapping by CMR to detect obstructive coronary artery disease and coronary microvascular dysfunction: validation against invasive coronary physiology. JACC Cardiovasc Imaging. 2019;12(10):1958–69.
36. Camaioni C, Knott KD, Augusto JB, Seraphim A, Rosmini S, Ricci F, et al. Inline perfusion mapping provides insights into the disease mechanism in hypertrophic cardiomyopathy. Heart. 2020;106(11):824–9.
37. Hachamovitch R, Hayes SW, Friedman JD, Cohen I, Berman DS. Comparison of the short-term survival benefit associated with revascularization compared with medical therapy in patients with no prior coronary artery disease undergoing stress myocardial perfusion single photon emission computed tomography. Circulation. 2003;107(23):2900–7.
38. Wissmann L, Gotschy A, Santelli C, Tezcan KC, Hamada S, Manka R, et al. Analysis of spatiotemporal fidelity in quantitative 3D first-pass perfusion cardiovascular magnetic resonance. J Cardiovasc Magn Reson. 2017;19(1):11.
39. Nensa F, Bamberg F, Rischpler C, Menezes L, Poeppel TD, la Fougere C, et al. Hybrid cardiac imaging using PET/MRI: a joint position statement by the European Society of Cardiovascular Radiology (ESCR) and the European Association of Nuclear Medicine (EANM). Eur Radiol. 2018;28(10):4086–101.
40. Rahimtoola SH. A perspective on the three large multicenter randomized clinical trials of coronary bypass surgery for chronic stable angina. Circulation. 1985;72(6 Pt 2):V123–35.
41. Heusch G. Hibernating myocardium. Physiol Rev. 1998;78(4):1055–85.
42. Beanlands RS, Hendry PJ, Masters RG, deKemp RA, Woodend K, Ruddy TD. Delay in revascularization is associated with increased mortality rate in patients with severe left ventricular dysfunction and viable myocardium on fluorine 18-fluorodeoxyglucose positron emission tomography imaging. Circulation. 1998;98(19 Suppl):Ii51–6.
43. Di Carli MF, Davidson M, Little R, Khanna S, Mody FV, Brunken RC, et al. Value of metabolic imaging with positron emission tomography for evaluating prognosis in patients with coronary artery disease and left ventricular dysfunction. Am J Cardiol. 1994;73(8):527–33.
44. Schinkel AF, Poldermans D, Elhendy A, Bax JJ. Assessment of myocardial viability in patients with heart failure. J Nucl Med. 2007;48(7):1135–46.
45. Nensa F, Poeppel TD, Beiderwellen K, Schelhorn J, Mahabadi AA, Erbel R, et al. Hybrid PET/MR imaging of the heart: feasibility and initial results. Radiology. 2013;268(2):366–73.
46. Rischpler C, Langwieser N, Souvatzoglou M, Batrice A, van Marwick S, Snajberk J, et al. PET/MRI early after myocardial infarction: evaluation of viability with late gadolinium enhancement transmurality vs. 18F-FDG uptake. Eur Heart J Cardiovasc Imaging. 2015;16(6):661–9.
47. Priamo J, Adamopoulos D, Rager O, Frei A, Noble S, Carballo D, et al. Downstream indication to revascularization following hybrid cardiac PET/MRI: preliminary results. Nucl Med Commun. 2017;38(6):515–22.
48. Dall'Armellina E, Karia N, Lindsay AC, Karamitsos TD, Ferreira V, Robson MD, et al. Dynamic changes of edema and late gadolinium enhancement after acute myocardial infarction and their relationship to functional recovery and salvage index. Circ Cardiovasc Imaging. 2011;4(3):228–36.
49. Bulluck H, Hammond-Haley M, Fontana M, Knight DS, Sirker A, Herrey AS, et al. Quantification of both the area-at-risk and acute myocardial infarct size in ST-segment elevation myocardial infarction using T1-mapping. J Cardiovasc Magn Reson. 2017;19(1):57.
50. Kandler D, Lucke C, Grothoff M, Andres C, Lehmkuhl L, Nitzsche S, et al. The relation between hypointense core, microvascular obstruction and intramyocardial haemorrhage in acute reperfused myocardial infarction assessed by cardiac magnetic resonance imaging. Eur Radiol. 2014;24(12):3277–88.
51. Bulluck H, Dharmakumar R, Arai AE, Berry C, Hausenloy DJ. Cardiovascular magnetic resonance in acute ST-segment-elevation myocardial infarction: recent advances, controversies, and future directions. Circulation. 2018;137(18):1949–64.
52. Bulluck H, White SK, Frohlich GM, Casson SG, O'Meara C, Newton A, et al. Quantifying the area at risk in reperfused ST-segment-elevation myocardial infarction patients using hybrid cardiac positron emission tomography-magnetic resonance imaging. Circ Cardiovasc Imaging. 2016;9(3):e003900.
53. Grothoff M, Elpert C, Hoffmann J, Zachrau J, Lehmkuhl L, de Waha S, et al. Right ventricular injury in ST-elevation myocardial infarction: risk stratification by visualization of wall motion, edema, and delayed-enhancement cardiac magnetic resonance. Circ Cardiovasc Imaging. 2012;5(1):60–8.
54. Di Carli MF, Prcevski P, Singh TP, Janisse J, Ager J, Muzik O, et al. Myocardial blood flow, function, and metabolism in repetitive stunning. J Nucl Med. 2000;41(7):1227–34.
55. Fukuoka Y, Nakano A, Uzui H, Amaya N, Ishida K, Arakawa K, et al. Reverse blood flow-glucose

metabolism mismatch indicates preserved oxygen metabolism in patients with revascularised myocardial infarction. Eur J Nucl Med Mol Imaging. 2013;40(8):1155–62.

56. Spinelli L, Imbriaco M, Nappi C, Nicolai E, Giugliano G, Ponsiglione A, et al. Early cardiac involvement affects left ventricular longitudinal function in females carrying alpha-galactosidase A mutation: role of hybrid positron emission tomography and magnetic resonance imaging and speckle-tracking echocardiography. Circ Cardiovasc Imaging. 2018;11(4):e007019.
57. Nappi C, Altiero M, Imbriaco M, Nicolai E, Giudice CA, Aiello M, et al. First experience of simultaneous PET/MRI for the early detection of cardiac involvement in patients with Anderson-Fabry disease. Eur J Nucl Med Mol Imaging. 2015;42(7):1025–31.
58. Knott KD, Augusto JB, Nordin S, Kozor R, Camaioni C, Xue H, et al. Quantitative myocardial perfusion in Fabry disease. Circ Cardiovasc Imaging. 2019;12(7):e008872.
59. Trivieri MG, Dweck MR, Abgral R, Robson PM, Karakatsanis NA, Lala A, et al. (18)F-sodium fluoride PET/MR for the assessment of cardiac amyloidosis. J Am Coll Cardiol. 2016;68(24):2712–4.
60. Manabe O, Yoshinaga K, Ohira H, Masuda A, Sato T, Tsujino I, et al. The effects of 18-h fasting with low-carbohydrate diet preparation on suppressed physiological myocardial (18)F-fluorodeoxyglucose (FDG) uptake and possible minimal effects of unfractionated heparin use in patients with suspected cardiac involvement sarcoidosis. J Nucl Cardiol. 2016;23(2):244–52.
61. von Olshausen G, Hyafil F, Langwieser N, Laugwitz KL, Schwaiger M, Ibrahim T. Detection of acute inflammatory myocarditis in Epstein Barr virus infection using hybrid 18F-fluoro-deoxyglucose-positron emission tomography/magnetic resonance imaging. Circulation. 2014;130(11):925–6.
62. Nensa F, Poeppel TD, Krings P, Schlosser T. Multiparametric assessment of myocarditis using simultaneous positron emission tomography/magnetic resonance imaging. Eur Heart J. 2014;35(32):2173.
63. Greulich S, Deluigi CC, Gloekler S, Wahl A, Zurn C, Kramer U, et al. CMR imaging predicts death and other adverse events in suspected cardiac sarcoidosis. JACC Cardiovasc Imaging. 2013;6(4):501–11.
64. Youssef G, Leung E, Mylonas I, Nery P, Williams K, Wisenberg G, et al. The use of 18F-FDG PET in the diagnosis of cardiac sarcoidosis: a systematic review and metaanalysis including the Ontario experience. J Nucl Med. 2012;53(2):241–8.
65. Birnie DH, Sauer WH, Bogun F, Cooper JM, Culver DA, Duvernoy CS, et al. HRS expert consensus statement on the diagnosis and management of arrhythmias associated with cardiac sarcoidosis. Heart Rhythm. 2014;11(7):1305–23.
66. Slart R, Glaudemans A, Lancellotti P, Hyafil F, Blankstein R, Schwartz RG, et al. A joint procedural position statement on imaging in cardiac sarcoidosis: from the Cardiovascular and Inflammation & Infection Committees of the European Association of Nuclear Medicine, the European Association of Cardiovascular Imaging, and the American Society of Nuclear Cardiology. J Nucl Cardiol. 2018;25(1):298–319.
67. Schneider S, Batrice A, Rischpler C, Eiber M, Ibrahim T, Nekolla SG. Utility of multimodal cardiac imaging with PET/MRI in cardiac sarcoidosis: implications for diagnosis, monitoring and treatment. Eur Heart J. 2014;35(5):312.
68. Wada K, Niitsuma T, Yamaki T, Masuda A, Ito H, Kubo H, et al. Simultaneous cardiac imaging to detect inflammation and scar tissue with (18) F-fluorodeoxyglucose PET/MRI in cardiac sarcoidosis. J Nucl Cardiol. 2016;23(5):1180–2.
69. White JA, Rajchl M, Butler J, Thompson RT, Prato FS, Wisenberg G. Active cardiac sarcoidosis: first clinical experience of simultaneous positron emission tomography—magnetic resonance imaging for the diagnosis of cardiac disease. Circulation. 2013;127(22):e639–41.
70. Wicks EC, Menezes LJ, Barnes A, Mohiddin SA, Sekhri N, Porter JC, et al. Diagnostic accuracy and prognostic value of simultaneous hybrid 18F-fluorodeoxyglucose positron emission tomography/magnetic resonance imaging in cardiac sarcoidosis. Eur Heart J Cardiovasc Imaging. 2018;19(7):757–67.
71. Hanneman K, Kadoch M, Guo HH, Jamali M, Quon A, Iagaru A, et al. Initial experience with simultaneous 18F-FDG PET/MRI in the evaluation of cardiac sarcoidosis and myocarditis. Clin Nucl Med. 2017;42(7):e328–34.
72. Dweck MR, Abgral R, Trivieri MG, Robson PM, Karakatsanis N, Mani V, et al. Hybrid magnetic resonance imaging and positron emission tomography with fluorodeoxyglucose to diagnose active cardiac sarcoidosis. JACC Cardiovasc Imaging. 2018;11(1):94–107.
73. Cheng L, Ma L, Schoenhagen P, Ye H, Lou X, Gao Y, et al. Comparison of three-dimensional volume-targeted thin-slab FIESTA magnetic resonance angiography and 64-multidetector computed tomographic angiography for the identification of proximal coronary stenosis. Int J Cardiol. 2013;167(6):2969–76.
74. Chen MY, Bandettini WP, Shanbhag SM, Vasu S, Booker OJ, Leung SW, et al. Concordance and diagnostic accuracy of vasodilator stress cardiac MRI and 320-detector row coronary CTA. Int J Cardiovasc Imaging. 2014;30(1):109–19.
75. Bettencourt N, Chiribiri A, Schuster A, Ferreira N, Sampaio F, Pires-Morais G, et al. Direct comparison of cardiac magnetic resonance and multidetector computed tomography stress-rest perfusion imaging for detection of coronary artery disease. J Am Coll Cardiol. 2013;61(10):1099–107.

76. Bettencourt N, Ferreira ND, Leite D, Carvalho M, Ferreira WDS, Schuster A, et al. CAD detection in patients with intermediate-high pre-test probability: low-dose CT delayed enhancement detects ischemic myocardial scar with moderate accuracy but does not improve performance of a stress-rest CT perfusion protocol. JACC Cardiovasc Imaging. 2013;6(10):1062–71.
77. Donati OF, Scheffel H, Stolzmann P, Baumuller S, Plass A, Leschka S, et al. Combined cardiac CT and MRI for the comprehensive workup of hemodynamically relevant coronary stenoses. AJR Am J Roentgenol. 2010;194(4):920–6.
78. Scheffel H, Stolzmann P, Alkadhi H, Azemaj N, Plass A, Baumueller S, et al. Low-dose CT and cardiac MR for the diagnosis of coronary artery disease: accuracy of single and combined approaches. Int J Cardiovasc Imaging. 2010;26(5):579–90.
79. Groothuis JG, Beek AM, Brinckman SL, Meijerink MR, van den Oever ML, Hofman MB, et al. Combined non-invasive functional and anatomical diagnostic work-up in clinical practice: the magnetic resonance and computed tomography in suspected coronary artery disease (MARCC) study. Eur Heart J. 2013;34(26):1990–8.
80. von Spiczak J, Manka R, Gotschy A, Oebel S, Kozerke S, Hamada S, et al. Fusion of CT coronary angiography and whole-heart dynamic 3D cardiac MR perfusion: building a framework for comprehensive cardiac imaging. Int J Cardiovasc Imaging. 2018;34(4):649–60.
81. Danad I, Szymonifka J, Twisk JWR, Norgaard BL, Zarins CK, Knaapen P, et al. Diagnostic performance of cardiac imaging methods to diagnose ischaemia-causing coronary artery disease when directly compared with fractional flow reserve as a reference standard: a meta-analysis. Eur Heart J. 2017;38(13):991–8.
82. Ronnow Sand NP, Nissen L, Winther S, Petersen SE, Westra J, Christiansen EH, et al. Prediction of coronary revascularization in stable angina: comparison of FFRCT with CMR stress perfusion imaging. JACC Cardiovasc Imaging. 2020;13(4):994–1004.
83. Rizvi A, Han D, Danad I, Ó Hartaigh B, Lee JH, Gransar H, et al. Diagnostic performance of hybrid cardiac imaging methods for assessment of obstructive coronary artery disease compared with stand-alone coronary computed tomography angiography: a meta-analysis. JACC Cardiovasc Imaging. 2018;11(4):589–99.
84. Abadia AF, van Assen M, Martin SS, Vingiani V, Griffith LP, Giovagnoli DA, et al. Myocardial extracellular volume fraction to differentiate healthy from cardiomyopathic myocardium using dual-source dual-energy CT. J Cardiovasc Comput Tomogr. 2020;14(2):162–7.
85. Ohta Y, Kitao S, Yunaga H, Watanabe T, Mukai-Yatagai N, Kishimoto J, et al. Quantitative evaluation of non-ischemic dilated cardiomyopathy by late iodine enhancement using rapid kV switching dual-energy computed tomography: a feasibility study. J Cardiovasc Comput Tomogr. 2019;13(2):148–56.
86. Lee HJ, Im DJ, Youn JC, Chang S, Suh YJ, Hong YJ, et al. Myocardial extracellular volume fraction with dual-energy equilibrium contrast-enhanced cardiac CT in nonischemic cardiomyopathy: a prospective comparison with cardiac MR imaging. Radiology. 2016;280(1):49–57.
87. Sidhu MS, Ghoshhajra BB, Uthamalingam S, Kilcullen N, Engel LC, Medina HM, et al. Clinical experiences of delayed contrast enhancement with cardiac computed tomography: case series. BMC Res Notes. 2013;6:2.
88. Takaoka H, Funabashi N, Ozawa K, Uehara M, Sano K, Komuro I, et al. Improved diagnosis of detection of late enhancement in left ventricular myocardium using 2nd generation 320-slice CT reconstructed with FIRST in non-ischemic cardiomyopathy. Int Heart J. 2018;59(3):542–9.
89. Ko SM, Hwang SH, Lee HJ. Role of cardiac computed tomography in the diagnosis of left ventricular myocardial diseases. J Cardiovasc Imaging. 2019;27(2):73–92.
90. Hutton BF, Occhipinti M, Kuehne A, Mathe D, Kovacs N, Waiczies H, et al. Development of clinical simultaneous SPECT/MRI. Br J Radiol. 2018;91(1081):20160690.
91. Lamb J, Holland JP. Advanced methods for radiolabeling multimodality nanomedicines for SPECT/MRI and PET/MRI. J Nucl Med. 2018;59(3):382–9.
92. Klocke FJ, Baird MG, Lorell BH, Bateman TM, Messer JV, Berman DS, et al. ACC/AHA/ASNC guidelines for the clinical use of cardiac radionuclide imaging—executive summary: a report of the American College of Cardiology/American Heart Association Task Force on Practice Guidelines (ACC/AHA/ASNC Committee to revise the 1995 Guidelines for the Clinical Use of Cardiac Radionuclide Imaging). J Am Coll Cardiol. 2003;42(7):1318–33.
93. Underwood SR, Anagnostopoulos C, Cerqueira M, Ell PJ, Flint EJ, Harbinson M, et al. Myocardial perfusion scintigraphy: the evidence. Eur J Nucl Med Mol Imaging. 2004;31(2):261–91.
94. Knuuti J, Kajander S, Maki M, Ukkonen H. Quantification of myocardial blood flow will reform the detection of CAD. J Nucl Cardiol. 2009;16(4):497–506.
95. Hamon M, Fau G, Nee G, Ehtisham J, Morello R. Meta-analysis of the diagnostic performance of stress perfusion cardiovascular magnetic resonance for detection of coronary artery disease. J Cardiovasc Magn Reson. 2010;12:29.
96. Hedeer F, Palmer J, Arheden H, Ugander M. Gated myocardial perfusion SPECT underestimates left ventricular volumes and shows high variability compared to cardiac magnetic resonance imaging—a comparison of four different commercial automated software packages. BMC Med Imaging. 2010;10:10.

97. Schwitter J, Wacker CM, Wilke N, Al-Saadi N, Sauer E, Huettle K, et al. MR-IMPACT II: magnetic resonance imaging for myocardial perfusion assessment in coronary artery disease trial: perfusion-cardiac magnetic resonance vs. single-photon emission computed tomography for the detection of coronary artery disease: a comparative multicentre, multivendor trial. Eur Heart J. 2013;34(10):775–81.
98. Greenwood JP, Maredia N, Younger JF, Brown JM, Nixon J, Everett CC, et al. Cardiovascular magnetic resonance and single-photon emission computed tomography for diagnosis of coronary heart disease (CE-MARC): a prospective trial. Lancet. 2012;379(9814):453–60.
99. Gibbons RJ, Verani MS, Behrenbeck T, Pellikka PA, O'Connor MK, Mahmarian JJ, et al. Feasibility of tomographic 99mTc-hexakis-2-methoxy-2--methylpropyl-isonitrile imaging for the assessment of myocardial area at risk and the effect of treatment in acute myocardial infarction. Circulation. 1989;80(5):1277–86.
100. Ugander M, Soneson H, Engblom H, van der Pals J, Erlinge D, Heiberg E, et al. Quantification of myocardium at risk in myocardial perfusion SPECT by co-registration and fusion with delayed contrast-enhanced magnetic resonance imaging—an experimental ex vivo study. Clin Physiol Funct Imaging. 2012;32(1):33–8.
101. Nordlund D, Kanski M, Jablonowski R, Koul S, Erlinge D, Carlsson M, et al. Experimental validation of contrast-enhanced SSFP cine CMR for quantification of myocardium at risk in acute myocardial infarction. J Cardiovasc Magn Reson. 2017;19(1):12.
102. Sorensson P, Heiberg E, Saleh N, Bouvier F, Caidahl K, Tornvall P, et al. Assessment of myocardium at risk with contrast enhanced steady-state free precession cine cardiovascular magnetic resonance compared to single-photon emission computed tomography. J Cardiovasc Magn Reson. 2010;12:25.
103. Dilsizian V, Bonow RO, Epstein SE, Fananapazir L. Myocardial ischemia detected by thallium scintigraphy is frequently related to cardiac arrest and syncope in young patients with hypertrophic cardiomyopathy. J Am Coll Cardiol. 1993;22(3):796–804.
104. Cecchi F, Olivotto I, Gistri R, Lorenzoni R, Chiriatti G, Camici PG. Coronary microvascular dysfunction and prognosis in hypertrophic cardiomyopathy. N Engl J Med. 2003;349(11):1027–35.
105. Terai H, Shimizu M, Ino H, Yamaguchi M, Uchiyama K, Oe K, et al. Changes in cardiac sympathetic nerve innervation and activity in pathophysiologic transition from typical to end-stage hypertrophic cardiomyopathy. J Nucl Med. 2003;44(10):1612–7.
106. Zhao C, Shuke N, Okizaki A, Yamamoto W, Sato J, Ishikawa Y, et al. Comparison of myocardial fatty acid metabolism with left ventricular function and perfusion in cardiomyopathies: by 123I-BMIPP SPECT and 99mTc-tetrofosmin electrocardiographically gated SPECT. Ann Nucl Med. 2003;17(7):541–8.
107. Pennell DJ, Sechtem UP, Higgins CB, Manning WJ, Pohost GM, Rademakers FE, et al. Clinical indications for cardiovascular magnetic resonance (CMR): consensus panel report. Eur Heart J. 2004;25(21):1940–65.
108. Yamanari H, Kakishita M, Fujimoto Y, Hashimoto K, Kiyooka T, Katayama Y, et al. Effect of regional myocardial perfusion abnormalities on regional myocardial early diastolic function in patients with hypertrophic cardiomyopathy. Heart Vessel. 1997;12(4):192–8.
109. Yuki H, Utsunomiya D, Shiraishi S, Takashio S, Sakamoto F, Tsuda N, et al. Correlation of left ventricular dyssynchrony on gated myocardial perfusion SPECT analysis with extent of late gadolinium enhancement on cardiac magnetic resonance imaging in hypertrophic cardiomyopathy. Heart Vessel. 2018;33(6):623–9.
110. Sazonova SI, Ilyushenkova JN, Lishmanov YB, Batalov RE, Sazonov AE, Larionova LA, et al. Assessment of radiological techniques application possibility for non-invasive diagnostics of latent inflammatory processes in myocardium in patients with atrial fibrillation. Ann Nucl Med. 2016;30(10):738–48.
111. Niederkohr RD, Daniels C, Raman SV. Concordant findings on myocardial perfusion SPECT and cardiac magnetic resonance imaging in a patient with myocarditis. J Nucl Cardiol. 2008;15(3):466–8.
112. Kataoka S, Momose M, Fukushima K, Serizawa N, Suzuki A, Kondo C, et al. Regional myocardial damage and active inflammation in patients with cardiac sarcoidosis detected by non-invasive multi-modal imaging. Ann Nucl Med. 2017;31(2):135–43.

Hybrid Imaging Using Single Photon Emission Computed Tomography

4

G. Ross Farris, Ami E. Iskandrian, Fadi G. Hage, and Pradeep Bhambhvani

Abbreviations

AC	Attenuation correction
CAC	Coronary calcium score
CAD	Coronary artery disease
CCTA	Coronary computed tomography angiography
COR	Class of recommendation
CT	Computed tomography
EF	Ejection fraction
LOE	Level of evidence
LV	Left ventricle (ventricular)
MBF	Myocardial blood flow
MPI	Myocardial perfusion imaging
SPECT	Single photon emission computed tomography

G. R. Farris · F. G. Hage P. Bhambhvani
University of Alabama at Birmingham, Birmingham Veteran's Affairs Medical Center, Birmingham, AL, USA
e-mail: Grfarris1@uabmc.edu; Fhage@uabmc.edu; Pbhambhvani@uabmc.edu

A. E. Iskandrian (✉)
Division of Cardiovascular Disease, University of Alabama at Birmingham, Birmingham, AL, USA
e-mail: aiskand@uab.edu; aiskandrian@uabmc.edu

4.1 Introduction

According to the Oxford English Dictionary, the word "hybrid" has its origin in 1595–1605 from Latin "hybrida." Examples include the offspring of two animals or plants of different breeds, varieties, or species; cross-breeding of two unlike cultures or traditions; a hybrid of the academic and business worlds; a word composed of different languages and things that are powered by more than one source such as hybrid automobiles.

Hybrid imaging may refer to using a single imaging modality in multiple ways or combining separate imaging modalities together, sequentially or simultaneously. An example of the former would be combining first-pass radionuclide ventriculography using a multi-crystal gamma camera and single photon emission computed tomography (SPECT) perfusion imaging using the Anger gamma camera. Another example would be doing coronary artery calcium scoring (CAC) and coronary computed tomography angiography (CCTA) during the same series of scans. Examples of the latter include SPECT plus coronary calcium score or SPECT plus CCTA. There are many examples of hybrid imaging using positron emission tomography (PET) either alone or with CT or magnetic resonance imaging, which will not be discussed here. CT attenuation-correction of SPECT images could be considered as a third type of hybrid imaging, using one modality to enhance another.

F. Nudi et al. (eds.), *Hybrid Cardiac Imaging for Clinical Decision-Making*,
https://doi.org/10.1007/978-3-030-99391-7_4

This chapter will focus on hybrid cardiac imaging with SPECT/CT for readers with expertise in SPECT. As such, this chapter will not cover procedural aspects of imaging which are discussed in many guidelines [1–3]. The focus will be on the indications, value, and pitfalls of SPECT/CT. The hybrid PET/CT, PET/MRI and their use in a variety of disorders such as CAD, microvascular disorders, viability assessment, amyloid heart disease, sarcoid heart disease, endocarditis, and device infections will not be discussed in detail in this chapter.

4.1.1 Hybrid SPECT/CT and PET/CT

CT is often used in combination with SPECT or PET to provide a patient-specific attenuation-correction map (CT-AC). There are many advantages to this technique of AC over line-source attenuation correction including lack of interference with emission data and lack of decay of the radioactive source. CT-AC increases the diagnostic accuracy compared to non-AC SPECT by reducing the number of false-positive perfusion defects caused by soft tissue attenuation resulting in an improvement in confidence in scan interpretation [4]. Part of the advantage of PET perfusion over SPECT perfusion imaging is thought to be because PET studies are routinely done with AC while only a minority of SPECT studies are performed with AC for a variety of reasons.

Simultaneous assessment of coronary anatomy and physiology can be obtained in a single study by utilizing hybrid PET/CT or SPECT/CT. Hybrid SPECT/CT systems are commercially available but more expensive than standalone SPECT systems [5]. These hybrid systems can assess the presence and severity of coronary artery disease (CAD) using coronary artery calcification (CAC) score and/or coronary CT angiography (CCTA) [6, 7].

4.1.2 SPECT/CT MPI with CAC

The principle limitation of SPECT (or PET MPI) is the lack of sensitivity for the detection of nonobstructive CAD. MPI relies on regional perfusion abnormalities caused by flow limiting stenosis in the coronary arteries. However, patients may have mild CAD that would benefit from aggressive medical or lifestyle interventions that are not detected using these techniques because the lesions are not "hemodynamically" significant. The addition of CAC and/or CCTA scanning mitigates this limitation and has been one of the reasons for advocating hybrid imaging. The other limitation of MPI that could be mitigated with the use of CCTA is its well-known tendency to underestimate the extent of multi-vessel disease and the possibility of missing left main disease when accompanied by right coronary artery disease resulting in parallel hemodynamic effects on both sides of the coronary distribution that leads to what is colloquially known as balanced ischemia.

The frequency and severity of abnormal stress SPECT-MPI studies have progressively decreased over the past two decades, to the point that a large proportion (approximately 90%) of current studies are normal [8, 9]. Some of these patients with normal perfusion by SPECT-MPI may have CAD (more commonly non-flow limiting coronary atherosclerosis). A 2004 study evaluating over 1100 patients with normal SPECT-MPI studies found that 78% had abnormal CAC, and >30% had CAC scores >400, indicating extensive atherosclerosis [10]. The use of CAC or CCTA may lead to intensification of medical management in such patients as the improved understanding of the patient's risk can lead to improved treatment adherence [11].

The addition of CAC scanning to SPECT-MPI may also improve risk stratification. The combination of CAC and MPI abnormalities is more predictive than either alone since each assesses a different aspect of coronary disease. Each increment of CAC correlates with a rising event rate just as each increment in perfusion defect size (PDS) [12]. SPECT has excellent short- and medium-term prognostic predictive value (there are nevertheless few studies on long-term prognostication), while CAC may be a good discriminator of long-term risk.

Some have suggested that an additional benefit of hybrid MPI and CAC is an increase in certainty in scan interpretation and detection of hemodynamically significant stenosis. This may be helpful when assessing patients with borderline MPI abnormalities or discordant results between MPI and clinical or ECG stress responses [10]. The extent of CAC abnormality is a more powerful predictor of obstructive CAD than traditional CAD risk factors [13]. In the absence of CAC, borderline or discordant findings can be weighed towards normal in reporting and management recommendations. In the presence of extensive CAC, borderline and discordant tests can raise suspicion for obstructive or even high-risk CAD [14]. The reader can find a more detailed discussion on CAC in Sect. 4.1.6, which deals with computed tomography. The pertinent parts of ACC/AHA and ESC guidelines related to the use of CAC are summarized in Tables 4.1, 4.2, 4.3, and 4.4.

4.1.3 SPECT-MPI with CCTA

Combined coronary CT angiography (CCTA) and MPI could be done sequentially (sequential) at the same time and on the same system or serially (serial) on two different systems and at different times. (see also Chaps. 1–6). Examples of hybrid SPECT and CCTA are shown in Figs. 4.1 and 4.2.

A summary of the studies on this hybrid approach is provided in Table 4.5. The sequential protocol has the advantage of more precise registration than fused images using the serial protocol. A disadvantage of the sequential protocol is that patients are committed to both studies regardless of the results of the first study, while the serial protocol allows incorporation of the results from the first set of images (SPECT or CCTA) into the decision-making process and then deciding whether the second study is indeed necessary. The advantages and disadvantages of both protocols are listed in Table 4.6.

One of the often-quoted reasons for using hybrid SPECT/CCTA is the fear that a normal MPI may be due to balanced ischemia. Recent data suggest that measuring stress and rest myocardial blood flow (MBF) may be a valid alternative (discussed elsewhere in this book) [30]. A consensus statement from the American Society of Cardiology and the Society of Nuclear

Table 4.1 Summary of American guidelines regarding CAC

	COR	LOE	Recommendation
2019 ACC/AHA Guideline on the Primary Prevention of Cardiovascular Disease [15]	IIa	B-NR	In adults at intermediate risk (≥7.5%–<20% 10-year ASCVD risk) or selected adults at borderline risk (5%–<7.5% 10-year ASCVD risk), if risk-based decisions for preventive interventions (e.g., statin therapy) remain uncertain, it is reasonable to measure a coronary artery calcium score to guide clinician–patient risk discussion
2018 AHA/ACC/AACVPR/AAPA/ABC/ACPM/ADA/AGS/APhA/ASPC/NLA/PCNA Guideline on the Management of Blood Cholesterol [16]	IIa	B-NR	In intermediate risk (≥7.5%–<20% 10-year ASCVD risk) adults or selected borderline risk (5%–<7.5% 10-year ASCVD risk) adults in whom a coronary artery calcium score is measured for the purpose of making a treatment decision, AND If the coronary artery calcium score is zero, it is reasonable to withhold statin therapy and reassess in 5–10 years, as long as higher risk conditions are absent (e.g., diabetes, family history of premature CHD, cigarette smoking); If coronary artery calcium score is 1–99, it is reasonable to initiate statin therapy for patients ≥55 years of age; If coronary artery calcium score is 100 or higher or in the 75th percentile or higher, it is reasonable to initiate statin therapy, irrespective of age
2012 ACCF/AHA/ACP/AATS/PCNA/SCAI/STS guideline for the Diagnosis and Management of Patients With Stable Ischemic Heart Disease [17]	IIb	C	For patients with a low to intermediate pretest probability of obstructive IHD, noncontrast cardiac CT to determine the CAC score may be considered

ASCVD atherosclerotic cardiovascular disease, *CHD* coronary heart disease, *CAC* coronary artery calcium, *NR* not specifically reviewed

Table 4.2 Coronary artery calcium measurement candidates who might benefit from knowing their coronary artery calcium score is zero [15]

1.	Patients reluctant to initiate statin who wish to understand their risk and potential for benefit more precisely
2.	Patients concerned about the need to reinstitute statin therapy after discontinuation for statin-associated symptoms
3.	Older patients (men 55–80 years of age; women 60–80 years of age) with low burden of risk factors who question whether they would benefit from statin therapy
4.	Middle-aged adults (40–55 years of age) with pooled cohort equation-calculated 10-year risk of ASCVD 5–<7.5% with factors that increase their ASCVD risk, although they are in a borderline risk group

Table 4.3 ACCF/SCCT/ACR/AHA/ASE/ASNC/NASCI/SCAI/SCMR 2010 appropriate use criteria for cardiac computed tomography [18]

1. Appropriate	
(a)	Asymptomatic patient, first scan, intermediate risk
(b)	Asymptomatic patient, first scan, low risk, positive family history
2. Uncertain	
(a)	Asymptomatic patient, repeat scan, 0 calcium score >5 years prior
(b)	Asymptomatic patient, first scan, high risk
3. Inappropriate	
(a)	Asymptomatic patient, repeat scan, Positive <2 years prior
(b)	Asymptomatic patient, first scan, low risk, no family history of CAD

Table 4.4 Summary of European Society of Cardiology (ESC) guidelines including COR/LOE

1. 2019 ESC Guidelines on diabetes, pre-diabetes, and cardiovascular diseases developed in collaboration with the EASD [19]	
(a)	CAC score with CT may be considered as a risk modifier in the CV risk assessment of asymptomatic patients with DM at moderate risk. (IIb/B)
2. 2019 ESC/EAS Guidelines for the management of dyslipidemias: lipid modification to reduce cardiovascular risk [20]	
(a)	CAC score assessment with CT may be considered as a risk modifier in the CV risk assessment of asymptomatic individuals at low or moderate risk (IIb/B)

Medicine and Molecular Imaging Cardiovascular Council suggests that PET-MBF is rapidly being incorporated into routine clinical practice [31]. However, increased costs, lack of cyclotron/generator availability, and lack of expertise and familiarity with PET may limit the widespread adoption of such techniques [32]. Nevertheless, the use of PET-MBF is on the rise.

An exciting and emerging area of interest in SPECT is the quantification of absolute MBF using the newer generation of solid state or Cadmium Zinc Telluride (CZT) detector cameras. Due to lower costs and the fact that SPECT systems are already in place across the world, methods to determine absolute MBF with SPECT systems are highly appealing [33]. The combination of SPECT-MPI and SPECT-MBF could be viewed as another example of hybrid imaging using the same technology but different methods of acquisition and processing (Fig. 4.3). As with PET, abnormal MBF by SPECT could be due to coronary stenosis or microvascular disease, or both. In some of these patients, CAC or CCTA is required just as when using PET.

Solid state detector cameras have improved sensitivity, spatial, temporal, and energy resolution compared to previous camera types [34, 35]. This allows for the improved and easier dynamic acquisition of images, which is required to evaluate absolute MBF [19, 33]. Animal and human studies have shown that MBF measurements using solid state detector SPECT cameras and either ^{201}Thallium or ^{99m}Technetium correlate with MBF measurements obtained with microspheres and PET tracers [19, 20]. Giubbinn et al. built on this by demonstrating a reasonable correlation between MBF and myocardial flow reserve (MFR) measured by N13NH3-PET and 99m Tc-tetrofosmin CZT SPECT [31]. This remains an area of active research and widespread interest in the field.

CCTA is increasingly being used as a first-line test for patients with suspected CAD. This was recently recommended in the 2019 European Society of Cardiology Guidelines for the diagnosis and management of chronic coronary syn-

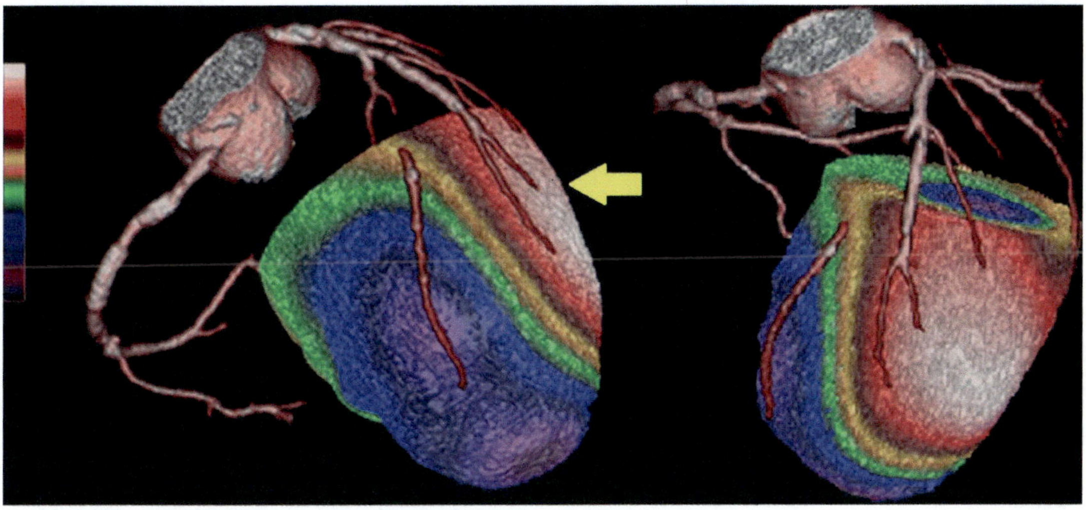

Fig. 4.1 This is an example of hybrid CCTA/SPECT-MPI in an older man presenting with angina and multiple risk factors for atherosclerotic cardiovascular disease. The CCTA images reveal a chronic total occlusion of the mid LAD (yellow arrow). The SPECT-MPI images reveal severe ischemia in the anterior wall (red and white area) [21]

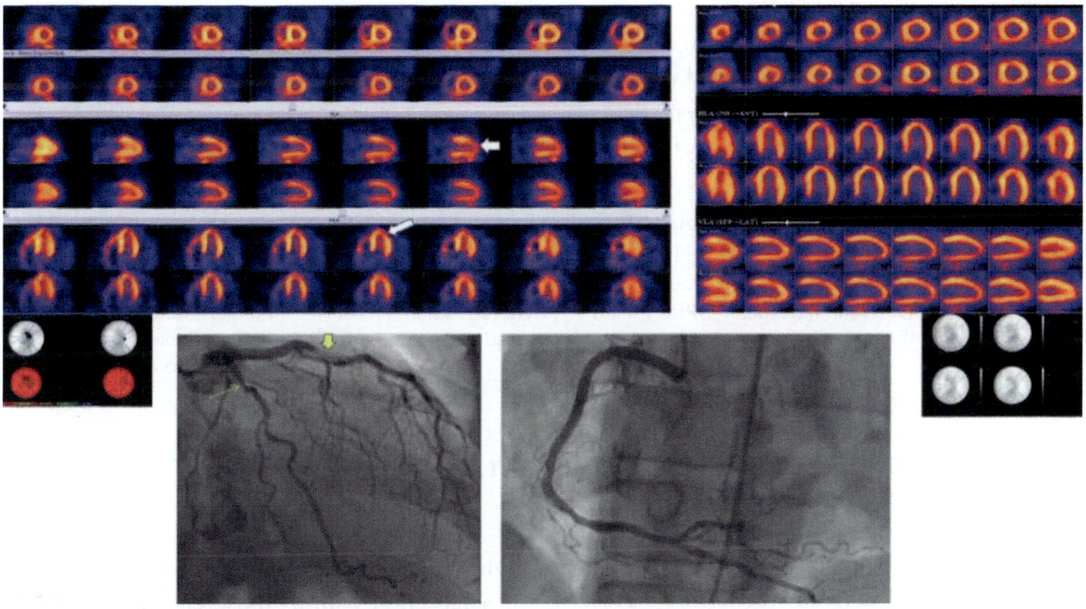

Fig. 4.2 These images show the benefit of attenuation correction (AC) by CT. The upper left panel shows conventional camera images with AC (top rows) and without AC (lower rows). The short white arrow indicates an anteroapical perfusion defect. The long white arrow indicates an apical perfusion defect. The quantification is shown below the figures. The upper right panel shows CZT images obtained upright (top rows) and supine (bottom rows). The quantification showing no perfusion defect is shown below. The center panels reveal a coronary angiogram with critical mid LAD stenosis (short yellow arrow) and a LCX lesion (long yellow arrow). There was no obstructive disease in the RCA [22]

Table 4.5 Summary of results using hybrid SPEC/CCTA

Author/ reference	# pts	Modality	Reference	Results
Sloma, et al. [23]	*N* = 35	Standalone CCTA + SPECT	ICA	Improved sensitivity and specificity with SPECT/CT vs CCTA or SPECT alone
Gaemperli et al. [24]	*N* = 38	Standalone CCTA + SPECT	ICA	Hybrid imaging added diagnostic information on the functional relevance of coronary artery lesions
Santana et al. [25]	*N* = 50	Standalone CCTA + SPECT	ICA	Hybrid imaging provided incremental diagnostic information compared to MPI alone or side-by-side MPI-CCTA for the diagnosis of obstructive CAD and for localization of CAD to the left anterior descending coronary artery
Rispler et al. [26]	*N* = 56	Hybrid SPECT/ CCTA	ICA	Hybrid imaging improved sensitivity, specificity, NPV, PPV when compared to CCTA alone
Schaap et al. [27]	*N* = 98	Hybrid SPECT/ CCTA	ICA + FFR	Hybrid imaging improved sensitivity, specificity, NPV, PPV
Schaap et al. [28]	*N* = 205	Hybrid SPECT/ CCTA	ICA + FFR	Hybrid SPECT/CCTA imaging has a substantially higher yield than standalone SPECT or CCTA in the diagnostic workup of patients suspected of significant CAD
Liga et al. [29]	*N* = 252	Standalone CCTA + SPECT/ PET	ICA + FFR	Hybrid imaging improved the localization of disease and NPV, PPV

ICA invasive coronary angiography, *FFR* fractional flow reserve, *NPV* negative predictive value, *PPV* positive predictive value

Table 4.6 Advantages/limitations of serial vs. sequential hybrid imaging

Approach	Definition	Example	Advantages	Disadvantages
True simultaneous	Same machine, same time	PET/MRI	More convenient for patient and staff, decreased motion artifacts	More complex hardware and software
Pseudo simultaneous	Same machine, sequentially obtained[a]	SPECT/CT, PET/CT	More convenient for patient and staff	Possible respiratory motion mismatch, artifacts
Sequential	Different machine, different time	SPECT + CT	Reduced radiation/cost (if second exam not needed)	Longer exam, increased staff workload, increased radiation dose

[a] e.g., CT followed by SPECT during the same imaging session

dromes (Table 4.7) [36]. The most recent ACC/AHA and NICE guidelines also acknowledge the merits of CCTA (Tables 4.8 and 4.9). CCTA when combined with physiological measurements such as CT-derived fraction flow reserve (FFR) may overcome the important limitation of this technique in patients with apparent intermediate stenoses.

4.1.4 Other Applications of SPECT/ CT

Hybrid imaging can also play a role in the setting of acute chest pain as those encountered in the emergency departments. A variety of methods have been used to risk stratify these patients (a large number of methods indicates that none is

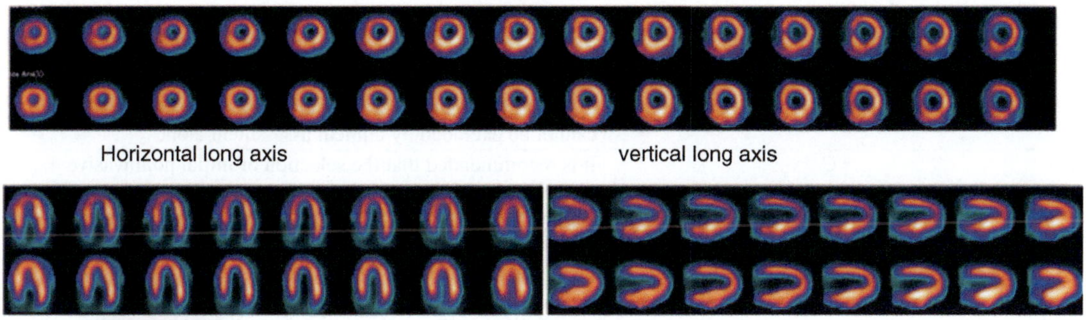

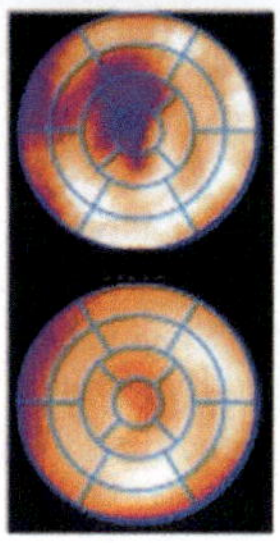

Quantitative myocardial blood flow (^{99m}Tc-Tetrofosmin–CZT with AC)

	Rest (ml/min/g)	Stress (ml/min/g)	MFR (stress/rest)
LAD	0.39	1.37	3.53
LCX	0.42	1.91	4.49
RCA	0.46	1.95	4.23
Global LV	0.42	1.67	4.00

Fig. 4.3 Attenuation corrected- CZT measurement of myocardial blood flow. There is a severe reversible perfusion defect in the anterior wall. Quantitative measurement shows a markedly reduced MBF of the LAD during stress [31]

ideal!) but clearly some may benefit from hybrid SPECT/CAC or SPECT/CCTA (Fig. 4.4). One potential avenue for hybrid imaging is the prediction of vulnerable plaques that may signify impending ACS. Small studies have established that hybrid 18F-NaF PET/CT can identify vulnerable coronary lesions [32, 39]. As this technology and the surrounding expertise progress, our understanding of the pathophysiology of CAD, atherosclerosis, and risk stratification will all improve [40].

Another group that may benefit from hybrid imaging involves those with heart failure to determine the underlying etiology and the status of myocardial viability (Fig. 4.5) [42]. New onset heart failure is a common cause of both inpatient and outpatient cardiac consultation. Heart failure is commonly divided into subgroups, and one of the most common differentiators is the presence or absence of significant CAD. In patients who have CAD, it is important to determine the severity of the disease, both in terms of area affected and the degree of severity within the affected area.

Multiple trials have examined myocardial viability studies and revascularization. A substudy of the STITCH Trial, a nonblinded trial that randomized 1212 patients to medical therapy with or without coronary artery bypass surgery (CABG), included the 601 participants that underwent myocardial viability studies via SPECT or with dobutamine stress echo (DSE) [43]. Patients in the viability subgroup were randomized to medical therapy with or without coronary artery bypass surgery (CABG). There was an association of increased survival in the patients with viable myocardium, but this association became statistically nonsignificant after multivariate adjustment. The study was limited by lack of randomization due to viability and, more importantly, absence of information on viability in the majority of patients in the study resulting in the high likelihood of selection bias. Additionally, a high percentage of patients in the viability subgroup had single vessel disease, who may not routinely undergo viability assessment in routine practice. The HEART trial also randomized patients with heart failure with reduced ejection

Table 4.7 2019 ESC Guidelines for the diagnosis and management of chronic coronary syndromes [36]

COR	LOE	Recommendation
I	B	Noninvasive functional imaging for myocardial ischemia or coronary CTA is recommended as the initial test to diagnose CAD in symptomatic patients in whom obstructive CAD cannot be excluded by clinical assessment alone
I	C	It is recommended that the selection of initial noninvasive diagnostic test is done based on the clinical likelihood of CAD and other patient characteristics that influence test performance, local expertise, and the availability of tests
I	B	Functional imaging for myocardial ischemia is recommended if coronary CTA has shown CAD of uncertain functional significance or is not diagnostic
IIa	C	Coronary CTA should be considered as an alternative to invasive angiography if another noninvasive test is equivocal or nondiagnostic
III	C	Coronary CTA is not recommended when extensive coronary calcification, irregular heart rate, significant obesity, inability to cooperate with breath-hold commands, or any other conditions make obtaining good image quality unlikely
III	C	Coronary calcium detection by CT is not recommended to identify individuals with obstructive CAD
I	B	Risk stratification, preferably using stress imaging or coronary CTA (if permitted by local expertise and availability), or alternatively exercise stress ECG (if significant exercise can be performed and the ECG is amenable to the identification of ischaemic changes), is recommended in patients with suspected or newly diagnosed CAD
IIa	B	If coronary CTA is available for event risk stratification, additional stress imaging should be performed before the referral of a patient with few/no symptoms for ICA
III	C	Coronary CTA is not recommended as a routine follow-up test for patients with established CAD
I	C	Invasive angiography or coronary CTA is recommended in patients with characteristic episodic resting angina and ST-segment changes, which resolve with nitrates and/or calcium antagonists, to determine the extent of underlying coronary disease
IIb	C	In high-risk asymptomatic adults (with diabetes, a strong family history of CAD, or when previous risk-assessment tests suggest a high risk of CAD), functional imaging or coronary CTA may be considered for cardiovascular risk assessment
III	C	In low-risk nondiabetic asymptomatic adults, coronary CTA or functional imaging for ischemia are not indicated for further diagnostic assessment
IIa	C	Coronary CTA should be considered as an alternative to coronary angiography before valve intervention in patients with severe valvular heart disease and low probability of CAD
IIb	B	In asymptomatic adults (age > 40 years) with diabetes, functional imaging or coronary CTA may be considered for advanced cardiovascular risk assessment

Table 4.8 2012 ACCF/AHA/ACP/AATS/PCNA/SCAI/STS guideline for the diagnosis and management of patients with stable ischemic heart disease [17]

COR	LOE	Recommendation
IIa	B	CCTA is reasonable for patients with a low to intermediate pretest probability of IHD who are incapable of at least moderate physical functioning or have disabling comorbidity
IIa	C	CCTA is reasonable for patients with an intermediate pretest probability of IHD who (a) have continued symptoms with prior normal test findings, (b) have inconclusive results from prior exercise or pharmacological stress testing, or c) are unable to undergo stress with nuclear MPI or echocardiography
IIa	C	CCTA can be useful as a first-line test for risk assessment in patients with SIHD who are unable to exercise to an adequate workload regardless of the interpretability of ECG
IIa	C	CCTA can be useful for risk assessment in patients with SIHD who have an indeterminate result from functional testing
IIb	B	CCTA might be reasonable for patients with an intermediate pretest probability of IHD who have at least moderate physical functioning or no disabling comorbidity
IIb	B	CCTA may be reasonable for risk assessment in patients with SIHD who are able to exercise to an adequate workload but have an uninterpretable ECG
IIb	C	CCTA might be considered for risk assessment in patients with SIHD unable to undergo stress imaging or as an alternative to invasive coronary angiography when functional testing indicates a moderate- to high-risk results and knowledge of angiographic coronary anatomy is unknown
IIb	B	CCTA for assessment of patency of CABG or of coronary stents 3 mm or larger in diameter might be reasonable in patients with known SIHD who have new or worsening symptoms not consistent with UA, irrespective of ability to exercise. (Level of Evidence)
IIb	B	CCTA might be reasonable in patients with known SIHD who have new or worsening symptoms not consistent with UA, irrespective of ability to exercise, in the absence of known moderate or severe calcification or if the CCTA is intended to assess coronary stents less than 3 mm in diameter
III	C	Pharmacological stress imaging (nuclear MPI, echocardiography, or CMR) or CCTA is not recommended for risk assessment in patients with SIHD who are able to exercise to an adequate workload and have an interpretable ECG
III	C	A request to perform either (a) more than 1 stress imaging study or (b) a stress imaging study and a CCTA at the same time is not recommended for risk assessment in patients with SIHD
III	B	CCTA should not be performed for assessment of native coronary arteries with known moderate or severe calcification or with coronary stents less than 3 mm in diameter in patients with known SIHD who have new or worsening symptoms not consistent with UA, irrespective of ability to exercise
III	C	Nuclear MPI, echocardiography, or CMR, with either exercise or pharmacological stress or CCTA is not recommended for follow-up assessment in patients with SIHD, if performed more frequently than at (a) 5-year intervals after CABG or (b) 2-year intervals after PCI

Table 4.9 NICE clinical guideline 95: Recent-onset chest pain of suspected cardiac origin: assessment and diagnosis [37]

Section	Recommendation
1.3.4.3	Offer 64-slice (or above) CT coronary angiography if: • clinical assessment indicates typical or atypical angina or • clinical assessment indicates non-anginal chest pain but 12-lead resting ECG has been done and indicates ST-T changes or Q waves.
1.3.5.1	Offer noninvasive functional imaging for myocardial ischemia if 64-slice (or above) CT coronary angiography has shown CAD of uncertain functional significance or is nondiagnostic

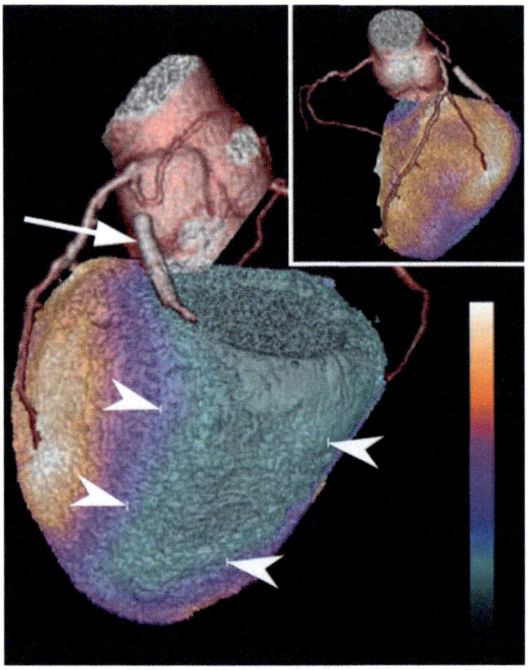

Fig. 4.4 3D volume-rendered fusion image generated from a CCTA and SPECT-MPI at rest. The arrow indicates an occluded stent in the proximal LCX. The arrowheads highlight the associated myocardial scar [38]

fraction and demonstrated viable myocardium by DSE to medical therapy versus medical therapy plus surgical revascularization with CABG [44]. This trial showed that medical therapy was noninferior to medical therapy plus CABG, but it was underpowered due to slow recruitment and loss of funding leading to much lower enrollment than expected. The PARR-2 trial evaluated the efficacy of FDG-PET-assisted management vs standard care without PET imaging in the risk stratification and identification of patients who would benefit from revascularization [45]. This study did not show a difference in the composite endpoint of cardiac death, MI, or cardiac rehospitalization. However, it was limited due to poor adherence to the imaging recommended therapeutic strategy. Despite the disappointing results of the above trials, American and European guidelines still recommend viability testing prior to revascularization with a 2a and 2b class of recommendations, respectively [46, 47].

The role of hybrid imaging in assessing myocardial viability has not yet been established but is intuitively attractive. It is important to note that in clinical practice, providers routinely evaluate coronary artery anatomy using invasive or, less commonly, noninvasive coronary angiography in association with perfusion imaging to plan clinical management. The role of hybrid imaging in this regard is an area of active ongoing research, especially regarding hybrid PET studies. The Alternative Imaging Modalities in Ischemic Heart Failure (AINI-HF) trial is ongoing and seeks to compare advanced cardiac imaging with PET/CT or CMR with standard viability imaging with SPECT.

Once CAD has been ruled out, it is important to assess for other etiologies of heart failure, as this can influence treatment decisions. The 2013 ACCF/AHA Heart Failure Guideline recommends assessing for rheumatologic diseases or amyloidosis if there is appropriate clinical suspicion [46]. The guidelines also note that cardiac sarcoidosis is underdiagnosed, especially in patients without known systemic sarcoidosis.

The Heart Rhythm Society (HRS) released an Expert Consensus Statement on The Diagnosis and Management of Arrhythmias Associated with Cardiac Sarcoidosis in 2014 [48]. This

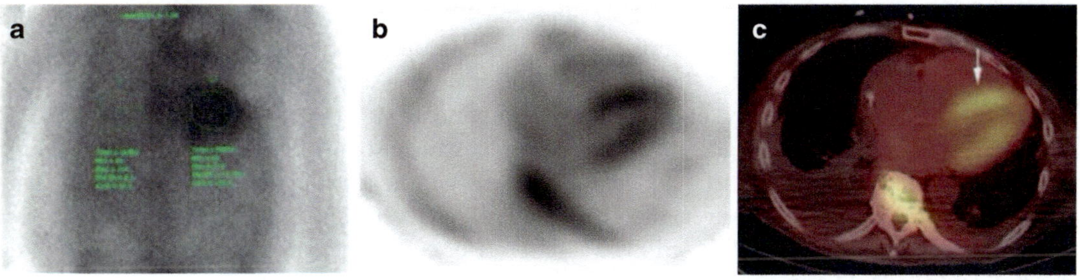

Fig. 4.5 Planar (**a**), axial SPECT (**b**), and axial SPECT/CT (**c**) images of a patient with a positive 99m-Tc-PYP scan suggestive of transthyretin cardiac amyloidosis. There is prominent left ventricular myocardial tracer uptake (arrow) and decreased rib uptake. The heart to contralateral ratio is elevated at 1.56 [41]

guideline recommended screening sarcoidosis patients by history, ECG, and echocardiography for signs of cardiac involvement. It recommended patients that screened positive then undergo advanced imaging such as cardiac magnetic resonance (CMR) or FDG-PET. Recent work by Wicks et al. showed that simultaneous hybrid 18F-FDG PET and CMR was superior to either modality alone [42]. Older guidelines mention the utility of SPECT imaging for cardiac sarcoidosis, particularly resting perfusion abnormalities that do not fit a coronary artery distribution. However, SPECT has largely been replaced by PET in this area due to improved sensitivity and spatial resolution [49].

Cardiac amyloidosis is a clinically underdiagnosed entity of increased interest recently due to the emergence of effective treatments. Patients with light chain amyloidosis may see improvement in survival by a decade or more by receiving appropriate chemotherapy [41, 50]. Patients diagnosed with transthyretin cardiac amyloidosis now have emerging treatment options [51]. Cardiac amyloidosis is thought to be underdiagnosed due to the difficulty of making the diagnosis. Tissue biopsy is invasive and echocardiographic findings have low specificity [41]. However, nuclear methods are emerging due to their ability to both diagnose cardiac amyloidosis and differentiate light chain amyloidosis from transthyretin amyloidosis [52]. Some authors advocate for a multimodality imaging approach to diagnosing cardiac amyloidosis [53, 54]. Given the benefits of multimodality imaging, it is reasonable to expect a role for hybrid imaging to emerge. An example of a positive 99m-Tc-PYP scan with hybrid SPECT/CT images is seen in Fig. 4.5.

4.1.5 Current Guidelines

The 2012 ACCF/AHA/ACP/AATS/PCNA/SCAI/STS Guidelines for the diagnosis and management of patients with stable ischemic heart disease [17] briefly discusses hybrid imaging. While no recommendations are made, the guidelines note that hybrid imaging provides more information than either test alone and may add value as well as guide therapeutic decision-making.

The ACCF/AHA/ASE/ASNC/HFSA/HRS/SCAI/SCCT/SCMR/STS 2013 Multimodality Appropriate Use Criteria for the Detection and Risk Assessment of Stable Ischemic Heart Disease do not provide recommendations or criteria for hybrid imaging [55]. However, Sect. 4.2 of this document provides criteria regarding sequential testing, which is relevant to hybrid imaging. The following sequences of tests are recognized as appropriate within 90 days of each other: CCTA following abnormal MPI, Stress MPI, stress echocardiography, or stress CMR following CCTA showing obstructive CAD, and stress MPI or stress echocardiography following CAC with a score greater than 100. In sequential testing more than 90 days apart, the appropriateness depends on the presence and stability of symptoms. In patients with new or worsening symptoms, the criteria are the same as above. In asymptomatic or stable patients, no further testing is recognized as appropriate.

The 2013 European Society of Cardiology (ESC) Guidelines on the management of stable CAD do not make a specific recommendation regarding hybrid imaging. However, they make the following statement: "Hybrid SPECT/CT, PET/CT and PET/CMR imaging are now available at a few selected centers. Hybrid imaging is a novel technique combining functional and anatomical aspects, which holds much promise for future clinical application. The limited evidence available today indicates a higher diagnostic accuracy, as compared with single techniques. Initial reports also point to the prognostic value of hybrid imaging" [56].

The 2014 ESC/European Association for Cardio-Thoracic Surgery (EACTS) Guidelines on myocardial revascularization recommend hybrid imaging as a class IIa (LOE B) recommendation in symptomatic intermediate risk patients with suspected CAD "Hybrid imaging may be reasonable in symptomatic intermediate risk patients with suspected CAD" [49]. The 2018 ESC/EACTS Guidelines on myocardial revascularization do not mention hybrid imaging [47].

The 2019 ESC Guidelines for the diagnosis and management of chronic coronary syndromes do not comment on or recommend hybrid imaging [36].

4.1.6 Hybrid Imaging: When and Why?

It is generally agreed upon that the answer as to which test, when and why is never an easy one despite the many guidelines. The central theme however remains the same and that is the patient's interest comes first and then local resources and expertise. The options are no test, a single test (plenty to choose from!), and hybrid techniques. The decline in the number of abnormal tests results (especially large ischemia) that mirrors the decline in overall mortality from CAD at least in developed countries puts a high burden for choosing wisely. This has become even more important with recent results from ISCHEMIA trial which soon might influence future guidelines and hence reimbursement concerns, especially in the United States [57].

But certain generalizations might be in order based on current evidence

1. CAC is a useful screening test and hence patients with a low probability of CAD and 0 calcium score might not need further testing (of note in the United States CAC is out of pocket expense to the patients though it is not prohibitively expensive!).
2. Nonimaging treadmill or bicycle exercise could be used in some patients and provide useful data for patient management.
3. Single modality imaging (SPECT, PET, CCTA, Stress echocardiography) might be the backbone for most patients because of convenience, cost, and availability.
4. Serial or sequential hybrid imaging with SPECT/CCTA might be very useful in patients with equivocal test results by a single modality, when the test result disagrees with clinical judgment, or in specific patient scenarios rather than broadly. This cautious recommendation takes into consideration the added cost to the health system if all patients should undergo hybrid imaging that will unlikely be feasible even if recommended because of lack of resources).
5. MBF by PET (but do not discount SPECT) is rapidly gaining momentum in patient care especially if the new F-18 tracer (Flurpiridaz) is approved and may influence the choice of imaging modality and the need for hybrid imaging.
6. It is important to keep in mind that guidelines reflect different sets of expectations. Take for example the ESC guidelines; it is hard to believe that all members of the European Union have a uniform policy, resources, and reimbursement mandates.

4.2 Safety

It is important to consider the safety profile of any test or procedure to be performed on a patient. The main risks associated with SPECT-MPI are the risk of the stressor, either exercise or pharmacologic, and the risk of radiation. The risks of the various CT techniques are related to radiation exposure (least with CAC). There is an additional risk associated with contrast dye in the studies that require CCTA. Table 4.10 examines the radiation doses of the various modalities.

There are numerous ways to reduce radiation doses with SPECT. The stress portion could be performed first (known as stress-first imaging), allowing for the rest portion to be omitted if the stress images are normal (known as stress-only imaging) thereby simplifying the test and reducing the radiation exposure considerably. Due to the advent of better cameras, low dose stress protocols are now in place in many centers, further reducing the radiation dose. Hybrid imaging techniques, such as CCTA followed by stress MPI only if there is an abnormality identified, offer a low radiation method to obtain both anatomic and functional data.

Table 4.10 Radiation doses of various imaging modalities and protocols [1, 6, 58]

Modality/Protocol	Dose 1 (mSv)	Dose 2 (mSv)	Total dose (mSv)
Tc-99m Stress-only	4.0–8.0	N/A	4.0–8.0
Tc-99m Rest/Stress 1 day	1.2–2.3	4.0–8.0	5.2–10.3
Tc-99m Stress/Rest 1 day	4.0–8.0	1.2–2.3	6.3–10.3
Tl-201 Rest/redistribution (viability)	10.3–20.7	N/A	10.3–20.7
Coronary CT Angiography (CCTA)	12.0	N/A	12.0
Coronary Artery Calcium (CAC) Scoring	3.0		3.0
CT Attenuation Correction (CT-AC)	0.1–1.0	N/A	0.1–1.0

4.2.1 Incidental Findings

An incidental finding may be defined as any abnormality that is not related to the illness that prompted the use of diagnostic imaging test [51]. As the imaging field of view of the cardiovascular CT usually includes portions of the lungs, pleura, mediastinum, chest wall, bones, upper abdomen, and thoracic aorta, incidental findings are possible. Common extracardiac findings discovered by cardiac CT include pulmonary nodules, emphysema, bronchiectasis, pleural effusion, diaphragmatic hernia, liver nodule or cyst, liver steatosis, aortic dilatation, adenopathy, and many others [52]. The prevalence of non-cardiac incidental findings ranges from 8 to 69% depending on the type of CT protocol used and the age of the population imaged [53] (Fig. 4.6).

Hybrid imaging may lead to increased incidental findings when compared to a single imaging modality, due to more information being obtained. Incidental findings seen on cardiac CT scans were first discussed in the literature by Hunold et al. in 2001 [54]. They examined 1812 consecutive patients who were evaluated for CAC by electron beam CT scanning. All scans were assessed for non-coronary findings using a tissue window. 52% of the patients were found to have extra-coronary findings. Of these, 71% were cardiac in nature, including aortic disease though 90% of the aortic diseases was only in various

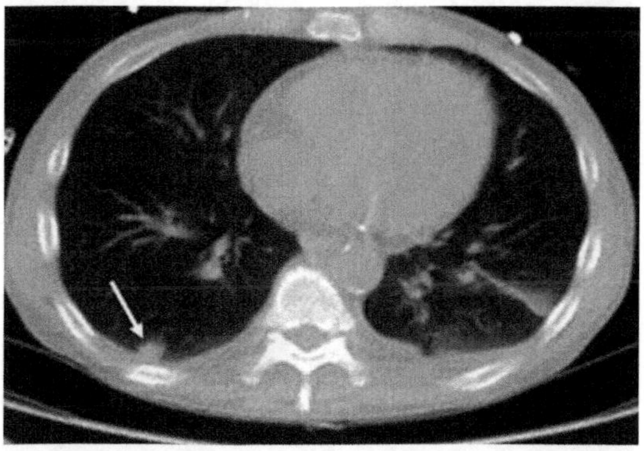

Fig. 4.6 This is a CT performed for attenuation correction in a man undergoing MPI. A 1.3 cm lung nodule was identified in the right lower lobe. Biopsy revealed squamous cell carcinoma [59]

stage of calcification. However, there were 41 patients with aortic ectasia, 11 with aortic aneurysms, and 3 patients were found to have carcinoma (two bronchial, one esophageal).

Following this, Goetze et al. reported on the abnormal findings detected on low dose, low resolution CT used for attenuation correction of SPECT studies [17]. They retrospectively examined 200 patients and found a total of 234 abnormalities in 119 of the patients. Twenty five of these were considered major findings, and included coronary calcification, dilated ascending aorta, pericardial effusion, lung nodules, infiltrates, masses, breast calcification, and a probable pericardial cyst. Only 16 of the 25 findings were previously known.

Incidental extracardiac findings are also seen with SPECT imaging [60]. While many are benign, these can have clinical importance [61]. Tc-99m sestamibi, which is commonly used for MPI, was also used to image a number of tumors including breast cancer, lung cancer, hepatocellular carcinoma, thyroid cancer, lymphoma, thymoma, parathyroid tumors, and sarcoma [62–66]. Incidental cardiac findings have also been reported, including pericardial effusion and dextrocardia [60, 67]. An example of an important tumor-related extra cardiac finding is seen in Fig. 4.7.

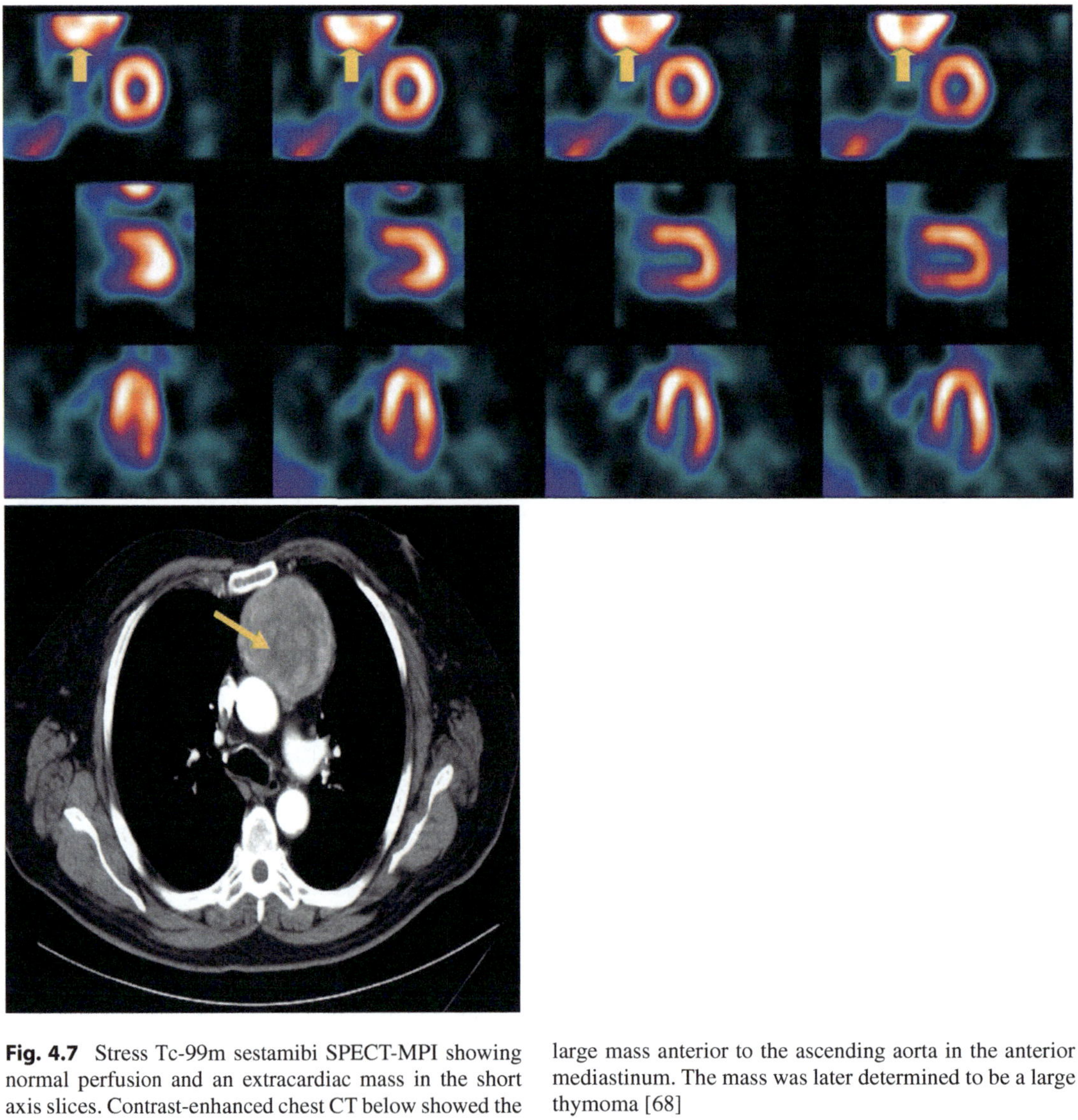

Fig. 4.7 Stress Tc-99m sestamibi SPECT-MPI showing normal perfusion and an extracardiac mass in the short axis slices. Contrast-enhanced chest CT below showed the large mass anterior to the ascending aorta in the anterior mediastinum. The mass was later determined to be a large thymoma [68]

The 2010 ACCF/ACR/AHA/NASCI/SAIP/SCAI/SCCT consensus statement on CCTA states that incidental findings may be divided into two categories. First, there are benign findings that do not require any additional imaging or follow-up. The second category is clinically significant findings that are potentially important and require further investigation. This category can be further divided into indeterminant or potentially significant findings that require additional testing and major findings requiring prompt evaluation and management. Using this classification, up to 25% of additional findings are reported to be potentially significant and up to 11% are reported to be major findings [69].

The discovery of incidental findings often leads to additional testing, even when the findings are likely benign. These tests are expensive and often expose the patient to additional radiation [56]. This testing is driven by the desire to differentiate benign findings from serious findings and may be precipitated by the fear of litigation and/or blame for missing important pathology. Additional imaging is often the next step in the evaluation of an incidental finding. Primary care office visits, subspecialist referrals, diagnostic and therapeutic procedures, and hospitalizations are also common [57]. These interventions are costly to the patient and society.

It is important to note that the entirety of the thorax is rarely imaged in cardiac CT. The superior and inferior borders of the heart serve as landmarks for the image [60]. Due to the small field of few, the lung apices and possibly the lung bases are excluded, leaving only ~10% of the lung tissue to be visualized [61]. Additionally, the number of slices in the z-axis is often reduced in order to limit radiation exposure.

There are numerous practice models in the United States established to deal with incidental findings. Certainly, many locations have either cardiology or radiology read all cardiac scans and have protocols regarding follow-up for incidental findings. Some practices have a cooperative relationship between radiology and cardiology, and the cardiologists read the cardiac portion of the examinations and the radiologists "overread" to assess for missed incidental findings. It is imperative that both cardiology and radiology trainees are taught to systematically assess all images in order to identify and diagnose incidental findings, although this is not currently routine in many training programs. The practice is likely entirely different out the United States, but the basic principles hold true that the reader should account and report incidental findings

Generally, it is the responsibility of the ordering provider to inform the patient of the results of a test. This includes unexpected or incidental results. Many institutions have policies in place that ensure high-risk findings be discussed between the reader and the ordering provider. Our preference is that major unexpected findings that require urgent attention be conveyed verbally rather than solely in the written report.

4.3 Pitfalls

There are drawbacks to hybrid cardiac imaging, in addition to the advantages listed above. These include increased cost, the potential for increased radiation exposure, and the requirement for more complex software and hardware to obtain the data. There are also additional opportunities for artifacts to arise, such as misregistration. One example of this is motion-related misregistration of SPECT and CT, where activity over the lungs is assigned a lower attenuation score and then is interpreted as a perfusion defect. If not detected, this leads to a false-positive result. However, we believe the overall advantages of hybrid cardiac imaging outweigh the pitfalls in selected patients.

4.4 Training the Next Generation of Imagers

Rapid advances in the technology and application of echocardiography, nuclear cardiology, CT, and cardiac magnetic resonance have led to new challenges in training new cardiovascular imaging specialists and in maintaining the competence of imagers in practice in the United States. This has led to considerable debate about the future of cardiovascular imaging training. One has to understand that most SPECT studies in the United States are performed and interpreted by cardiologists while most CCTA are performed and interpreted by radiologists. In Europe, this varies considerably from one country to another. The interpretation of hybrid imaging may involve a new paradigm of training and licensing, at least in the United States.

First, the chief limitation in training the imagers of the future is the finite amount of time available for training. The standard cardiology fellowship is 36 months long, and during this time trainees must acquire the knowledge and skills necessary to practice cardiology in the modern area. While it is possible for cardiologists in academic medical centers to become hyperspecialized with mastery of select areas, this is not possible in many practice settings. Many smaller practices will require well-rounded cardiologists with competence across the spectrum of cardiology. The current model is that the development of expertise within individual imaging modalities is obtained independently [70]. This means the time required to obtain expertise in each modality exceeds what is available in general cardiology fellowship and will likely require additional imaging fellowships.

4.5 Conclusion

It is an exciting time in the realm of cardiac imaging. New techniques and new applications of older techniques are constantly emerging. Identifying the best use of each modality and how they can be used together to maximize knowledge gained while minimizing cost is an important challenge for both clinicians and researchers.

References

1. Henzlova MJ, Duvall WL, Einstein AJ, Travin MI, Verberne HJ. ASNC imaging guidelines for SPECT nuclear cardiology procedures: stress, protocols, and tracers. J Nucl Cardiol. 2016;23(3):606–39.
2. Iskandrian A, Garcia E. Nuclear cardiac imaging. Principles and applications. 5th ed. Oxford: Oxford University Press; 2016.
3. Hage F. Myocardial perfusion imaging (MPI): performance, potential risks and outcomes. Hauppauge: Nova Science Publishers; 2018.
4. Garcia EV. SPECT attenuation correction: an essential tool to realize nuclear cardiology's manifest destiny. J Nucl Cardiol. 2007;14(1):16–24.
5. Iskandrian AE, Dilsizian V, Garcia EV, Beanlands RS, Cerqueira M, Soman P, et al. Myocardial perfusion imaging: lessons learned and work to be done-update. J Nucl Cardiol. 2018;25(1):39–52.
6. Dorbala S, Di Carli MF, Delbeke D, Abbara S, DePuey EG, Dilsizian V, et al. SNMMI/ASNC/SCCT guideline for cardiac SPECT/CT and PET/CT 1.0. J Nucl Med. 2013;54(8):1485–507.
7. Harrington R, Walsh R, Fuster V. Hurst's the heart. 14th ed. McGraw-Hill Education: New York; 2017.
8. Rozanski A, Gransar H, Hayes SW, Min J, Friedman JD, Thomson LE, et al. Temporal trends in the frequency of inducible myocardial ischemia during cardiac stress testing: 1991 to 2009. J Am Coll Cardiol. 2013;61(10):1054–65.
9. Iskandrian AE, Hage FG. Declining frequency of ischemia detection using stress myocardial perfusion imaging. J Am Coll Cardiol. 2013;61(10):1066–8.
10. Berman DS, Wong ND, Gransar H, Miranda-Peats R, Dahlbeck J, Hayes SW, et al. Relationship between stress-induced myocardial ischemia and atherosclerosis measured by coronary calcium tomography. J Am Coll Cardiol. 2004;44(4):923–30.
11. Berman DS, Rozanski A. Value-based imaging: combining coronary artery calcium with myocardial perfusion imaging. J Nucl Cardiol. 2016;23(5):939–41.
12. Engbers EM, Timmer JR, Ottervanger JP, Mouden M, Knollema S, Jager PL. Prognostic value of coronary artery calcium scoring in addition to single-photon emission computed tomographic myocardial perfusion imaging in symptomatic patients. Circ Cardiovasc Imaging. 2016;9(5):e003966.
13. Budoff MJ, Diamond GA, Raggi P, Arad Y, Guerci AD, Callister TQ, et al. Continuous probabilistic prediction of angiographically significant coronary artery disease using electron beam tomography. Circulation. 2002;105(15):1791–6.
14. Akincioglu C, Belhocine T, Gambhir S, Romsa J, Chouraiki G, Kribs S, et al. Complementary roles of low-dose SPECT-CT and high-resolution volume CT for detection of coronary artery disease. Clin Nucl Med. 2008;33(4):285–7.
15. Arnett DK, Blumenthal RS, Albert MA, Buroker AB, Goldberger ZD, Hahn EJ, et al. 2019 ACC/AHA guideline on the primary prevention of cardiovascular disease: a report of the American College of Cardiology/American Heart Association task force on clinical practice guidelines. Circulation. 2019;140(11):e596–646.
16. Grundy SM, Stone NJ, Bailey AL, Beam C, Birtcher KK, Blumenthal RS, et al. 2018 AHA/ACC/AACVPR/AAPA/ABC/ACPM/ADA/AGS/APhA/ASPC/NLA/PCNA guideline on the management of blood cholesterol: a report of the American College of Cardiology/American Heart Association task

force on clinical practice guidelines. Circulation. 2019;139(25):e1082–e143.
17. Fihn SD, Gardin JM, Abrams J, Berra K, Blankenship JC, Dallas AP, et al. 2012 ACCF/AHA/ACP/AATS/PCNA/SCAI/STS guideline for the diagnosis and management of patients with stable ischemic heart disease: a report of the American College of Cardiology Foundation/American Heart Association Task Force on Practice Guidelines, and the American College of Physicians, American Association for Thoracic Surgery, Preventive Cardiovascular Nurses Association, Society for Cardiovascular Angiography and Interventions, and Society of Thoracic Surgeons. J Am Coll Cardiol. 2012;60(24):e44–e164.
18. Taylor AJ, Cerqueira M, Hodgson JM, Mark D, Min J, O'Gara P, et al. ACCF/SCCT/ACR/AHA/ASE/ASNC/NASCI/SCAI/SCMR 2010 appropriate use criteria for cardiac computed tomography. A report of the American College of Cardiology Foundation Appropriate Use Criteria Task Force, the Society of Cardiovascular Computed Tomography, the American College of Radiology, the American Heart Association, the American Society of Echocardiography, the American Society of Nuclear Cardiology, the North American Society for Cardiovascular Imaging, the Society for Cardiovascular Angiography and Interventions, and the Society for Cardiovascular Magnetic Resonance. J Am Coll Cardiol. 2010;56(22):1864–94.
19. Wells RG, Marvin B, Poirier M, Renaud J, deKemp RA, Ruddy TD. Optimization of SPECT measurement of myocardial blood flow with corrections for attenuation, motion, and blood binding compared with PET. J Nucl Med. 2017;58(12):2013–9.
20. Wells RG, Timmins R, Klein R, Lockwood J, Marvin B, deKemp RA, et al. Dynamic SPECT measurement of absolute myocardial blood flow in a porcine model. J Nucl Med. 2014;55(10):1685–91.
21. Nudi F, Biondi-Zoccai G, Romagnoli A, Schillaci O, Nudi A, Versaci F. Hybrid anatomo-functional imaging of coronary artery disease: beneficial irrespective of its core components. J Nucl Cardiol. 2019;26(3):752–62.
22. Jameria ZA, Abdallah M, Fernandez-Ulloa M, O'Donnell R, Dwivedi AK, Washburn E, et al. Analysis of stress-only imaging, comparing upright and supine CZT camera acquisition to conventional gamma camera images with and without attenuation correction, with coronary angiography as a reference. J Nucl Cardiol. 2018;25(2):540–9.
23. Slomka PJ, Cheng VY, Dey D, Woo J, Ramesh A, Van Kriekinge S, et al. Quantitative analysis of myocardial perfusion SPECT anatomically guided by coregistered 64-slice coronary CT angiography. J Nucl Med. 2009;50(10):1621–30.
24. Gaemperli O, Schepis T, Valenta I, Husmann L, Scheffel H, Duerst V, et al. Cardiac image fusion from stand-alone SPECT and CT: clinical experience. J Nucl Med. 2007;48(5):696–703.
25. Santana CA, Garcia EV, Faber TL, Sirineni GK, Esteves FP, Sanyal R, et al. Diagnostic performance of fusion of myocardial perfusion imaging (MPI) and computed tomography coronary angiography. J Nucl Cardiol. 2009;16(2):201–11.
26. Rispler S, Keidar Z, Ghersin E, Roguin A, Soil A, Dragu R, et al. Integrated single-photon emission computed tomography and computed tomography coronary angiography for the assessment of hemodynamically significant coronary artery lesions. J Am Coll Cardiol. 2007;49(10):1059–67.
27. Schaap J, Kauling RM, Boekholdt SM, Nieman K, Meijboom WB, Post MC, et al. Incremental diagnostic accuracy of hybrid SPECT/CT coronary angiography in a population with an intermediate to high pre-test likelihood of coronary artery disease. Eur Heart J Cardiovasc Imaging. 2013;14(7):642–9.
28. Schaap J, de Groot JA, Nieman K, Meijboom WB, Boekholdt SM, Kauling RM, et al. Added value of hybrid myocardial perfusion SPECT and CT coronary angiography in the diagnosis of coronary artery disease. Eur Heart J Cardiovasc Imaging. 2014;15(11):1281–8.
29. Liga R, Vontobel J, Rovai D, Marinelli M, Caselli C, Pietila M, et al. Multicentre multi-device hybrid imaging study of coronary artery disease: results from the EValuation of INtegrated Cardiac Imaging for the Detection and Characterization of Ischaemic Heart Disease (EVINCI) hybrid imaging population. Eur Heart J Cardiovasc Imaging. 2016;17(9):951–60.
30. Di Carli MF, Dorbala S, Curillova Z, Kwong RJ, Goldhaber SZ, Rybicki FJ, et al. Relationship between CT coronary angiography and stress perfusion imaging in patients with suspected ischemic heart disease assessed by integrated PET-CT imaging. J Nucl Cardiol. 2007;14(6):799–809.
31. Giubbini R, Bertoli M, Durmo R, Bonacina M, Peli A, Faggiano I, et al. Comparison between the summed difference score and myocardial blood flow measured by 13N-ammonia. J Nucl Cardiol. 2018;25(5):1621–8.
32. Marchesseau S, Seneviratna A, Sjöholm AT, Qin DL, Ho JXM, Hausenloy DJ, et al. Hybrid PET/CT and PET/MRI imaging of vulnerable coronary plaque and myocardial scar tissue in acute myocardial infarction. J Nucl Cardiol. 2018;25(6):2001–11.
33. Ito Y, Katoh C, Noriyasu K, Kuge Y, Furuyama H, Morita K, et al. Estimation of myocardial blood flow and myocardial flow reserve by 99mTc-sestamibi imaging: comparison with the results of [15O]H2O PET. Eur J Nucl Med Mol Imaging. 2003;30(2):281–7.
34. Slomka PJ, Patton JA, Berman DS, Germano G. Advances in technical aspects of myocardial perfusion SPECT imaging. J Nucl Cardiol. 2009;16(2):255–76.
35. Bocher M, Blevis IM, Tsukerman L, Shrem Y, Kovalski G, Volokh L. A fast cardiac gamma camera with dynamic SPECT capabilities: design, system validation and future potential. Eur J Nucl Med Mol Imaging. 2010;37(10):1887–902.

36. Knuuti J, Wijns W, Saraste A, Capodanno D, Barbato E, Funck-Brentano C, et al. 2019 ESC guidelines for the diagnosis and management of chronic coronary syndromes. Eur Heart J. 2020;41(3):407–77.
37. (UK) NCGCfAaCC. Chest pain of recent onset: assessment and diagnosis of recent onset chest pain or discomfort of suspected cardiac origin. 2010.
38. Gaemperli O, Kaufmann PA. Hybrid cardiac imaging: more than the sum of its parts? J Nucl Cardiol. 2008;15(1):123–6.
39. Joshi NV, Vesey AT, Williams MC, Shah AS, Calvert PA, Craighead FH, et al. 18F-fluoride positron emission tomography for identification of ruptured and high-risk coronary atherosclerotic plaques: a prospective clinical trial. Lancet. 2014;383(9918):705–13.
40. Bing R, Driessen RS, Knaapen P, Dweck MR. The clinical utility of hybrid imaging for the identification of vulnerable plaque and vulnerable patients. J Cardiovasc Comput Tomogr. 2019;13(5):242–7.
41. Andrikopoulou E, Bhambhvani P. Nuclear imaging of cardiac amyloidosis. J Nucl Cardiol. 2019;26(2):505–8.
42. Wicks EC, Menezes LJ, Barnes A, Mohiddin SA, Sekhri N, Porter JC, et al. Diagnostic accuracy and prognostic value of simultaneous hybrid 18F-fluorodeoxyglucose positron emission tomography/magnetic resonance imaging in cardiac sarcoidosis. Eur Heart J Cardiovasc Imaging. 2018;19(7):757–67.
43. Bonow RO, Maurer G, Lee KL, Holly TA, Binkley PF, Desvigne-Nickens P, et al. Myocardial viability and survival in ischemic left ventricular dysfunction. N Engl J Med. 2011;364(17):1617–25.
44. Cleland JG, Calvert M, Freemantle N, Arrow Y, Ball SG, Bonser RS, et al. The HEART failure revascularisation trial (HEART). Eur J Heart Fail. 2011;13(2):227–33.
45. Beanlands RS, Nichol G, Huszti E, Humen D, Racine N, Freeman M, et al. F-18-fluorodeoxyglucose positron emission tomography imaging-assisted management of patients with severe left ventricular dysfunction and suspected coronary disease: a randomized, controlled trial (PARR-2). J Am Coll Cardiol. 2007;50(20):2002–12.
46. Yancy CW, Jessup M, Bozkurt B, Butler J, Casey DE, Drazner MH, et al. 2013 ACCF/AHA guideline for the management of heart failure: a report of the American College of Cardiology Foundation/American Heart Association task force on practice guidelines. J Am Coll Cardiol. 2013;62(16):e147–239.
47. Neumann FJ, Sousa-Uva M, Ahlsson A, Alfonso F, Banning AP, Benedetto U, et al. 2018 ESC/EACTS Guidelines on myocardial revascularization. Eur Heart J. 2019;40(2):87–165.
48. Birnie DH, Sauer WH, Bogun F, Cooper JM, Culver DA, Duvernoy CS, et al. HRS expert consensus statement on the diagnosis and management of arrhythmias associated with cardiac sarcoidosis. Heart Rhythm. 2014;11(7):1305–23.
49. Hulten E, Aslam S, Osborne M, Abbasi S, Bittencourt MS, Blankstein R. Cardiac sarcoidosis-state of the art review. Cardiovasc Diagn Ther. 2016;6(1):50–63.
50. Madan S, Kumar SK, Dispenzieri A, Lacy MQ, Hayman SR, Buadi FK, et al. High-dose melphalan and peripheral blood stem cell transplantation for light-chain amyloidosis with cardiac involvement. Blood. 2012;119(5):1117–22.
51. Maurer MS, Schwartz JH, Gundapaneni B, Elliott PM, Merlini G, Waddington-Cruz M, et al. Tafamidis treatment for patients with transthyretin amyloid cardiomyopathy. N Engl J Med. 2018;379(11):1007–16.
52. Bokhari S, Castaño A, Pozniakoff T, Deslisle S, Latif F, Maurer MS. (99m)Tc-pyrophosphate scintigraphy for differentiating light-chain cardiac amyloidosis from the transthyretin-related familial and senile cardiac amyloidoses. Circ Cardiovasc Imaging. 2013;6(2):195–201.
53. Dorbala S, Cuddy S, Falk RH. How to image cardiac amyloidosis: a practical approach. JACC Cardiovasc Imaging. 2020;13(6):1368–83.
54. Alexanderson-Rosas E, Escudero-Salamanca M, Garcia-Diaz JA, Alvarez-Santana R, Cano-Zarate R, Mamani-Tito J, et al. Light-chain cardiac amyloidosis: a multimodality approach. J Nucl Cardiol. 2020;27(6):2432–5.
55. Wolk MJ, Bailey SR, Doherty JU, Douglas PS, Hendel RC, Kramer CM, et al. ACCF/AHA/ASE/ASNC/HFSA/HRS/SCAI/SCCT/SCMR/STS 2013 multimodality appropriate use criteria for the detection and risk assessment of stable ischemic heart disease: a report of the American College of Cardiology Foundation Appropriate Use Criteria Task Force, American Heart Association, American Society of Echocardiography, American Society of Nuclear Cardiology, Heart Failure Society of America, Heart Rhythm Society, Society for Cardiovascular Angiography and Interventions, Society of Cardiovascular Computed Tomography, Society for Cardiovascular Magnetic Resonance, and Society of Thoracic Surgeons. J Am Coll Cardiol. 2014;63(4):380–406.
56. Montalescot G, Sechtem U, Achenbach S, Andreotti F, Arden C, Budaj A, et al. 2013 ESC guidelines on the management of stable coronary artery disease: the task force on the management of stable coronary artery disease of the European Society of Cardiology. Eur Heart J. 2013;34(38):2949–3003.
57. Maron DJ, Hochman JS, Reynolds HR, Bangalore S, O'Brien SM, Boden WE, et al. Initial invasive or conservative strategy for stable coronary disease. N Engl J Med. 2020;382(15):1395–407.
58. Radiation dose in X-ray and CT exams; 2020. https://www.radiologyinfo.org/en/info.cfm?pg=safety-xray: radiologyinfo.org.
59. He BJ, Malm BJ, Carino M, Sadeghi MM. Prevalence and variability in reporting of clinically actionable incidental findings on attenuation-correction CT scans in a veteran population. J Nucl Cardiol. 2019;26(5):1688–93.

60. Muzaffar R, Raslan O, Ahmed F, Goldfarb L, Sterkel B, Osman MM. Incidental findings on myocardial perfusion SPECT images. J Nucl Med Technol. 2017;45(3):175–80.
61. Chatziioannou SN, Alfaro-Franco C, Moore WH, Alanis-Williams L, Dhekne RD, Ford PV. The significance of incidental noncardiac findings in Tc-99m sestamibi myocardial perfusion imaging: illustrated by a case. Tex Heart Inst J. 1999;26(3):229–31.
62. Bhambhvani P, Dubovsky E, Heo J, Iskandrian A. Incidental detection of hepatocellular carcinoma by SPECT myocardial perfusion imaging. J Nucl Cardiol. 2010;17(6):1116–7.
63. Waxman AD. The role of (99m)Tc methoxyisobutylisonitrile in imaging breast cancer. Semin Nucl Med. 1997;27(1):40–54.
64. Nishiyama Y, Kawasaki Y, Yamamoto Y, Fukunaga K, Satoh K, Takashima H, et al. Technetium-99m-MIBI and thallium-201 scintigraphy of primary lung cancer. J Nucl Med. 1997;38(9):1358–61.
65. Derebek E. Technetium-99m sestamibi uptake in hepatocellular carcinoma. Eur J Nucl Med. 1998;25(11):1587–8.
66. Williams KA, Hill KA, Sheridan CM. Noncardiac findings on dual-isotope myocardial perfusion SPECT. J Nucl Cardiol. 2003;10(4):395–402.
67. Bernasconi A, Azancot A, Simpson JM, Jones A, Sharland GK. Fetal dextrocardia: diagnosis and outcome in two tertiary centres. Heart. 2005;91(12):1590–4.
68. Farag AA, Hage FG. Incidentally found giant thymomas by SPECT myocardial perfusion imaging. J Nucl Cardiol. 2015;22(2):385–7.
69. Mark DB, Berman DS, Budoff MJ, Carr JJ, Gerber TC, Hecht HS, et al. ACCF/ACR/AHA/NASCI/SAIP/SCAI/SCCT 2010 expert consensus document on coronary computed tomographic angiography: a report of the American College of Cardiology Foundation task force on expert consensus documents. J Am Coll Cardiol. 2010;55(23):2663–99.
70. Marwick TH, Chandrashekhar Y, Narula J. Training in multimodality CV imaging: is there an inclusive model? JACC Cardiovasc Imaging. 2016;9(10):1235–7.

Hybrid Cardiac Imaging for the Specialist with Expertise in Computed Tomography

5

Jochen von Spiczak, Robert Manka, and Hatem Alkadhi

5.1 Introduction

In recent decades, cardiac CT has been established as an important noninvasive imaging modality in the diagnostic workup of patients with cardiovascular disease. Different pathologies can be assessed—including acute aortic syndrome, valvular heart disease, endocarditis, hypertrophic cardiomyopathy, pericardial disease, and congenital heart disease [1]. Since coronary artery disease (CAD) is the most important cardiovascular disease in terms of prevalence and mortality [2], this chapter will mainly concentrate on cardiac CT being used for the evaluation of CAD. In the context of CAD, recent guidelines [3] differentiate between acute (acute coronary syndrome, ACS) and chronic manifestation of the disease (chronic coronary syndrome, CCS). In the emergency setting of ACS, a timely diagnosis is of utmost importance to not prolong the time for interventional or surgical revascularization. For patients presenting with acute chest pain and low to intermediate clinical likelihood of ACS, cardiac CT might be used as a single modality test to rule out clinically significant CAD [4–6]. In CCS highest diagnostic accuracy is desirable to identify patients with coronary lesions that are likely to benefit from revascularization. In these patients, a multimodal multiparametric approach including cardiac CT might be favorable.

Noninvasive cardiac CT can assess different pathologic aspects of CAD. By use of native low-dose CT images of the heart, risk stratification is possible by means of coronary calcium scoring. Due to its high spatial resolution, coronary CT angiography (CTA) is well suited for the accurate anatomical depiction of coronary arteries and possible lumen narrowing. To also evaluate the hemodynamic relevance of such coronary stenoses, computing the fractional flow reserve (FFR) from CT images has been proposed. If CT images are acquired over multiple phases, the left ventricle (LV) can be segmented to evaluate the functional parameters of the heart (CT volumetry). For functional diagnostics of myocardial ischemia, dynamic stress CT perfusion can be applied. Ten to 15 min after contrast injection, CT late enhancement images can be acquired to assess myocardial fibrosis or scar. All aforementioned imaging parameters can be carried out within one single examination on the same CT scanner—therefore, we use the term "multiparametric" imaging.

J. von Spiczak (✉) · R. Manka
Institute for Diagnostic and Interventional Radiology, University Hospital Zurich, Zurich, Switzerland

Institute for Biomedical Engineering, University and ETH Zurich, Zurich, Switzerland
e-mail: jochen.vonspiczak@usz.ch; robert.manka@usz.ch

H. Alkadhi
Institute for Diagnostic and Interventional Radiology, University Hospital Zurich, Zurich, Switzerland
e-mail: hatem.alkadhi@usz.ch

F. Nudi et al. (eds.), *Hybrid Cardiac Imaging for Clinical Decision-Making*, https://doi.org/10.1007/978-3-030-99391-7_5

Cardiac CT not only provides different imaging parameters but is also the most widely used basis for being combined with a second independent and complementary imaging modality, which is called "multimodal" or "hybrid" imaging.[1] While coronary CTA provides detailed information on the anatomy and stenoses or occlusions of the coronary arteries, other modalities depict resulting myocardial ischemia (e.g., cardiac MRI stress perfusion, single-photon emission CT, SPECT, or positron emission tomography, PET) or myocardial scar (e.g., cardiac MRI late gadolinium enhancement, LGE).

5.1.1 Guidelines

In patients in whom CAD cannot be excluded by clinical assessment alone, noninvasive diagnostic tests are recommended (class of recommendation[2] I, level of evidence[3] B) [3]. Testing can be done either by functional testing (e.g., stress echocardiography, cardiac MRI, SPECT, or PET) or anatomical imaging of the coronary arteries by coronary CTA [3].

5.1.1.1 Applicability of Cardiac CT—Multiparametric Imaging

Before selecting cardiac CT as a noninvasive diagnostic test, clinical likelihood of the disease in the individual patient should be considered (class I, level C) [3]. The clinical likelihood—also called "pre-test probability"—can be estimated by clinical parameters including age, sex, and the nature of symptoms (e.g., typical/atypical chest pain, non-anginal symptoms, or dyspnea) [7]. The clinical pre-test probability is further modified by the presence of cardiovascular risk factors (dyslipidemia, diabetes, hypertension, smoking, and family history of CAD), resting or exercise electrocardiogram (ECG) changes, and LV dysfunction [3]. Compared to other noninvasive tests for the diagnostic workup of CAD, cardiac CT is particularly suitable for patients without known CAD and with low to intermediate pre-test probability of the disease [3, 8, 9]. Other preconditions for the application of cardiac CT are patient characteristics probably leading to high image quality, desirable information on atherosclerosis, local expertise, and availability of the modality [3, 8].

5.1.1.2 Applicability of Cardiac CT—Multimodal Imaging

According to current guidelines, multimodal imaging including more than one noninvasive imaging test is feasible for the comprehensive diagnostic workup of CCS [3, 8, 10]. Sequential imaging should be performed within 90 days of an abnormal or uncertain result in the first imaging test [10]. In particular, the combination of coronary CTA and one functional test is recommended if:

- results of coronary CTA are positive [10] or of uncertain functional significance [3],
- results of the initial noninvasive functional test are equivocal or nondiagnostic [3, 10].

5.1.2 Technical Considerations

What is special about cardiac CT in comparison to CT imaging of other organs? First, the heart is continuously moving due to the constant heartbeat. Within each heart cycle, the coronary arteries are in a relatively steady position for a very limited period of time only. This phase differs intra- and inter-individually and changes depend-

---

[1]The term "hybrid" imaging specifically describes the acquisition of images of the same body region with two different modalities at the same time and usually on the same scanner (e.g., CT/single-photon emission CT or CT/positron emission tomography). The word "multimodal" imaging is used in a broader sense and refers to different imaging modalities possibly acquired in independent examinations, still assessing complementary diagnostic information of the same pathology (e.g., CT coronary angiography and cardiac MRI stress perfusion).

[2]Class of recommendation: I, is recommended or is indicated, IIa/b, should/may be considered, and III, is not recommended.

[3]Level of evidence: A, data derived from multiple randomized clinical trials or meta-analyses, B, data derived from a single randomized clinical trial or large non-randomized studies, and C, consensus of opinion of the experts and/or small studies, retrospective studies, registries.

ing on the heart rate [11]. Second, the coronary arteries have a relatively small size of approximately 3 mm down to 1–1.5 mm in their distal segments. Therefore, the technical prerequisites for a successful cardiac CT examination include synchronization of data acquisition with the heart cycle by ECG triggering as well as a high temporal and high spatial resolution. State-of-the-art CT scanners are capable of temporal and spatial resolutions of below 100 ms and 0.3 mm, respectively [12].

5.1.2.1 Cardiac CT Acquisition Modes

Three different acquisition modes of cardiac CT have evolved over time [13]. They are differing in terms of ECG synchronization, heart cycle coverage, and level of radiation exposure [12, 14]:

1. In *spiral mode*, data is continuously acquired by a spiral scan with continuous, slow table movement during the entire heart cycle. After acquiring the raw data, heart phases can be selected for image reconstruction by using retrospective ECG gating. While spiral acquisitions provide data from all heart phases, the level of radiation is relatively high when the tube current is kept at its maximum during the entire heart cycle (approximately 10–20 mSv). To decrease the level of radiation, an ECG-based modulation of the tube current can be applied (so-called ECG pulsing, decreasing the tube current to 20% of the maximum current during most heart phases, resulting in approximately 5–10 mSv total radiation). This technique still allows to reconstruct images from all heart phases; however, phases acquired with reduced tube current exhibit higher image noise. While retrospectively ECG gated acquisition with ECG pulsing enables sufficient image quality in the case of high (>70/min) or irregular heartbeats, retrospective ECG triggering without tube current modulation is no longer used today.
2. In *sequential* or *step-and-shoot mode*, prospective ECG triggering is applied. Data acquisition (and associated X-ray radiation) is performed without table movement during predefined phases of the heart cycle only. Afterward, the table is moved along the z-axis to the next position and data acquisition is repeated during the same time points within the heart cycle. While this technique does not allow to reconstruct images from all heart phases, prospective ECG triggering yields lower levels of radiation (approximately 1–3 mSv). Due to the sequential nature of this acquisition mode, misalignment artifacts (also known as "stair-step artifacts") could arise [12].
3. *Flash* or *high-pitch-mode* is a special variant of prospective ECG gating that is available in modern dual-source CT scanners. The second tube detector subsystem is used to fill gaps in the projection data that arise when deploying a high pitch (>2) in single source CTs. Due to larger detector widths and high rotation speeds, such modern multidetector CTs are capable of imaging the entire heart within one diastolic resting period (approximately 0.25 s). Preconditions for high-pitch acquisition are a relatively low (<65/min) and very regular heartbeat. High-pitch coronary CTA using optimized protocols can reach very low levels of radiation (<0.5 mSv) [15].

5.2 Cardiac CT: Multiparametric Imaging

Within one single examination, multiple imaging parameters can be acquired on the same CT scanner. All these parameters cover different aspects of CAD as summarized in Table 5.1 and separately described in the following.

5.2.1 CT Calcium Scoring

CT calcium scoring is used to quantify the amount of calcification of the coronary vessels, which was found to be a valuable prognostic marker for cardiovascular outcome [16, 17]. Especially in asymptomatic patients, CT calcium scoring can be also used for planning primary prevention interventions such as statins and aspi-

Table 5.1 Imaging parameters assessing various pathologic aspects of chronic coronary syndrome in cardiac CT

Imaging parameter	Image acquisition	Pathologic aspect
CT calcium scoring	Native low-dose CT image	Risk stratification of patients with CCS, assessing the individual coronary calcium burden relative to a gender- and age-adjusted reference value
Coronary CTA	Contrast-enhanced ECG gated high spatial resolution CT angiography of the coronary arteries	Anatomical depiction of the coronary arteries as well as possible anomalies, lumen narrowing, or occlusion
CT-derived FFR	Post-processing of coronary CTA images based on computational fluid dynamics or machine learning	Hemodynamic relevance of coronary lesions
CT volumetry	Post-processing of coronary CTA images (only applicable if retrospective ECG gating is used)	Functional parameters of the LV including EDV, ESV, and LVEF
Dynamic stress CT perfusion	Contrast-enhanced myocardial first-pass perfusion under medical stress conditions (e.g., triggered by adenosine)	Myocardial hypoperfusion resulting from relevant coronary lesions
CT late enhancement	Contrast-enhanced images of the myocardium acquired 10–15 min after contrast injection	Myocardial fibrosis or scar (e.g., due to prior myocardial infarction)

All imaging parameters can be assessed on the same scanner within one single examination.
CCS chronic coronary syndrome, *CTA* CT angiography, *ECG* electrocardiogram, *EDV* end-diastolic volume, *ESV* end-systolic volume, *FFR* fractional flow reserve, *LV* left ventricle, *LVEF* left ventricular ejection fraction

rin [16]. Different scores were proposed for the quantification of coronary calcifications:

For calculating the *Agatston score* [18], the area of calcium plaques (defined by attenuation values >130 Hounsfield units [HU]) is multiplied by a density factor depending on the plaque's maximum HU value (i.e., factor 1–4 for maximum HU values of 130–199, 200–299, 300–399, and ≥400, respectively). The idea of the density factor is that regions with higher CT attenuation contribute more strongly to the resulting score. Even though the Agatston score is not well reproducible due to its susceptibility to moving artifacts and image noise, it is still the most widely used scoring system for coronary calcification.

The *volume score* simply calculates the plaque volume by multiplying the number of voxels with an attenuation >130 HU with the voxel volume (i.e., in-plane resolution × slice thickness). The volume score shows better reproducibility but is prone to partial volume effects.

The *mass score* aims to estimate the true mass of calcium hydroxyapatite in a coronary lesion. Therefore, the plaque volume is multiplied by its average HU value and a calibration factor. The calibration factor depends on the CT scanner as well as the protocol and must therefore be derived from phantom measurements. Due to its complexity, the mass score has not been widely adopted in clinical routine.

More recently, the *calcium density score* [19] was defined as the Agatston score divided by the total plaque area. The result reflects the average Agatston density factor (ranging from 1 to 4, see above). It was found that for subjects with similar calcium volume, the calcium density holds an additional prognostic value. More particularly, higher density scores were found to be associated with lower cardiovascular risk [17, 19].

The coronary calcium burden correlates well with the probability of adverse cardiovascular events (e.g., myocardial infarctions) in the future. For the interpretation of the coronary calcium scores, the score of an individual patient is usually compared to the score of gender- and age-matched asymptomatic comparison group [20–22]. Patients with a calcium score above the

75th percentile have a significantly increased risk of adverse cardiovascular events and may benefit from aggressive lipid reduction therapy [23].

5.2.2 Coronary CT Angiography

Due to its high spatial resolution, coronary CTA using an intravenously administered iodine contrast agent can accurately depict the anatomy of coronary arteries, coronary walls, and pathological lumen narrowing [24].

Image acquisition should be performed in a mid-inspiration position because deep inspiration by the patient is often combined with "pressing" that leads to an intrathoracic pressure rise and subsequently insufficient coronary contrast. Since high intravenous injection rates (4–6 mL/s) are necessary for coronary CTA, a large-lumen cannula (at least 18 G) should be chosen. ECG leads should be attached outside the examination volume to avoid imaging artifacts.

Premedication for coronary CTA includes nitroglycerin and optionally beta blockers. For both drugs contraindications apply (Table 5.2). Nitroglycerin induces a dilatation of the epicardial arteries and is therefore an absolute necessity for diagnostic image quality. Beta blockers can be used in patients with higher and/or irregular heartbeat as well as for CT systems with lower detector width (equal to or below 64 detector lines).

Analysis of coronary CTA should be performed by a trained radiologist. Besides the axially acquired original images, perpendicular and/or curved multiplanar reformations (MPRs) of the coronary vessels are used for interpretation (as illustrated in Figs. 5.1 and 5.2). Besides curved MPRs, also reconstructions perpendicular to the vessel lumen can be used to more precisely estimate and/or measure the percentage of lumen narrowing of coronary lesions. When reporting results from coronary CTA, one should follow applicable naming conventions—in particular regarding the notation of coronary vessels and their branches [25]. To further standardize coronary CTA reporting, the Coronary Artery Disease Reporting and Data System (CAD-RADS) can be used [26], which was found to offer incremental value [27].

Coronary CTA is characterized by a high sensitivity [28] and excellent negative predictive value [29, 30]. Accordingly, a negative result in coronary CTA is correlated with an extremely good prognosis regarding adverse cardiac events [31, 32]. However, specificity of coronary CTA is lower. The latter can be increased by adding comprehensive functional information as is done in a multimodal imaging approach [33].

Table 5.2 Premedication for coronary CTA along with their most important characteristics

Premedication	Nitroglycerin	Beta blocker
Objective	Dilatation of epicardial coronary arteries	Adjustment of a high and/or irregular heartbeat
Administration	• Sublingual spray • 0.8–1.2 mg glycerol trinitrat spray • 4–12 min before the examination (usually given before the calcium scoring)	• Metoprolol 50 mg p.o. (45–60 min before image acquisition) • Metoprolol 2.5–16 mg i.v. (on the CT table directly before image acquisition)
Contraindications	• Severe aortic stenosis • Hypertrophic obstructive cardiomyopathy (HOCM) • Severe hypotension • Use of phosphodiesterase inhibitors (Sildenafil, e.g., Viagra®)	• Decompensated heart failure • Bronchial asthma • Systolic blood pressure < 100 mmHg • Heart rate < 60/min • Use of other drugs causing AV conduction delay

If no contraindications exist, nitroglycerin should always be given before coronary CTA image acquisition, because resulting coronary dilatation is a prerequisite for diagnostic image quality. The use of beta blockers on the other hand is not mandatory. Itst use depends on the individual patient, the CT scanner, and the locally established imaging protocols. Exemplary values are listed, please refer to proper medical instructions before use

AV atrioventricular, *i.v.* intravenously, *p.o.* per os

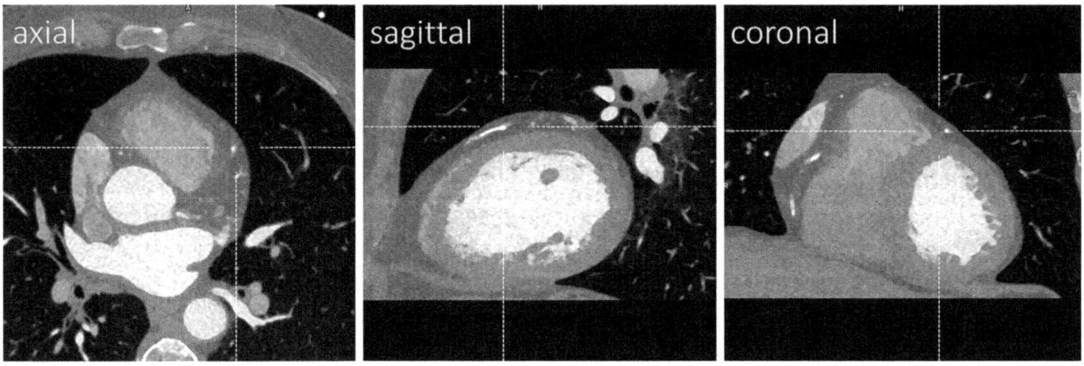

Fig. 5.1 Multiplanar reformations (MPR) of coronary CT angiography. Images of a 59-year-old male patient with severe three-vessel disease are shown. While the axial slices correspond to the originally acquired image data, the sagittal and coronal images are reformations computed from the original dataset. By using such MPRs, a coronary vessel can be assessed in different geometries following its anatomical course (in this example: left anterior descending)

5.2.3 CT-Derived FFR

FFR is a functional marker assessing the hemodynamic relevance of coronary stenoses. It is defined as the pressure distal to a stenosis as a fraction of the pressure before the stenosis (thus, the FFR value expresses the maximal perfusion in the presence of a stenosis relative to the maximally expected value under normal conditions). In invasive coronary angiography (ICA), FFR values can be derived from intracoronary pressure measurements performed during pharmacologically induced vasodilatation [34, 35]. In a large randomized multicenter study (Fractional Flow Reserve versus Angiography for Multivessel Evaluation, FAME) the role of FFR in patients with multivessel CCS was evaluated; showing that routine FFR significantly reduces mortality and myocardial infarction [36, 37].

To also estimate the hemodynamic relevance of coronary lesions without necessitating an invasive procedure, computing FFR values from noninvasive coronary CTA has been proposed. Large prospective multicenter trials evaluating the novel technique (DeFACTO [38], DISCOVER-FLOW [39], NXT [40]) proved high diagnostic accuracy for the detection of coronary lesions causing myocardial ischemia. All aforementioned studies used a proprietary algorithm applying computational fluid dynamics (CFD) for computing FFR values [41]. Recently, a novel technique was introduced calculating FFR values from coronary CTA based on machine learning (ML) [42]. The ML model was trained on a large database of synthetically generated coronary anatomies. Comparing the ML and CFD approaches, equal diagnostic accuracy at significantly shorter processing times was found [43, 44]. An example of a coronary tree with CT-derived FFR values is shown in Fig. 5.3.

5.2.4 CT Volumetry

LV functional parameters are an important aspect in the diagnostic workup of patients suffering from CCS and are known to hold substantial prognostic information [45]. Functional parameters include LV end-diastolic volume (EDV), end-systolic volume (ESV), and ejection fraction (EF = (EDV − ESV)/EDV). Even though results from CT volumetry were found to correlate well with the reference standard of cardiac MRI [46–48], less invasive methods like echocardiography and cardiac MRI are usually preferred as primary methods for the evaluation of functional cardiac parameters. Still, whenever coronary CTA data are acquired using retrospective ECG gating, image data inherently contain information of

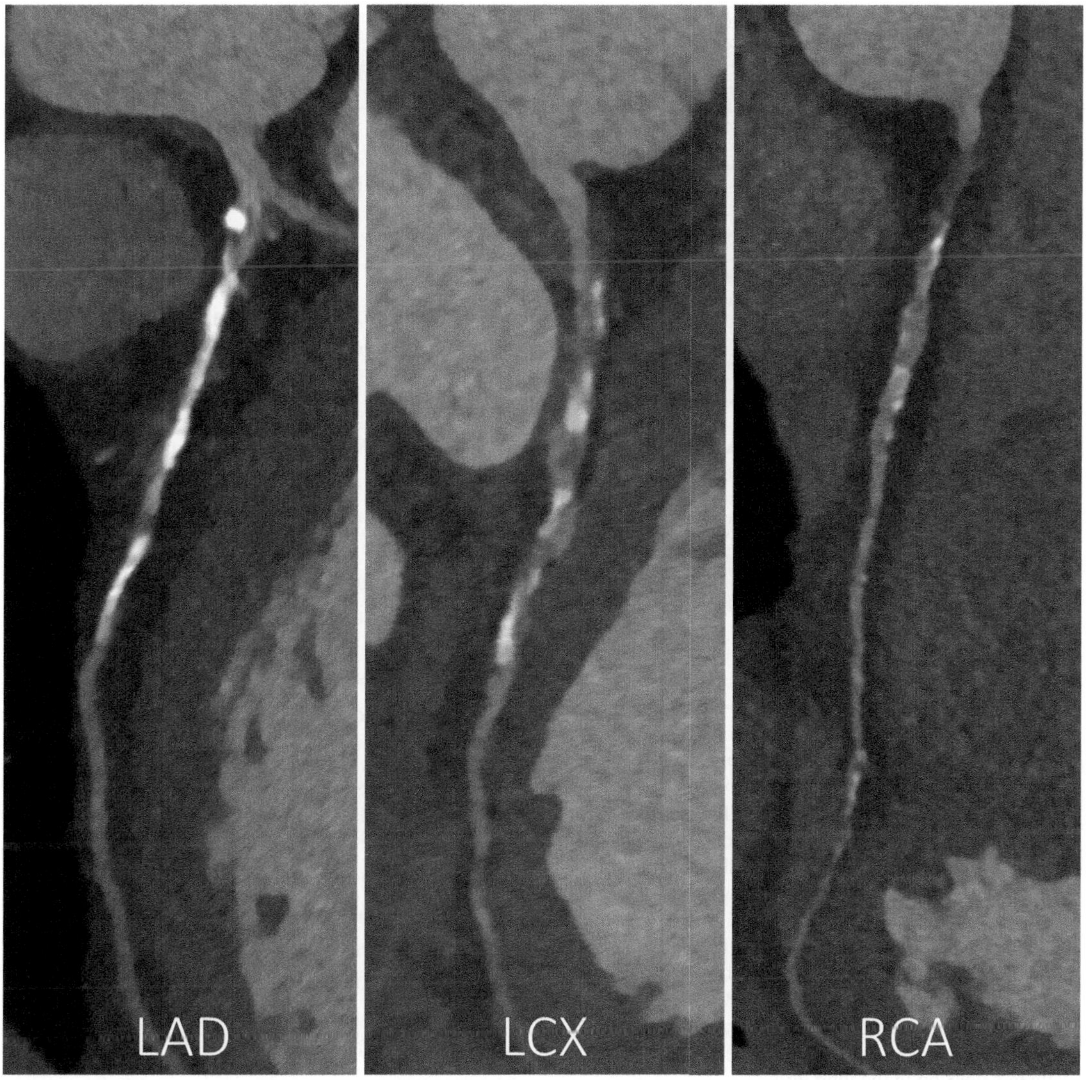

Fig. 5.2 Curved multiplanar reformations (curved MPR) of coronary CT angiography. Images of a 59-year-old male patient with severe three-vessel disease are shown (same patient as in Fig. 5.1). Curved MPRs are following the course of each vessel so that one can evaluate the coronary arteries over their full length. One major limitation of coronary CT angiography can be seen in this example: coronary CT angiography is perfect for ruling out coronary artery disease in patients with a low pre-test probability of the disease, but in a positive case, it does not provide information regarding the physiologic impact of identified lesions and is a poor predictor of resulting myocardial ischemia. In such case, subsequent testing with a complementary image modality providing information on resulting perfusion deficits might be favorable (cf. Figure 5.5). *LAD* left anterior descending artery, *LCX* left circumflex artery, *RCA* right coronary artery

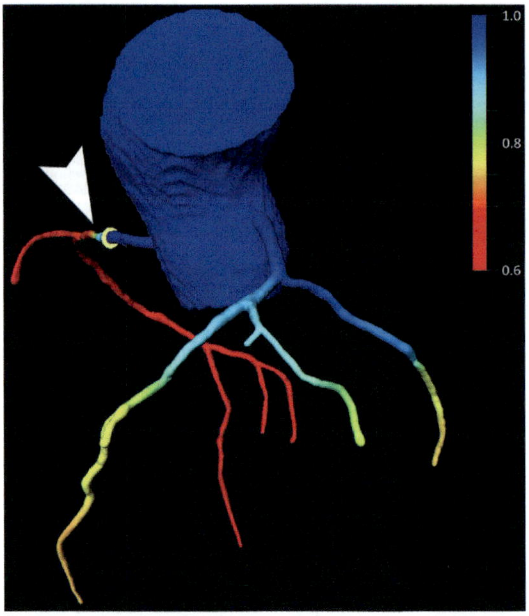

Fig. 5.3 CT-derived fractional flow reserve (FFR). The coronary tree with color-coded FFR values derived from coronary CT angiography of a 65-year-old male patient is shown. CT data were acquired 13 years after heart transplant due to ischemic dilatative cardiomyopathy. A relevant stenosis of the proximal right coronary artery (RCA, marked by arrowhead ➤) leads to an FFR drop in the distal parts of the vessel. The left anterior descending (LAD) and left circumflex (LCX) artery are showing intermediate CT-derived FFR values. All findings were confirmed by invasive coronary angiography (proximal RCA: 70–80% stenosis, mid LAD: wall irregularities, mid LCX: 50% stenosis). Diffuse lumen restrictions could possibly be explained by cardiac allograft vasculopathy—a disease with characteristic fibrotic proliferation and intimal thickening of the coronary arteries that many heart transplant recipients develop in the long term

different time points in the cardiac cycle to measure global LV functional parameters with high accuracy.

5.2.5 Dynamic Stress CT Perfusion

Similar to stress perfusion imaging by MRI or PET, dynamic stress CT perfusion acquires a series of CT images after injection of a contrast agent during pharmacological hyperemia [49]. To be able to acquire dynamic images of the entire LV during first-pass perfusion, the LV must be covered within 1 or 2 acquisitions—a prerequisite that restricts dynamic CT perfusion to the latest generation wide-detector CT systems or second/third generation dual-source CT systems [49, 50]. By measuring attenuation changes over time, myocardial perfusion parameters can be calculated in a quantitative fashion and be displayed as volumetric perfusion maps.

A typical scan protocol including dynamic stress CT perfusion is illustrated in Fig. 5.4. Initial CT calcium scoring and coronary CTA are followed by a 10–15 min delay to allow for sufficient contrast washout. Coronary artery dilatation and resulting myocardial hyperemia are induced by continuous intravenous administration of adenosine (140–210 μg/kg body weight/min). During adenosine stress, the patient's heart rate, blood pressure, and symptoms (e.g., angina, dyspnea, cough) are constantly monitored. After

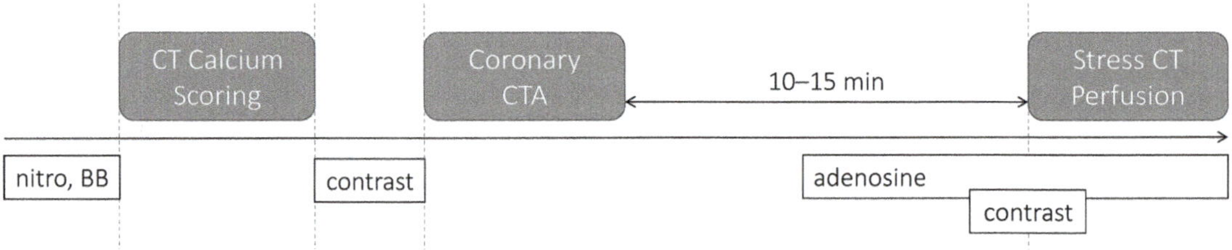

Fig. 5.4 Scan protocol including dynamic stress CT perfusion. After performing a native low-dose calcium scan and coronary CT angiography under rest conditions, dynamic stress CT perfusion images are acquired under pharmacologically induced hyperemia. A 10–15 min delay between both scans is required for contrast medium washout. *adenosine*, intravenously administered adenosine; *BB*, beta blocker; *contrast*, contrast medium; *nitro*, nitroglycerin

3 min of adenosine administration, a compact iodine contrast bolus is injected through a separate intravenous cannula followed by a saline flush. CT perfusion imaging starts just before the contrast bolus reaches the right ventricle. During a 30 s breath hold, the CT table continuously moves back and forth and a set of 10–15 low-dose datasets covering the entire LV is acquired. Adenosine administration is stopped directly after the scan.

Combining the acquired time-attenuation curves (TAC) of the myocardium with the arterial input function (AIF) derived from a sample volume in the descending aorta, myocardial blood flow (MBF) through each voxel can be calculated [51, 52]. For analyzing the acquired data, MBF values are visualized as color-coded volumetric maps and/or bulls-eye plots. The reading clinician can then sample manually drawn regions-of-interest or report MBF per myocardial segment using the 17-segment American Heart Association (AHA) model [53]. Dynamic stress CT perfusion was found to permit robust discrimination between hemodynamically relevant stenoses and coronary lesions not causing ischemia [54].

5.2.6 CT Late Enhancement

Myocardial viability can be assessed by nuclear imaging or by cardiac MRI late gadolinium enhancement (LGE) [55]. Cardiac MRI LGE highlights accumulation of gadolinium-based contrast agent in areas of myocardial fibrosis or scar (caused by inflammation or infarction, respectively). Since iodine-based CT contrast agents show pharmacokinetics similar to those of gadolinium chelates, the same principle may be used for myocardial CT late enhancement imaging. It has been shown that CT late enhancement can characterize areas of irreversibly damaged myocardium with contrast patterns similar to cardiac MRI [56, 57]. CT late enhancement not only correlates well with cardiac MRI during different stages of infarction (i.e., acute, subacute, and chronic stages) [58, 59] but also reliably depicts the transmurality of subendocardial infarction [60]. The latter is an important parameter for rating the viability of the affected tissue and thus helps with the identification of coronary lesions that are likely to benefit from revascularization.

It must be emphasized that the aforementioned papers have studied CT late enhancement in animal models only. While CT late enhancement has not yet found its way into clinical routine, some preliminary studies have evaluated its applicability in human subjects as well [61–64]. As compared to cardiac MRI, CT late enhancement seems to systematically underestimate the size of myocardial infarction [61, 63].

5.2.7 CT Multiparametric Image Fusion

As we have seen above, coronary CTA offers excellent sensitivity and an almost perfect negative predictive value for diagnostics of CAD. However, in the case of a positive result, coronary CTA does not provide information regarding the physiological impact of the identified lesions and poorly predicts myocardial ischemia. It was found that the combination of coronary CTA and myocardial CT perfusion offers incremental value over any of the two imaging parameters alone [65–67].

To ease intuitive interpretation of a combined coronary CTA/CT perfusion imaging approach, first attempts to three-dimensionally fuse both imaging parameters have been made [68, 69]. Three-dimensional (3D) image fusion helps to accurately correlate coronary lesions to resulting areas of myocardial hypoperfusion without the need to mentally co-register them within the complex cardiac anatomy [68, 69].

When combining coronary CTA with subsequent myocardial CT perfusion, one should always consider the inherently increased level of radiation. Compared to subsequent radionuclide perfusion imaging, the combination of the two CT imaging parameters may offer advantages in terms of simplicity, convenience due to its single-test nature, as well as cost and dose savings [69]. However, in patients eligible for cardiac MRI perfusion imaging, a multimodality approach combining coronary CTA with MRI perfusion might still be favorable [68].

5.3 Cardiac CT: Multimodal Imaging

As discussed above, cardiac CT covers different pathologic aspects of CAD through its multiple imaging parameters. Moreover, coronary CTA is the most widely used morphological basis for multimodal cardiac imaging combining information from two independent, but comprehensive diagnostic tests. While coronary CTA accurately depicts the coronary anatomy and possible coronary lesions, image data from other modalities can further characterize the myocardium (regarding myocardial ischemia, edema, fibrosis, or scar). The combination of coronary CTA with subsequent myocardial perfusion imaging (MPI) is of particular interest in order to determine the hemodynamic significance of coronary stenoses.

Since all alternative imaging modalities are being discussed in detail in other chapters of this book, only a short overview is given at this point. Advantages and disadvantages of the different modalities compared to cardiac CT are noted. Moreover, possible contact points with cardiac CT are emphasized.

5.3.1 CT/Echocardiography

Echocardiography is a cardiological test that is inexpensive, radiation-free, and widely available. On the downside, echocardiography is highly dependent on the examiner's experience and therefore less reproducible than other imaging modalities. The combination of coronary CTA with echocardiography might be of particular interest in the emergency setting of patients with acute chest pain if relevant CAD cannot be excluded by coronary CTA and additional MPI would considerably prolong the time to diagnosis [70]. Three-dimensional fusion of coronary CTA and longitudinal strain values derived from 3D echocardiography was developed and showed promising results [70].

5.3.2 CT/SPECT

SPECT is based on the perfusion-dependent radionuclide uptake in cardiac myocytes, which can be detected by gamma cameras. While not being affected by cardiac arrhythmia, disadvantages of SPECT include its low spatial resolution and the application of ionizing radiation. Hybrid SPECT/CT scanners can acquire anatomical and functional data within the same examination [71]. Three-dimensional superposition of SPECT segments onto cardiac CT anatomy eases the correlation between coronary stenoses and perfusion defects [72].

5.3.3 CT/PET

Compared to SPECT, PET offers higher spatial resolution, accurate attenuation correction, and lower levels of radiation due to shorter half-life periods and favorable pharmacokinetic properties of the utilized radionuclides. PET has also the ability to quantify myocardial blood flow in absolute terms [73]. Disadvantages of the modality include higher costs and limited availability. Modern hybrid PET/CT systems are equipped with multislice CT, which allows for combined coronary CTA and PET imaging within one examination [74].

5.3.4 CT/MRI

Cardiac MRI can answer questions regarding morphology, function, ischemia, and viability within one examination. While cardiac MRI can rule out relevant CAD with similar accuracy as CT or PET [75], it does not involve ionizing radiation. Therefore, fusion of coronary CTA and cardiac MRI might be a favorable approach to multimodal cardiac imaging, because it applies as low radiation as possible while allowing for both accurate assessment of coronary stenoses and hypoperfusion. First studies taking this approach showed promising results [76–78] but had the limitation of incomplete LV coverage due to two-dimensional image acquisition of standard MRI perfusion sequences. Fusion of coronary CTA with newly developed whole-heart dynamic

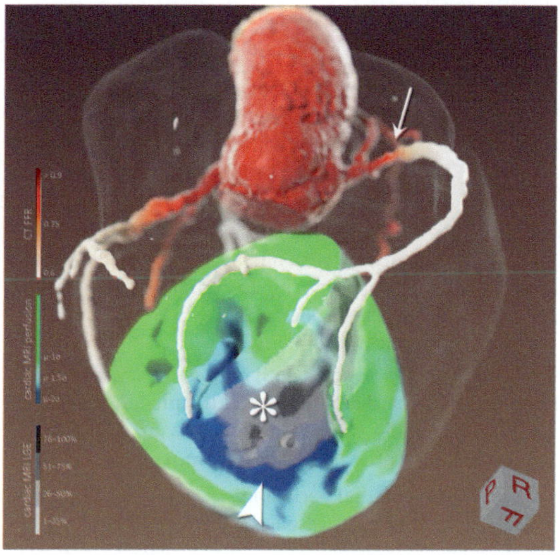

Fig. 5.5 Multimodal multiparametric three-dimensional image fusion. Cardiac CT and MRI data of a 59-year-old male patient with severe three-vessel disease are shown (same patient as in Figs. 5.1 and 5.2). Severe stenosis of the proximal right coronary artery (marked by arrow →) leads to pathologic CT-derived fractional flow reserve (FFR) values. Hypoperfusion of the inferior heart wall (marked by arrow head ➤, color-coded MRI perfusion data) has already led to myocardial scar of greater extent (marked by asterisk *, transmurality derived from MRI late gadolinium enhancement, LGE)

3D cardiac MR perfusion sequences enables coverage of the entire LV from base to apex [79]. A recent study proposed 3D image fusion of cardiac CT and MRI including information on anatomy, coronary stenoses, hemodynamic impact, ischemia, and infarction [80] as exemplarily illustrated in Fig. 5.5.

5.4 Discussion

5.4.1 Number of Cases Undergoing Cardiac CT Multimodal Imaging

For diagnostic workup of CCS, a two-step diagnostic approach combining coronary CTA and subsequent MPI is feasible according to current guidelines (cf. paragraph 5.1.1.2). However, the actual number of patients undergoing both imaging tests in clinical routine is still low. Several studies that reported the number of cases undergoing coronary CTA in combination with cardiac MRI as an additional functional test are listed in Table 5.3. In summary, less than 5% of study patients underwent both complementary examinations.

5.4.2 Advantages of Cardiac CT Multimodal Imaging

In contrast to the low number of patients undergoing multimodal diagnostic workup including coronary CTA in today's clinical routine, studies investigating the benefit of multimodal imaging for CCS reported added diagnostic value in a higher number of cases.

A study determining individual coronary supply territories found an extremely high number of cases that do not match standard supply territories as assumed by the 17-segment AHA model (23% and 67% of discordant cases in a per-segment and per-patient analysis, respectively) [83]. In line with this finding, multiple studies have reported incremental diagnostic value of multimodal imaging and/or 3D image fusion including coronary CTA as listed in Table 5.4. A recent meta-analysis comparing multimodal imaging of CCS with stand-alone coronary CTA found unchanged sensitivity but significantly improved specificity [33]. This result might be of particular importance when considering the fact that 59% of patients with one positive imaging test do not show obstructive CAD in ICA and do not need revascularization [88]. Since ICA adds major costs and implies the risk of adverse events, multimodal cardiac imaging including coronary CTA may serve as a gatekeeper for ICA, especially in complicated cases and higher risk patients.

Table 5.3 Number of patients undergoing coronary CT angiography and cardiac MRI as an additional functional test

Reference	*N*	Study	Results
Bruder et al., J Am Coll Cardiol, 2009 [81]	11,040	EuroCMR registry [81]	1.8%[a] of patients undergoing cardiac MRI had a previous coronary CTA, while 0.8%[b] with an initial cardiac MRI were referred to subsequent coronary CTA
Moschetti et al., J Cardiovasc Magn Reson, 2012 [82]	2717	Separately analyzed sub-cohort of the EuroCMR registry regarding cost-effectiveness [82]	6% of initial stress cardiac MRI were inconclusive and necessitated additional testing, leading to coronary CTA in 13% of these cases (i.e., 0.8% of the initial patient population)
von Spiczak et al., Radiol Cardiothorac Imaging, 2020 [80]	434	Study on multimodal multiparametric fusion imaging in CCS	17 patients with both coronary CTA and cardiac MRI were identified in a total of 434 screened patients (i.e., 3.9% of the initial patient population)

Cardiac MRI was chosen as one exemplary imaging modality assessing myocardial perfusion.
CCS chronic coronary syndrome, *CTA* CT angiography, *EuroCMR* European Cardiovascular Magnetic Resonance
[a]Total number, not subdivided by pathology
[b]Specific for CCS

Table 5.4 Incremental diagnostic value of a multimodal imaging approach including coronary CT angiography

Reference	*N*	Modalities	Results
van Werkhoven et al., Heart, 2010 [84]	53	CT and MRI (2D readout)	Complementary diagnostic information in 26% (14/53) of cases
Groothuis et al., Eur Heart J, 2013 [85]	192	CT and MRI (2D readout)	Significantly improved specificity and overall accuracy; the combined strategy provided an alternative diagnosis in 10% (19/192) of cases
Gaemperli et al., J Nucl Med, 2007 [86]	38	CT and SPECT (3D fusion)	Incremental diagnostic information by 3D image fusion in 32% (12/38) of cases
Liga et al., Eur Heart J Cardiovasc Imaging, 2016 [87]	252	CT and SPECT/PET (3D fusion)	Reassignment of perfusion defect by 3D fusion in 18% (45/252) of cases
Donati et al., Invest Radiol, 2011 [77]	27	CT and MRI (3D fusion)	Refinement or reassignment by 3D image fusion in 19% (5/27) of cases
von Spiczak et al., Int J Cardiovasc Imaging, 2018 [79]	23	CT and MRI (3D fusion)	Refinement or rejudgement by 3D image fusion in 26% (6/23) of cases

The first two papers studied multimodal imaging with conventional two-dimensional readout. The next four papers reported diagnostic improvements by multimodal imaging with three-dimensional image fusion.
2D two-dimensional, *3D* three-dimensional, *PET* positron emission tomography, *SPECT* single-photon emission computed tomography

5.5 Conclusion

In today's clinical routine, cardiac CT is often used as a valuable tool in the noninvasive diagnostic workup of many cardiovascular pathologies, most importantly CAD.

In cardiac CT *multiparametric* imaging, coronary CTA is the most important imaging parameter. It accurately depicts the anatomy and possible stenoses of the coronary arteries and is characterized by its high sensitivity and its excellent negative predictive value. Other CT imaging parameters include CT calcium scoring as a prognostic marker in CCS, CT-derived FFR to assess the hemodynamic relevance of coronary lesions, CT volumetry to evaluate the LV function, as well as CT perfusion and late enhancement to detect myocardial ischemia and infarction, respectively.

In cardiac CT *multimodal* imaging, coronary CTA is often used to depict the anatomy and to assess coronary stenoses, while a second modality (i.e., PET, SPECT, or MRI) evaluates resulting ischemia or scars of the myocardium. By co-registration of the two (or more) modalities and subsequent 2D overlay or 3D rendering, culprit lesions can be correlated to resulting areas of myocardial hypoperfusion or scar with a high degree of certainty. We have seen that all pathological aspects of CCS could be combined in a common 3D scene as demonstrated in a recent study.

The number of CCS patients undergoing cardiac CT multimodal imaging in clinical routine remains low. However, studies have constantly shown that combining cardiac CT with other imaging modalities can yield complementary diagnostic information in a relevant percentage of cases. Specificity and diagnostic accuracy can be significantly increased. By that, multimodal multiparametric cardiac imaging including cardiac CT may serve as a gatekeeper for invasive procedures or surgery, especially in complicated cases of cardiovascular disease.

Conflict of Interest None.

Funding Disclosure None.

References

1. Al-Mallah MH, Aljizeeri A, Villines TC, Srichai MB, Alsaileek A. Cardiac computed tomography in current cardiology guidelines. J Cardiovasc Comput Tomogr. 2015;9:514–23.
2. Benjamin EJ, Muntner P, Alonso A, Bittencourt MS, Callaway CW, Carson AP, et al. Heart disease and stroke Statistics-2019 update: a report from the American Heart Association. Circulation. 2019;139:e56–e528.
3. Knuuti J, Wijns W, Saraste A, Capodanno D, Barbato E, Funck-Brentano C, et al. 2019 ESC guidelines for the diagnosis and management of chronic coronary syndromes. Eur Heart J. 2020;41:407–77.
4. Hoffmann U, Bamberg F, Chae CU, Nichols JH, Rogers IS, Seneviratne SK, et al. Coronary computed tomography angiography for early triage of patients with acute chest pain: the ROMICAT (Rule Out Myocardial Infarction using Computer Assisted Tomography) trial. J Am Coll Cardiol. 2009;53:1642–50.
5. Linde JJ, Kelbæk H, Hansen TF, Sigvardsen PE, Torp-Pedersen C, Bech J, et al. Coronary CT angiography in patients with non-ST-segment elevation acute coronary syndrome. J Am Coll Cardiol. 2020;75:453–63.
6. van Velzen JE, de Graaf FR, Kroft LJ, de Roos A, Reiber JHC, Bax JJ, et al. Performance and efficacy of 320-row computed tomography coronary angiography in patients presenting with acute chest pain: results from a clinical registry. Int J Cardiovasc Imaging. 2012;28:865–76.
7. Juarez-Orozco LE, Saraste A, Capodanno D, Prescott E, Ballo H, Bax JJ, et al. Impact of a decreasing pre-test probability on the performance of diagnostic tests for coronary artery disease. Eur Heart J Cardiovasc Imaging. 2019;20:1198–207.
8. Saraste A, Barbato E, Capodanno D, Edvardsen T, Prescott E, Achenbach S, et al. Imaging in ESC clinical guidelines: chronic coronary syndromes. Eur Heart J. 2019;20:1187–97.
9. Haase R, Schlattmann P, Gueret P, Andreini D, Pontone G, Alkadhi H, et al. Diagnosis of obstructive coronary artery disease using computed tomography angiography in patients with stable chest pain depending on clinical probability and in clinically important subgroups: meta-analysis of individual patient data. BMJ. 2019;365:l1945.
10. Wolk MJ, Bailey SR, Doherty JU, Douglas PS, Hendel RC, Kramer CM, et al. ACCF/AHA/ASE/ASNC/HFSA/HRS/SCAI/SCCT/SCMR/STS 2013 multimodality appropriate use criteria for the detection and risk assessment of stable ischemic heart disease: a report of the American College of Cardiology Foundation Appropriate Use Criteria Task Force, American Heart Association, American Society of Echocardiography, American Society of Nuclear Cardiology, Heart Failure Society of America, Heart Rhythm Society, Society for Cardiovascular Angiography and

Interventions, Society of Cardiovascular Computed Tomography, Society for Cardiovascular Magnetic Resonance, and Society of Thoracic Surgeons. J Am Coll Cardiol. 2014;63:380–406.
11. Araoz PA, Kirsch J, Primak AN, Braun NN, Saba O, Williamson EE, et al. Optimal image reconstruction phase at low and high heart rates in dual-source CT coronary angiography. Int J Cardiovasc Imaging. 2009;25:837–45.
12. Machida H, Tanaka I, Fukui R, Shen Y, Ishikawa T, Tate E, et al. Current and novel imaging techniques in coronary CT. Radiographics. 2015;35:991–1010.
13. Ajlan AM, Heilbron BG, Leipsic J. Coronary computed tomography angiography for stable angina: past, present, and future. Can J Cardiol. 2013;29:266–74.
14. Bastarrika G, Lee YS, Huda W, Ruzsics B, Costello P, Schoepf UJ. CT of coronary artery disease. Radiology. 2009;253:317–38.
15. Gordic S, Desbiolles L, Sedlmair M, Manka R, Plass A, Schmidt B, et al. Optimizing radiation dose by using advanced modelled iterative reconstruction in high-pitch coronary CT angiography. Eur Radiol. 2016;26:459–68.
16. Greenland P, Blaha MJ, Budoff MJ, Erbel R, Watson KE. Coronary calcium score and cardiovascular risk. J Am Coll Cardiol. 2018;72:434–47.
17. Sandfort V, Bluemke DA. CT calcium scoring. History, current status and outlook. Diagn Interv Imaging. 2017;98:3–10.
18. Agatston AS, Janowitz WR, Hildner FJ, Zusmer NR, Viamonte M, Detrano R. Quantification of coronary artery calcium using ultrafast computed tomography. J Am Coll Cardiol. 1990;15:827–32.
19. Criqui MH, Denenberg JO, Ix JH, McClelland RL, Wassel CL, Rifkin DE, et al. Calcium density of coronary artery plaque and risk of incident cardiovascular events. JAMA. 2014;311:271–8.
20. Raggi P, Callister TQ, Cooil B, He ZX, Lippolis NJ, Russo DJ, et al. Identification of patients at increased risk of first unheralded acute myocardial infarction by electron-beam computed tomography. Circulation. 2000;101:850–5.
21. Hoff JA, Chomka EV, Krainik AJ, Daviglus M, Rich S, Kondos GT. Age and gender distributions of coronary artery calcium detected by electron beam tomography in 35,246 adults. Am J Cardiol. 2001;87:1335–9.
22. McClelland RL, Chung H, Detrano R, Post W, Kronmal RA. Distribution of coronary artery calcium by race, gender, and age: results from the multiethnic study of atherosclerosis (MESA). Circulation. 2006;113:30–7.
23. Mitchell JD, Fergestrom N, Gage BF, Paisley R, Moon P, Novak E, et al. Impact of statins on cardiovascular outcomes following coronary artery calcium scoring. J Am Coll Cardiol. 2018;72:3233–42.
24. von Ballmoos MW, Haring B, Juillerat P, Alkadhi H. Meta-analysis: diagnostic performance of low-radiation-dose coronary computed tomography angiography. Ann Intern Med. 2011;154:413–20.
25. Leipsic J, Abbara S, Achenbach S, Cury R, Earls JP, Mancini GJ, et al. SCCT guidelines for the interpretation and reporting of coronary CT angiography: a report of the Society of Cardiovascular Computed Tomography Guidelines Committee. J Cardiovasc Comput Tomogr. 2014;8:342–58.
26. Cury RC, Abbara S, Achenbach S, Agatston A, Berman DS, Budoff MJ, et al. CAD-RADS™: Coronary Artery Disease—Reporting and Data System: an expert consensus document of the Society of Cardiovascular Computed Tomography (SCCT), the American College of Radiology (ACR) and the North American Society for Cardiovascular Imaging (NASCI). Endorsed by the American College of Cardiology. J Am Coll Radiol JACR. 2016;13:1458–1466.e9.
27. Bittner DO, Mayrhofer T, Budoff M, Szilveszter B, Foldyna B, Hallett TR, et al. Prognostic value of coronary CTA in stable chest pain: CAD-RADS, CAC, and cardiovascular events in PROMISE. JACC Cardiovasc Imaging. 2020;13:1534–45.
28. Gueret P, Deux J-F, Bonello L, Sarran A, Tron C, Christiaens L, et al. Diagnostic performance of computed tomography coronary angiography (from the Prospective National Multicenter Multivendor EVASCAN Study). Am J Cardiol. 2013;111:471–8.
29. Menke J, Kowalski J. Diagnostic accuracy and utility of coronary CT angiography with consideration of unevaluable results: a systematic review and multivariate Bayesian random-effects meta-analysis with intention to diagnose. Eur Radiol. 2016;26:451–8.
30. Knuuti J, Ballo H, Juarez-Orozco LE, Saraste A, Kolh P, Rutjes AWS, et al. The performance of non-invasive tests to rule-in and rule-out significant coronary artery stenosis in patients with stable angina: a meta-analysis focused on post-test disease probability. Eur Heart J. 2018;39:3322–30.
31. Hadamitzky M, Freissmuth B, Meyer T, Hein F, Kastrati A, Martinoff S, et al. Prognostic value of coronary computed tomographic angiography for prediction of cardiac events in patients with suspected coronary artery disease. JACC Cardiovasc Imaging. 2009;2:404–11.
32. Min JK, Dunning A, Lin FY, Achenbach S, Al-Mallah M, Budoff MJ, et al. Age- and sex-related differences in all-cause mortality risk based on coronary computed tomography angiography findings results from the international multicenter CONFIRM (Coronary CT Angiography Evaluation for Clinical Outcomes: An International Multicenter Registry) of 23,854 patients without known coronary artery disease. J Am Coll Cardiol. 2011;58:849–60.
33. Rizvi A, Han D, Danad I, Ó Hartaigh B, Lee JH, Gransar H, et al. Diagnostic performance of hybrid cardiac imaging methods for assessment of obstructive coronary artery disease compared with stand-alone coronary computed tomography angiography: a meta-analysis. JACC Cardiovasc Imaging. 2018;11:589–99.

34. Pijls NH, van Son JA, Kirkeeide RL, De Bruyne B, Gould KL. Experimental basis of determining maximum coronary, myocardial, and collateral blood flow by pressure measurements for assessing functional stenosis severity before and after percutaneous transluminal coronary angioplasty. Circulation. 1993;87:1354–67.
35. De Bruyne B, Pijls NH, Paulus WJ, Vantrimpont PJ, Sys SU, Heyndrickx GR. Transstenotic coronary pressure gradient measurement in humans: in vitro and in vivo evaluation of a new pressure monitoring angioplasty guide wire. J Am Coll Cardiol. 1993;22:119–26.
36. Tonino PAL, De Bruyne B, Pijls NHJ, Siebert U, Ikeno F, van't Veer M, et al. Fractional flow reserve versus angiography for guiding percutaneous coronary intervention. N Engl J Med. 2009;360:213–24.
37. Pijls NHJ, Fearon WF, Tonino PAL, Siebert U, Ikeno F, Bornschein B, et al. Fractional flow reserve versus angiography for guiding percutaneous coronary intervention in patients with multivessel coronary artery disease: 2-year follow-up of the FAME (Fractional Flow Reserve Versus Angiography for Multivessel Evaluation) study. J Am Coll Cardiol. 2010;56:177–84.
38. Min JK, Leipsic J, Pencina MJ, Berman DS, Koo B-K, van Mieghem C, et al. Diagnostic accuracy of fractional flow reserve from anatomic CT angiography. JAMA. 2012;308:1237–45.
39. Koo B-K, Erglis A, Doh J-H, Daniels DV, Jegere S, Kim H-S, et al. Diagnosis of ischemia-causing coronary stenoses by noninvasive fractional flow reserve computed from coronary computed tomographic angiograms. Results from the prospective multicenter DISCOVER-FLOW (Diagnosis of Ischemia-Causing Stenoses Obtained Via Noninvasive Fractional Flow Reserve) study. J Am Coll Cardiol. 2011;58:1989–97.
40. Nørgaard BL, Leipsic J, Gaur S, Seneviratne S, Ko BS, Ito H, et al. Diagnostic performance of noninvasive fractional flow reserve derived from coronary computed tomography angiography in suspected coronary artery disease: the NXT trial (Analysis of Coronary Blood Flow Using CT Angiography: Next Steps). J Am Coll Cardiol. 2014;63:1145–55.
41. Taylor CA, Fonte TA, Min JK. Computational fluid dynamics applied to cardiac computed tomography for noninvasive quantification of fractional flow reserve: scientific basis. J Am Coll Cardiol. 2013;61:2233–41.
42. Itu L, Rapaka S, Passerini T, Georgescu B, Schwemmer C, Schoebinger M, et al. A machine-learning approach for computation of fractional flow reserve from coronary computed tomography. J Appl Physiol. 1985;2016(121):42–52.
43. Coenen A, Kim Y-H, Kruk M, Tesche C, De Geer J, Kurata A, et al. Diagnostic accuracy of a machine-learning approach to coronary computed tomographic angiography-based fractional flow reserve: result from the MACHINE consortium. Circ Cardiovasc Imaging. 2018;11:e007217.
44. Tesche C, De Cecco CN, Baumann S, Renker M, McLaurin TW, Duguay TM, et al. Coronary CT angiography-derived fractional flow reserve: machine learning algorithm versus computational fluid dynamics modeling. Radiology. 2018;288:64–72.
45. White HD, Norris RM, Brown MA, Brandt PW, Whitlock RM, Wild CJ. Left ventricular end-systolic volume as the major determinant of survival after recovery from myocardial infarction. Circulation. 1987;76:44–51.
46. Busch S, Johnson TRC, Wintersperger BJ, Minaifar N, Bhargava A, Rist C, et al. Quantitative assessment of left ventricular function with dual-source CT in comparison to cardiac magnetic resonance imaging: initial findings. Eur Radiol. 2008;18:570–5.
47. van der Vleuten PA, de Jonge GJ, Lubbers DD, Tio RA, Willems TP, Oudkerk M, et al. Evaluation of global left ventricular function assessment by dual-source computed tomography compared with MRI. Eur Radiol. 2009;19:271–7.
48. Juergens KU, Grude M, Maintz D, Fallenberg EM, Wichter T, Heindel W, et al. Multi–detector row CT of left ventricular function with dedicated analysis software versus MR imaging: initial experience. Radiology; 2004;230:403–410.
49. Nieman K, Balla S. Dynamic CT myocardial perfusion imaging. J Cardiovasc Comput Tomogr. 2020;14:303–6.
50. Varga-Szemes A, Meinel FG, De Cecco CN, Fuller SR, Bayer RR, Schoepf UJ. CT myocardial perfusion imaging. AJR Am J Roentgenol. 2015;204:487–97.
51. Mahnken AH, Klotz E, Pietsch H, Schmidt B, Allmendinger T, Haberland U, et al. Quantitative whole heart stress perfusion CT imaging as noninvasive assessment of hemodynamics in coronary artery stenosis: preliminary animal experience. Invest Radiol. 2010;45:298–305.
52. Bamberg F, Klotz E, Flohr T, Becker A, Becker CR, Schmidt B, et al. Dynamic myocardial stress perfusion imaging using fast dual-source CT with alternating table positions: initial experience. Eur Radiol. 2010;20:1168–73.
53. Cerqueira MD, Weissman NJ, Dilsizian V, Jacobs AK, Kaul S, Laskey WK, et al. Standardized myocardial segmentation and nomenclature for tomographic imaging of the heart. A statement for healthcare professionals from the Cardiac Imaging Committee of the Council on Clinical Cardiology of the American Heart Association. Circulation. 2002;105:539–42.
54. Rossi A, Wragg A, Klotz E, Pirro F, Moon JC, Nieman K, et al. Dynamic computed tomography myocardial perfusion imaging: comparison of clinical analysis methods for the detection of vessel-specific ischemia. Circ Cardiovasc Imaging. 2017;10:e005505.
55. Kim RJ, Wu E, Rafael A, Chen EL, Parker MA, Simonetti O, et al. The use of contrast-enhanced magnetic resonance imaging to identify reversible myocardial dysfunction. N Engl J Med. 2000;343:1445–53.

56. Gerber BL, Belge B, Legros GJ, Lim P, Poncelet A, Pasquet A, et al. Characterization of acute and chronic myocardial infarcts by multidetector computed tomography: comparison with contrast-enhanced magnetic resonance. Circulation. 2006;113:823–33.
57. Lardo AC, Cordeiro MAS, Silva C, Amado LC, George RT, Saliaris AP, et al. Contrast-enhanced multidetector computed tomography viability imaging after myocardial infarction: characterization of myocyte death, microvascular obstruction, and chronic scar. Circulation. 2006;113:394–404.
58. Mahnken AH, Bruners P, Kinzel S, Katoh M, Mühlenbruch G, Günther RW, et al. Late-phase MSCT in the different stages of myocardial infarction: animal experiments. Eur Radiol. 2007;17:2310–7.
59. Baks T, Cademartiri F, Moelker AD, Weustink AC, van Geuns R-J, Mollet NR, et al. Multislice computed tomography and magnetic resonance imaging for the assessment of reperfused acute myocardial infarction. J Am Coll Cardiol. 2006;48:144–52.
60. Brodoefel H, Klumpp B, Reimann A, Fenchel M, Heuschmid M, Miller S, et al. Sixty-four-MSCT in the characterization of porcine acute and subacute myocardial infarction: determination of transmurality in comparison to magnetic resonance imaging and histopathology. Eur J Radiol. 2007;62:235–46.
61. Nikolaou K, Sanz J, Poon M, Wintersperger BJ, Ohnesorge B, Rius T, et al. Assessment of myocardial perfusion and viability from routine contrast-enhanced 16-detector-row computed tomography of the heart: preliminary results. Eur Radiol. 2005;15:864–71.
62. Mahnken AH, Koos R, Katoh M, Wildberger JE, Spuentrup E, Buecker A, et al. Assessment of myocardial viability in reperfused acute myocardial infarction using 16-slice computed tomography in comparison to magnetic resonance imaging. J Am Coll Cardiol. 2005;45:2042–7.
63. Sanz J, Weeks D, Nikolaou K, Sirol M, Rius T, Rajagopalan S, et al. Detection of healed myocardial infarction with multidetector-row computed tomography and comparison with cardiac magnetic resonance delayed hyperenhancement. Am J Cardiol. 2006;98:149–55.
64. Nieman K, Shapiro MD, Ferencik M, Nomura CH, Abbara S, Hoffmann U, et al. Reperfused myocardial infarction: contrast-enhanced 64-section CT in comparison to MR imaging. Radiology. 2008;247:49–56.
65. Rocha-Filho JA, Blankstein R, Shturman LD, Bezerra HG, Okada DR, Rogers IS, et al. Incremental value of adenosine-induced stress myocardial perfusion imaging with dual-source CT at cardiac CT angiography. Radiology. 2010;254:410–9.
66. Ko BS, Cameron JD, Leung M, Meredith IT, Leong DP, Antonis PR, et al. Combined CT coronary angiography and stress myocardial perfusion imaging for hemodynamically significant stenoses in patients with suspected coronary artery disease: a comparison with fractional flow reserve. JACC Cardiovasc Imaging. 2012;5:1097–111.
67. Magalhães TA, Kishi S, George RT, Arbab-Zadeh A, Vavere AL, Cox C, et al. Combined coronary angiography and myocardial perfusion by computed tomography in the identification of flow-limiting stenosis—the CORE320 study: an integrated analysis of CT coronary angiography and myocardial perfusion. J Cardiovasc Comput Tomogr. 2015;9:438–45.
68. von Spiczak J, Manka R, Mannil M, Oebel S, Hamada S, Higashigaito K, et al. 3D fusion of coronary CT angiography and CT myocardial perfusion imaging: intuitive assessment of morphology and function. J Cardiovasc Comput Tomogr. 2017;11:437–43.
69. Patel AR, Maffessanti F, Patel MB, Kebed K, Narang A, Singh A, et al. Hemodynamic impact of coronary stenosis using computed tomography: comparison between noninvasive fractional flow reserve and 3D fusion of coronary angiography with stress myocardial perfusion. Int J Cardiovasc Imaging. 2019;35:1733–43.
70. Maffessanti F, Patel AR, Patel MB, Walter JJ, Mediratta A, Medvedofsky D, et al. Non-invasive assessment of the haemodynamic significance of coronary stenosis using fusion of cardiac computed tomography and 3D echocardiography. Eur Heart J Cardiovasc Imaging. 2017;18:670–80.
71. Gaemperli O, Kaufmann PA, Alkadhi H. Cardiac hybrid imaging. Eur J Nucl Med Mol Imaging. 2014;41(Suppl 1):S91–S103.
72. Gaemperli O, Schepis T, Kalff V, Namdar M, Valenta I, Stefani L, et al. Validation of a new cardiac image fusion software for three-dimensional integration of myocardial perfusion SPECT and stand-alone 64-slice CT angiography. Eur J Nucl Med Mol Imaging. 2007;34:1097–106.
73. Di Carli MF. PET perfusion and flow assessment: tomorrows' technology today. Semin Nucl Med. 2020;50:227–37.
74. Bengel FM, Higuchi T, Javadi MS, Lautamäki R. Cardiac positron emission tomography. J Am Coll Cardiol. 2009;54:1–15.
75. Takx RAP, Blomberg BA, El Aidi H, Habets J, de Jong PA, Nagel E, et al. Diagnostic accuracy of stress myocardial perfusion imaging compared to invasive coronary angiography with fractional flow reserve meta-analysis. Circ Cardiovasc Imaging. 2015;8:e002666.
76. Stolzmann P, Alkadhi H, Scheffel H, Hennemuth A, Kuehnel C, Baumueller S, et al. Image fusion of coronary CT angiography and cardiac perfusion MRI: a pilot study. Eur Radiol. 2010;20:1174–9.
77. Donati OF, Alkadhi H, Scheffel H, Kuehnel C, Hennemuth A, Wyss C, et al. 3D fusion of functional cardiac magnetic resonance imaging and computed tomography coronary angiography: accuracy and added clinical value. Invest Radiol. 2011;46:331–40.
78. Kirişli HA, Gupta V, Kirschbaum SW, Rossi A, Metz CT, Schaap M, et al. Comprehensive visualization of multimodal cardiac imaging data for assessment of coronary artery disease: first clinical results of the

SMARTVis tool. Int J Comput Assist Radiol Surg. 2012;7:557–71.
79. von Spiczak J, Manka R, Gotschy A, Oebel S, Kozerke S, Hamada S, et al. Fusion of CT coronary angiography and whole-heart dynamic 3D cardiac MR perfusion: building a framework for comprehensive cardiac imaging. Int J Cardiovasc Imaging. 2018;34:649–60.
80. von Spiczak J, Mannil M, Model H, Schwemmer C, Kozerke S, Ruschitzka F, et al. Multimodal multiparametric three-dimensional image fusion in coronary artery disease: combining the best of two worlds. Radiol Cardiothorac Imaging. 2020;2:e190116.
81. Bruder O, Schneider S, Nothnagel D, Dill T, Hombach V, Schulz-Menger J, et al. EuroCMR (European Cardiovascular Magnetic Resonance) registry: results of the German pilot phase. J Am Coll Cardiol. 2009;54:1457–66.
82. Moschetti K, Muzzarelli S, Pinget C, Wagner A, Pilz G, Wasserfallen J-B, et al. Cost evaluation of cardiovascular magnetic resonance versus coronary angiography for the diagnostic work-up of coronary artery disease: application of the European cardiovascular magnetic resonance registry data to the German, United Kingdom, Swiss, and United States health care systems. J Cardiovasc Magn Reson. 2012;14:35.
83. Ortiz-Pérez JT, Rodríguez J, Meyers SN, Lee DC, Davidson C, Wu E. Correspondence between the 17-segment model and coronary arterial anatomy using contrast-enhanced cardiac magnetic resonance imaging. JACC Cardiovasc Imaging. 2008;1:282–93.
84. van Werkhoven JM, Heijenbrok MW, Schuijf JD, Jukema JW, van der Wall EE, Schreur JHM, et al. Combined non-invasive anatomical and functional assessment with MSCT and MRI for the detection of significant coronary artery disease in patients with an intermediate pre-test likelihood. Heart. 2010;96:425–31.
85. Groothuis JGJ, Beek AM, Brinckman SL, Meijerink MR, van den Oever MLP, Hofman MBM, et al. Combined non-invasive functional and anatomical diagnostic work-up in clinical practice: the magnetic resonance and computed tomography in suspected coronary artery disease (MARCC) study. Eur Heart J. 2013;34:1990–8.
86. Gaemperli O, Schepis T, Valenta I, Husmann L, Scheffel H, Duerst V, et al. Cardiac image fusion from stand-alone SPECT and CT: clinical experience. J Nucl Med. 2007;48:696–703.
87. Liga R, Vontobel J, Rovai D, Marinelli M, Caselli C, Pietila M, et al. Multicentre multi-device hybrid imaging study of coronary artery disease: results from the EValuation of INtegrated cardiac Imaging for the Detection and Characterization of Ischaemic Heart Disease (EVINCI) hybrid imaging population. Eur Heart J Cardiovasc Imaging. 2016;17:951–60.
88. Patel MR, Peterson ED, Dai D, Brennan JM, Redberg RF, Anderson HV, et al. Low diagnostic yield of elective coronary angiography. N Engl J Med. 2010;362:886–95.

6 Hybrid Cardiac Imaging for the Invasive Cardiologist

Enrico Romagnoli, Francesco Burzotta, Cristina Aurigemma, and Carlo Trani

6.1 Introduction

Since its introduction in 1960, the coronary angiography (CA) has represented the gold standard for the diagnosis of coronary artery disease (CAD) [1]. CA allows direct and accurate assessment of coronary anatomy and quantification of luminal narrowing due to CAD with a spatial resolution up to 0.1 mm, still unrevealed for the assessment of distal coronary segments. Notwithstanding, the limit of a bidimensional representation and the extreme variability in coronary artery morphology, the use of a "standardized" approach based on multiple orthogonal views and quantitative measurements (QCA) do CA an objective and reproducible tool for CAD assessment [1].

Thus, it is common practice among cardiologists to give therapeutic indications for CAD on the basis of the severity of lumen narrowing observed at CA. Moreover, most historical pharmacological and interventional clinical studies defining guidelines recommendations for CAD treatment are based on CA assessment [2, 3]. While the advantage of CA-based management of CAD in the acute setting is evident, both in terms of safety and cost-effectiveness, in stable patients this approach is more controversial. Indeed, recent studies showed as prognosis of CAD would rely on total coronary plaque burden more than on single lesion severity, and the evolution of stenosis could depend on its composition (e.g., vulnerable pattern) more than on effective lumen narrowing [4]. Moreover, in stable patients, the clinical impact of severe stenosis at CA can vary considerably in terms of myocardial perfusion abnormalities according to several anatomical and functional factors [5, 6]. Thus, a plaque characterization based only on residual lumen could result inadequate especially in presence of lumen-preserving positive vessel remodeling (e.g., intermediate lesion). Likewise, dichotomous definition of "obstructive" or "non-obstructive" CAD according to stenosis percentage does not allow to identify high-risk patients who may benefit from more intensive preventive therapies.

Worldwide, CAD is responsible for 44% of cardiovascular disease events [7]. Thus, refining our current methods of CAD diagnosis, not only for early detection but also for individuating its predisposition to rapid evolution, remains a major interest in order to better individualize risk stratification. Accurate identification of high-risk CAD features is essential to optimize therapeutic strategies in order to reduce atherosclerosis pro-

E. Romagnoli (✉) · C. Aurigemma
Fondazione Policlinico Universitario Agostino Gemelli IRCCS, Rome, Italy

F. Burzotta · C. Trani
Fondazione Policlinico Universitario Agostino Gemelli IRCCS, Rome, Italy

Università Cattolica del Sacro Cuore, Rome, Italy

F. Nudi et al. (eds.), *Hybrid Cardiac Imaging for Clinical Decision-Making*,
https://doi.org/10.1007/978-3-030-99391-7_6

gression and the risk of future events. To overcome this challenge, great efforts have been made in developing new in vivo imaging modalities creating the possibility of a more comprehensive hybrid invasive approach. This chapter provides an overview of the techniques currently approved and used in the context of invasive diagnostic procedures to obtain hybrid CAD modeling.

6.2 Rationale for Hybrid Invasive Imaging Approach

Plaque analysis by means of CA is limited to residual luminal area, which accurateness can be strongly limited in case of suboptimal visualization due to vessel foreshortening or overlap with other coronary branches [8]. The introduction of dedicated software to make a 3D luminal reconstruction (3D QCA) merging data from the original angiographic projections, improved reproducibility, and accuracy of coronary obstruction evaluation, but did not solve the main limitations of this diagnostic approach [9, 10]. Indeed, CA does not provide any information about intrinsic plaque characteristics as dimension, composition, and evolution; all data that have been demonstrated to provide important prognostic information in several histological and clinical studies [11–13].

The better comprehension of individual CAD pathophysiology and detection of high-risk lesions that predispose to future cardiovascular events are the main goals of the hybrid imaging approach. Histological studies showed as plaques causing acute clinical events act with three principal mechanisms: plaque rupture, plaque erosion, and thrombosis in calcific nodules [14, 15]. Majority of these lesions have specific compositional features that together identify the so-called vulnerable plaque, also termed thin-capped fibroatheroma (TCFA). High plaque burden with large necrotic core, thin fibrous cap (defined <65 μm in thickness), positive vessel remodeling, macrophage infiltration (i.e., inflammation), cholesterol crystals, calcific nodules, and intra-plaque hemorrhages [14–17] are all features associated with an increased risk of acute coronary events. Notably, TCFA features are not necessarily correlated with severe stenosis at CA; this is consistent with the observation that myocardial infarction is often due to plaque rupture of nonobstructive lesions [11, 18]. Histological studies also revealed that the majority of events related to vulnerable plaques are clinically silent hesitating in spontaneous plaque healing and/or thrombus resolution. These observations moved the focus of imaging assessment from individual plaque to the whole disease activity across the coronary vasculature. Thus, the identification of TCFA features in the context of single plaque feeds hope that it could be possible to identify stenosis deserving treatment regardless of its severity at angiography. Whereas, the accurate individual evaluation of CAD burden would enable identification of patients requiring more aggressive therapies aiming to reduce the atherosclerosis progression [5].

Finally, diagnostic imaging modalities that can reliably describe the pattern of coronary atherosclerosis could also monitor changes of plaque morphology in response to intensive pharmacotherapy, also those currently undergoing preclinical or clinical evaluation (e.g., statin therapy) [19].

6.3 Adjuvant Imaging Techniques for Invasive Cardiologist

Although noninvasive imaging techniques are more indicated for a more complete valuation of CAD extension in the whole coronary vasculature, at the present invasive imaging techniques have higher spatial resolution and result more accurate in terms of tissue components differentiation and plaque architecture. Invasive imaging techniques are therefore frequently used as a research tool to better assess CAD, and its ability in high-risk plaque discrimination has been validated in several clinical studies [20, 21].

Table 6.1 reports the properties of invasive imaging techniques currently used in combination with coronary angiography. Intravascular ultrasound (IVUS) and optical coherence tomog-

Table 6.1 Main properties of the existing invasive imaging methodologies used in combination with coronary angiography

	Accurate lumen assessment	Outer wall dimension (plaque burden)	Accurate 3D coronary anatomy reconstruction	Plaque micro-components analysis	Plaque phenotype identification (vulnerable plaques)	Coronary flow physiology assessment	Correlation with histology	Clinically validated
IVUS	✓✓✓	✓✓✓	✓	✓✓	✓✓	✓	✓✓	✓✓✓
OCT	✓✓✓	✓	✓	✓✓✓	✓✓	✓	✓✓	✓✓
NIRS	×	×	×	✓	✓	×	✓✓	✓
CTCA	✓✓	✓✓✓	✓✓✓	✓	✓✓	✓	✓	✓

✓ weak to excellent ability of the modality to detect this specific parameter; × the modality is unable to detect this parameter or no data are available

IVUS intravascular ultrasound, *OCT* optical coherence tomography, *NIRS* near-infrared spectroscopy, *CTCA* computed tomography coronary angiography

raphy (OCT) are the imaging techniques more frequently utilized to integrate data obtained with CA. More recently also NIRS is emerging as a potential adjunctive tool for hybrid imaging in this context [12]. A brief mention deserves also the computed tomography coronary angiography (CTCA) that with its widespread use constitutes frequently the preliminary screening exams before CA. Albeit it is a noninvasive imaging tool, in its category it is nowadays the only technique applied to define the plaque characteristics and to evaluate atherosclerosis progression/regression [22, 23]. In daily practice data from CTCA are frequently used to guide the interpretation and treatment of stenosis observed at CA.

6.4 Intravasculr Ultrasound (IVUS)

Intravascular ultrasound (IVUS) is the first in vivo imaging modality used to assess both the lumen and the vessel wall contours of coronary arteries. Today it still represents the most widely used intravascular imaging modality and the most validated in clinical studies.

This imaging modality is based on the emission of sound waves by means of a piezoelectric transducer at a frequency of 20–70 MHz; the reflected waves are received, amplified, and converted into grey-scale images with an axial and lateral resolution of 70–200 μm and 200–250 μm, respectively [24]. Practically, the IVUS catheter is retracted over a standard 0.014″ guidewire according to automatic (0.5–1.0 mm/s) or manual pullback. The result is presented in the forms of cross-sectional images and longitudinal views allowing the identification of lumen, the outer vessel wall, and plaque burden (Fig. 6.1).

Initially, IVUS has been extensively used to assess coronary lesion severity and to obtain a proper measure of vessel size. Indeed, while in a CA-guided procedure the vessel size is inferred from the lumen of the nearest largest coronary segment (i.e., reference vessel diameter), using the IVUS is possible for a more accurate evaluation of the original vessel size using the media-to-media distance. Several studies demonstrated as coronary vessel size estimation significantly varies between CA and IVUS, especially in case of severe and diffuse disease [25, 26]. In a head-to-head comparison a difference ≥ 1.0 mm was found in 71% for vessel sizes <2.75 mm in diameter and in 49% for >2.75 mm, respectively [25]. Thus, the first clinical application of IVUS was the guidance for percutaneous coronary intervention in terms of stent size selection, stent expansion, and adequate stent strut apposition [27].

Recognizing the potential clinical implication of this imaging technique, in the following years, an effort was made to improve the resolution and details of images. Indeed, grey-scale IVUS did not allow the assessment of atheromatous plaque components: echo-lucent signal could be the

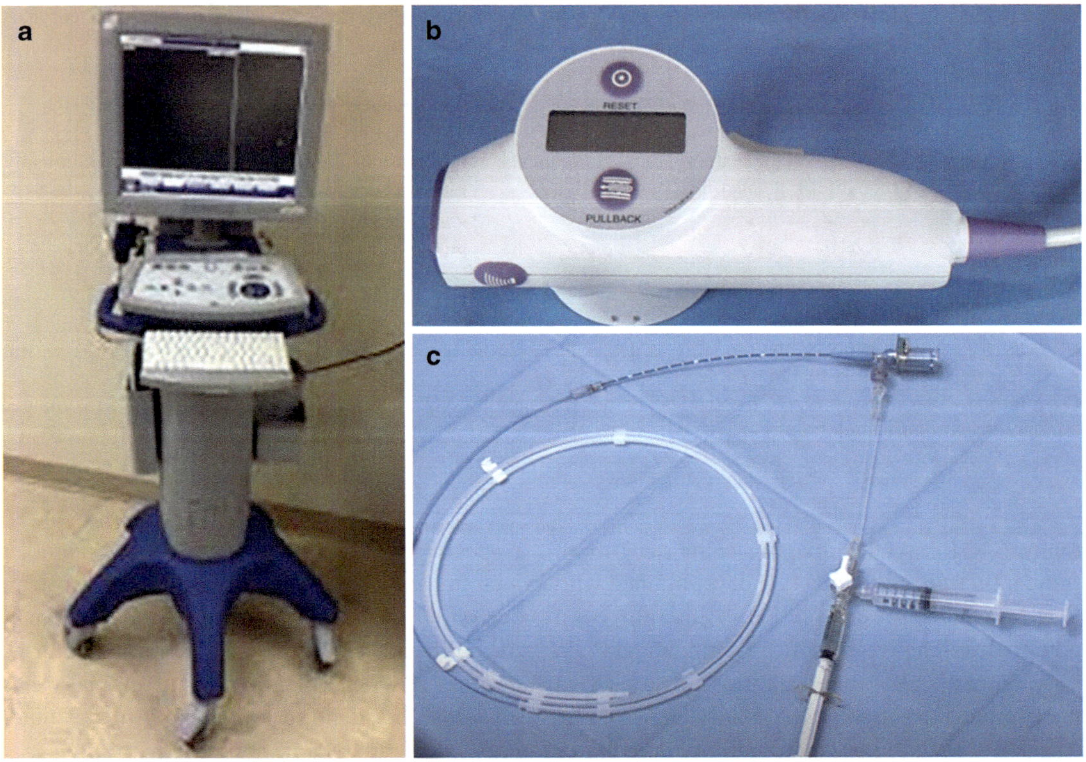

Fig. 6.1 IntraVascular Ultra Sound (IVUS) system (Volcano®, Philips, San Diego CA, USA) including console (**a**), mechanical rotation pullback device (**b**), and a 3.3F imaging catheter (**c**) containing optical fiber to deliver intravascular ultrasound (IVUS)

result of both a high lipid content or smooth cells hyperplasia, as well as acoustic shadow could be determined both by calcium deposit or necrotic tissue [28]. As a result, any attempt to describe plaque components or atherosclerosis evolution was strongly limited by a wide interobserver variability [29].

6.4.1 Plaque/Tissue Assessment

Grey-scale IVUS limitations have been partially addressed with the introduction of radiofrequency analysis of the IVUS backscatter signal. This approach, based on the measurement of the amplitude and the frequency of the IVUS signal, provides incremental information about plaque morphology and tissue components. The main processing systems adopting this approach are virtual histology (VH-IVUS) and integrated backscatter (IB-IVUS); at present, most clinical data has been generated with VH-IVUS which has been extensively used to assess plaque phenotype and study atherosclerotic evolution [11, 30, 31].

VH-IVUS utilizes a color code to identify four different plaque tissue components: white for dense calcium, dark green for fibrotic tissue, light green for fibro-fatty tissue, and red for necrotic core (Fig. 6.2). Albeit VH-IVUS studies showed an excellent correlation with histology [32], its accuracy sensibly decreases in detecting large necrotic core [33]. Indeed, also the latest VH-IVUS system (45 MHz) showed a 76.7% accuracy of IVUS-VH in detecting all tissue types [34]. Also, IB-IVUS showed a high agreement with histology in plaque tissue characterization [35],.in particular for the identification of

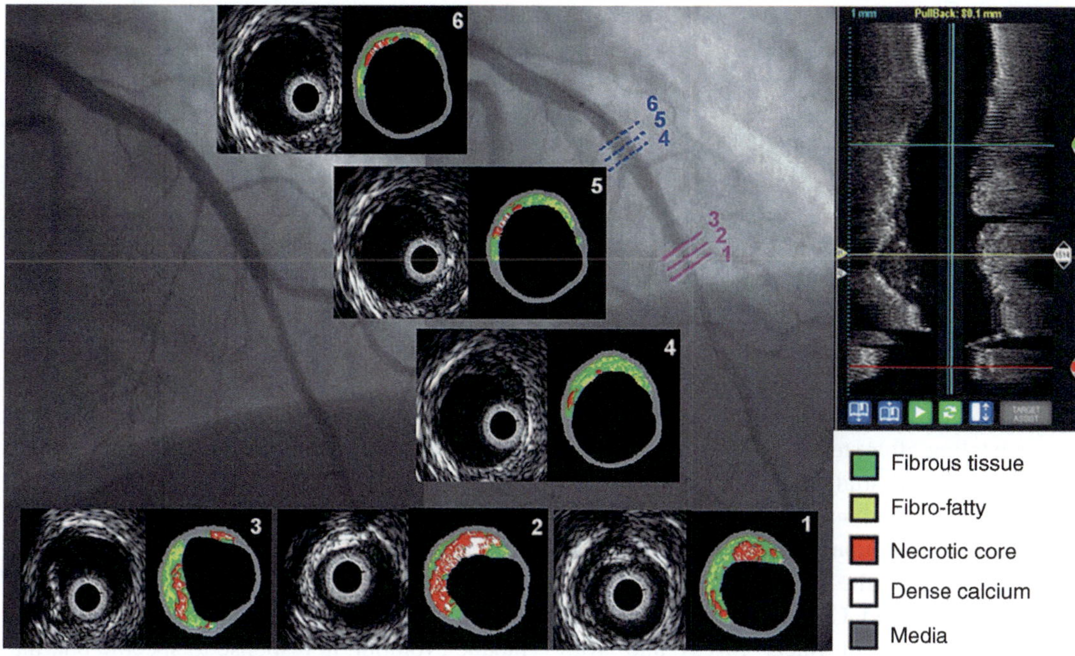

Fig. 6.2 Example of IVUS imaging application in patient with recent effort angina. Coronary angiography reveals intermediate stenosis in the mid-left anterior descending artery (*). Comparative analysis between GS-IVUS and VH-IVUS allows to differentiate fibrotic plaque (segments 4–6) from fibro-calcific plaque (segments 2 and 3) and vulnerable plaque (segment 1) according to the lipid content close to the lumen

lipid tissue of vulnerable plaques [36]. Nevertheless, albeit IB-IVUS showed higher accuracy in the assessment of plaque components when compared to VH-IVUS [37], it resulted less efficient when compared to OCT; thus, its use in clinical and research areas is limited [38].

Current IVUS probes provide high-resolution tomographic images of the coronary vessel. The detection of interface between media and adventitia and lumen contours allows an estimation of plaque burden expressed as the ratio between lumen area and vessel cross-sectional area. Moreover, VH-IVUS gives important information about prevalent plaque composition and may help in identifying plaque with complex morphology (e.g., necrotic core) that could be prone to rupture and progression. On the other hand, the low accuracy in complex lesions, the not infrequent presence of artifact, and the limited image resolution represent important limitations of an IVUS-based approach for the identification of vulnerable plaques.

6.4.2 Fluid-Dynamic Assessment

By means of fusion of angiography and IVUS images is possible to obtain an accurate vessel architecture and blood flow pattern reconstruction, but it requires the implementation of a specific protocol in the catheterization laboratory.

Coronary movements during cardiac cycles, extraction of the luminal position of IVUS probe during pullback, and the orientation of luminal contours onto luminal centreline are only examples of obstacles to overcome during the matching between these two imaging techniques.

The current validated approach is based on: (1) identification of luminal centreline using biplane angiography acquisition of target vessel including visualization of IVUS probe and lumen contours at the beginning and at the end of pullback; (2) identification of the end-diastolic IVUS frames using an ECG-gated acquisition; (3) sequential triangulation algorithm to place the IVUS borders perpendicular to the vessel centreline and correct their relative twist; (4) use of fiduciary anatomical landmark (e.g., side branch), visible with both imaging techniques, to align images orientation [39].

This complex and articulated method allows a reliable 3D coronary reconstruction in terms of vessel geometry, luminal definition, atheroma burden quantification, and endothelial shear stress (ESS) distribution [39]. This approach has been validated both in ex vivo and in vivo studies and broadly used to identify anatomical determinants of plaque progression and destabilization in native vessels and patterns of neointima healing after stent implantation [40, 41]. The only clinical study exploring the implications of local hemodynamic force on atherosclerotic disease evolution was the PREDICTION (The Prediction of the Progression of Coronary Artery Disease and Clinical Outcomes Using Vascular Profiling of Shear Stress and Wall Morphology) trial. In this study fusion of angiographic images and IVUS data was performed in order to reconstruct artery anatomy and blood flow pattern. According to the PREDICTION study, high plaque burden and low ESS identify lesions that will require treatment with a positive predictive value of 41% [42].

Still, in terms of ESS quantification, several limitations persist; indeed, the model currently used does not incorporate a side branch in the final reconstructed model. An alternative approach including the side branch reconstruction using ostium visualized on IVUS pullback and vessel geometry obtained with angiography has been proposed but required to be validated [43, 44].

6.4.3 Clinical Implication of CA-IVUS Hybrid Imaging

The good predictive accuracies of VH-IVUS for all tissue components supported the design of prospective large clinical studies in which VH-IVUS was utilized to identify vulnerable plaques. The VH-IVUS in Vulnerable Atherosclerosis (VIVA), including either stable and acute patients, identified TCFA and plaque burden ≥70% as the only plaque characteristics associated with following major cardiovascular events (MACE, composite of death, myocardial infarction, and unplanned revascularization) risk [31]. Consistently, also the PROSPECT (A Prospective Natural-History Study of Coronary Atherosclerosis) study reported plaque burden >70%, minimal luminal area <4.0 mm^2, and TCFA as an independent predictor of MACE; while non fibro-atheroma plaques appeared to be stable and clinically silent [11]. Finally, in the more recent ATHEROREMO-IVUS (The European Collaborative Project on Inflammation and Vascular Wall Remodelling in Atherosclerosis—Intravascular Ultrasound Study) study VH-TCFA and PB > 70% were identified as independent predictors of plaque-related MACE, including death and acute coronary syndromes [45].

The IVUS has been also applied to assess plaque evolution in response to specific pharmacological treatment. The Reversing Atherosclerosis with Aggressive Lipid Lowering (REVERSAL), the SATURN (Study of Coronary Atheroma by Intravascular Ultrasound: Effect of Rosuvastatin Versus Atorvastatin) and IBIS-4 (Integrated Biomarkers and Imaging Study-4) studies demonstrated as plaque regression is related to the lower level of low-density lipoprotein cholesterol (LDL-C) [46–48], providing the biological proof of correlation between high level of LDL-C and risk of future coronary events. The same beneficial effect on plaque composition has been observed in a trial evaluating the effect of blood pressure reduction and anti-atherosclerotic drug therapy. According to these studies, reduction in necrotic core and concomitant increase in fibrous tissue volumes are the expression of plaque stabilization [49–51].

6.5 Optical Coherence Tomography (OCT)

Albeit IVUS imaging improved the interpretation of CA findings in terms of vessel geometry reconstruction, plaque burden quantification, and intraluminal residual area, its introduction did not represent a significant improvement in the interpretation of plaque vulnerability. Indeed, the spatial resolution of IVUS did not allow the identification of vessel wall components or the micro-characteristics of complex plaques (Table 6.2).

Conversely, the Optical Coherence Tomography (OCT) technology with its unprecedented resolution approximates histology in the assessment of coronary vessel lumen and wall pathology. Utilized in interventional cardiology since late 1990s, this imaging modality utilizes echoes of near-infrared light to generate images of coronary arterial walls. The use of backscattered light instead of sound waves guarantees a superior spatial resolution (axial 10–15 μm and lateral resolution 20–30 μm) coupled with faster data acquisition (35 mm/s) but a limited penetration capacity (2–3 mm) [52].

Practically, the OCT catheter is advanced over a standard 0.014″ guidewire and an automated pullback is activated simultaneously with intracoronary contrast injection to eliminate scatter artifacts due to blood cells. The need for blood displacement constitutes also the main limitation of this technique: indeed, it causes a need for higher contrast dye volume (about 14–20 mL for any imaging acquisition) and limits its use in aorto-ostial segment (e.g., left main), where the incomplete vessel engagement by guiding catheter usually prevent adequate imaging acquisition (Fig. 6.3). Any attempt to replace contrast injection with other dyes (e.g., dextran or saline) failed in obtaining a good imaging quality or low rate of complications (e.g., arrhythmias).

Due to its safety in the context of coronary angiography [53], OCT is currently a powerful research tool used to assess plaque morphology and evaluate stenting procedure results. Current dedicated OCT software allows online revision both in axial (cross-section) and longitudinal views, and the 3D navigation in the vessel lumen (Fig. 6.4).

During the diagnostic phase, OCT contributes to the identification and interpretation of the culprit lesion, especially in the acute setting. Indeed, an expert eye could be able to identify the cause of acute coronary syndrome (e.g., plaque rupture or erosion) and differentiates the thrombus associated with the culprit lesion in white (platelet rich) or red (platelet poor) on the basis of backscatter and attenuation properties. Moreover, OCT has a proven efficacy in detecting vulnerable plaques [54, 55]. Indeed, OCT allows the evaluation of main histologic features of plaque vulnerability such as thin fibrous caps, large lipid cores, presence of macrophages [56], neovascularization [57], and micro-calcifications [58].

Table 6.2 Advantages and limitations of the existing invasive imaging methodologies in assessing plaque characteristics

	Plaque burden	Lipid tissue	Calcific tissue	Cap thickness	Macrophages	Cholesterol crystal	Neovessel	Thrombus
IVUS(-VH)	✓✓✓	✓	✓✓✓	✓	×	×	×	✓
OCT	✓✓	✓✓	✓✓	✓✓	✓	✓	✓	✓✓✓
NIRS	×	✓✓✓	×	×	×	×	×	×
IVUS-OCT	✓✓✓	✓✓✓	✓✓✓	✓✓	✓	✓	✓	✓✓✓
IVUS-NIRS	✓✓✓	✓✓✓	✓✓✓	×	×	×	×	✓
OCT-NIRS	✓✓	✓✓✓	✓✓	✓✓	✓	✓	✓	✓✓✓
OCT-NIRF	✓✓	✓✓	✓✓	✓✓	✓✓✓	✓	✓	✓✓✓
IVUS-NIRF	✓✓✓	✓	✓✓✓	×	✓✓✓	✓	✓	✓
IVPA-IVUS	✓✓✓	✓✓	✓✓✓	×	✓✓	×	×	✓

✓ *weak to* excellent ability of the modality to detect this specific parameter; × the modality is unable to detect this parameter or no data are available

IVUS intravascular ultrasound, *OCT* optical coherence tomography, *NIRS* near-infrared spectroscopy, *NIRF* near-infrared fluorescence, *IVPA* intravascular photoacoustic

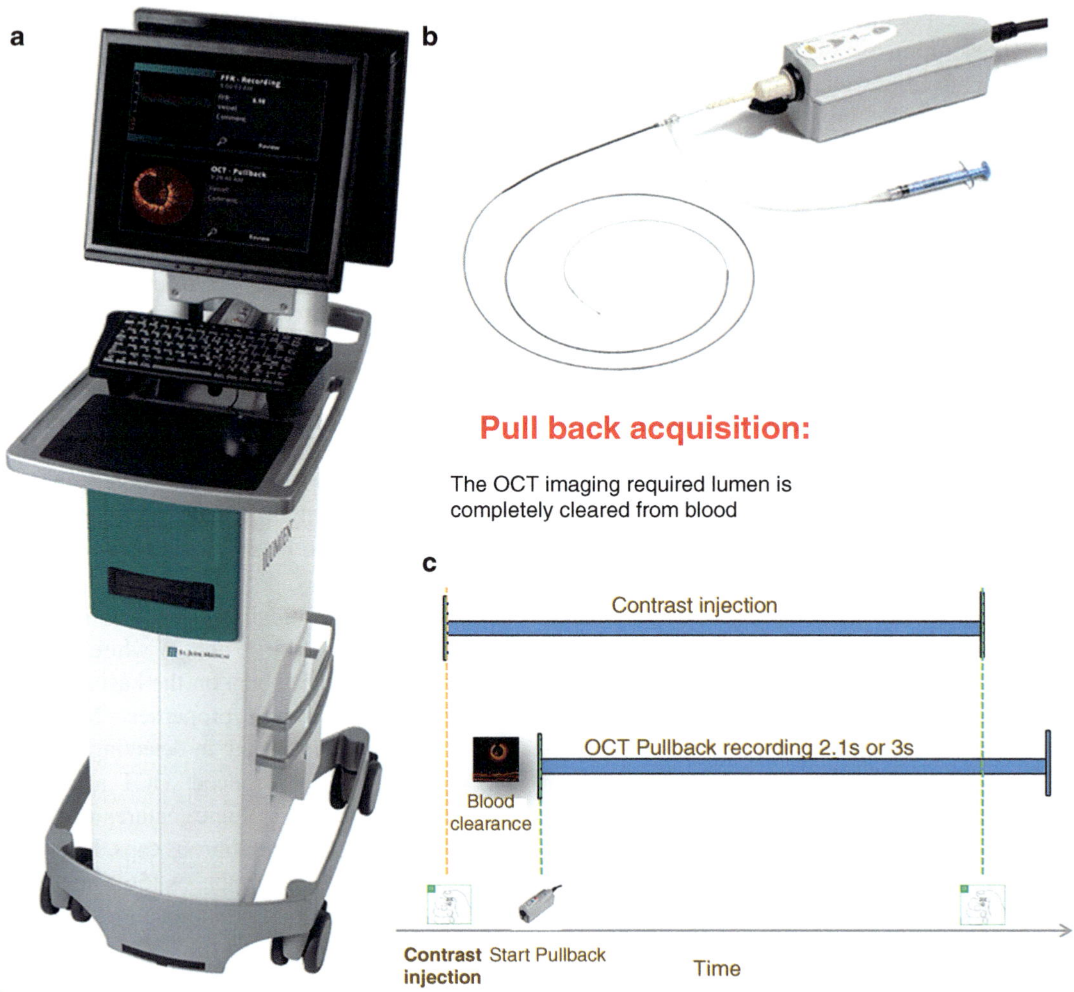

Fig. 6.3 Optical coherence tomography (OCT) system (OPTIS system, St. Jude Medical, St. Paul, MN, USA) including console (**a**), mechanical rotation pullback device and 2.7F imaging catheter (**b**). Differently from other invasive imaging technique, OCT requires complete blood displacement before acquisition by means of contrast dye injection (**c**)

6.5.1 Plaque/Tissue Assessment

Several studies have demonstrated a high correlation between OCT and histology for all tissue types [38]. Fibrous plaque appears as a signal-rich homogeneous lesion, fibro-calcific plaque as a signal-poor one with sharply demarcated borders, and lipid-rich plaque as a signal-poor lesion but with diffuse borders and sudden drop-off on OCT signal [21]. In particular, OCT is the preferred imaging technique to estimate the thickness of intima and media layers [59–62]. In particular, cap thickness is a strong predictor of plaque vulnerability and a value of ≤65 μm in thickness is the cut-off used to define TCFA. Nevertheless, there is no general agreement about the TCFA cut-off predicting higher rupture risk. In this context, the OCT could be also used to test the efficacy of pharmacological preventive treatment. Indeed, the OCT has been used to evaluate the effect of different statin therapy regimens on fibrous cap thickness evolution in culprit lesions [63].

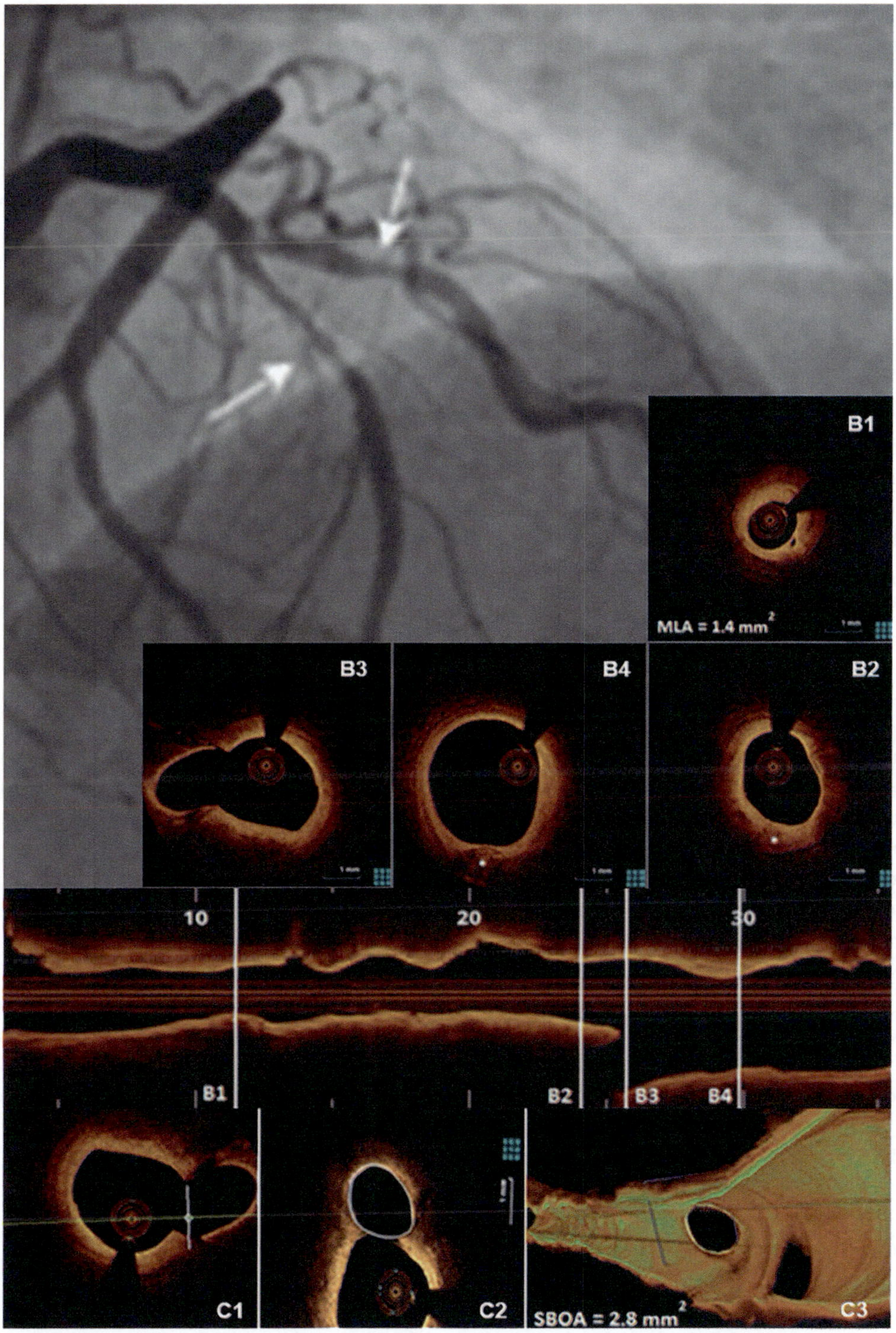

Fig. 6.4 Example of OCT imaging application in a patient with chronic stable angina. Coronary angiography reveals a severe stenosis at the level of mid-left anterior descending artery bifurcation (arrows). OCT imaging of the main vessel demonstrated a fibro-calcific plaque with MLA of 1.4 mm^2 (B1) distal to bifurcation, and small calcific deposits at level of bifurcation (B2, B4, asterisks). Side branch ostium area was estimated at 2.8 mm^2 using both cross-sectional and three-dimensional OCT cut-plane analyses (C1–C3)

On the other hand, OCT shows important limitations in the assessment of deeply embedded tissues. Indeed, OCT has a limited penetration (~2 mm) often preventing visualization of adventitia, especially in a larger or heavily diseased vessel [64, 65]. Thus, its accuracy sensibly decreases in presence of highly attenuating structures (e.g., thick fibrous cap) or backscattering elements (lipid or calcific nodules) [66].

Several comparison studies with histology confirmed the possibility to identify intra-plaque cellular components and active inflammation using OCT.

Thrombus—The OCT can be considered the gold standard for the detection and quantification of luminal thrombus. In particular, OCT is able to differentiate red and white thrombi with high sensitivity and specificity (90% and 88%, respectively): a high backscattering intraluminal mass with a shadowing behind defines a red thrombus, while a signal-rich low backscattering intraluminal mass is proper of white thrombi [67]. The association of thrombus with fibrous cap alteration or erupted calcific nodules is typically pathognomonic of destabilized plaques [68, 69]. Thus, the OCT showed higher accuracy in detecting culprit lesion for acute coronary events when compared to other invasive imaging techniques.

Macrophages—Macrophage accumulation appears at OCT as bright spots within the context of atherosclerotic plaque. The presence of high-intensity signal would be the expression of vascular inflammation, meaning of active atherosclerotic process. Macrophage in its activated form, the foam cell, can cause degradation of the extracellular components of the fibrous cap, leading to its weakening, thinning, and therefore favoring its rupture. Notwithstanding, several attempts, including also dedicated software [70, 71], OCT did not appear as accurate in macrophage identification as initially hypothesized. Nevertheless, most studies showed as the accuracy for detection of macrophage accumulation increased when bright spots are overlaying TCFA. In this context, macrophages' presence is associated with worse outcome [13].

Cholesterol Crystals—Cholesterol crystals represent a marker of vulnerable atherosclerotic lesions and appear at OCT like linear signal-rich steak usually within a lipid pool [58]. Cholesterol crystals could be responsible for mechanically induced fibrous cap rupture [72, 73]. However, the accuracy of cholesterol crystal identification has not been formally examined yet.

Neovascularization—Intravascular neovessel are defined as small black holes with a diameter ranging from 50 to 300 μm visible in three consecutive cross sections [74]. Nevertheless, the OCT had low sensitivity and specificity in detecting plaque neo-revascularization when compared to histology. Albeit potentially useful to study plaque evolution, the clinical significance of intra-plaque neo-revascularization is unknown [75].

6.5.2 Fluid-Dynamic Assessment

Fusion between CA images and OCT-based vessel reconstruction has been tested to define intravascular endothelial shear stress (ESS) patterns and understand the implication of hemodynamic forces on plaque micro-characteristics.

Adopting the same methodological approach proposed for the fusion of CA and IVUS fusion, computational fluid-dynamic models were calculated by merging data from biplane angiography and intraluminal plaque distribution [76–79]. Coronary blood flow (mL/s) was calculated directly from the time required for blood displacement during contrast dye injection, while ESS was calculated as the product of blood viscosity and the gradient of blood velocity at the wall. According to these models, coronary segments exposed to low ESS have a larger lipid burden, thinner fibrous cap, and higher incidence of TCFA [79].

These studies confirmed the possibility to obtain a geometrically correct vessel reconstruction and a high accuracy in the detection of segments exposed to low ESS. In particular, the presence of lower ESS was observed in the region of ruptured plaque suggesting a key role of flow patterns in the formation of vulnerable lesions [79]. This technique was also used to examine the correlation between flow forces and neo-intima or neo-atherosclerosis formation [80, 81].

However, this approach did not have broad diffusion in clinical practice or research field. Systole-diastole vessel variations, longitudinal movement of OCT probe during pullback, variable orientation of OCT frames [76], and presence of side branches not included in the OCT pullback [82, 83] are the main limitations of this methodology, still not adequately validated.

6.5.3 Clinical Implication of CA-OCT Hybrid Imaging

Being rupture/erosion of vulnerable plaques is the most frequent cause of the acute coronary syndrome, the possibility to identify plaques with such a vulnerable profile could represent a promising approach to prevent clinical events. Nevertheless, the clinical evidence favoring an OCT-based plaque assessment is limited to a few small studies [84, 85]. In particular, a recent prospective international registry showed that the risk of plaque progression is correlated with the number of OCT features of vulnerability. In this study collecting 1776 lipid plaques the simultaneous presence of MLA <3.5 mm^2, FCT <75 μm, lipid arc circumferential extension >180°, and macrophage infiltration was an independent predictor of 1-year event. Thus, this registry suggests the possibility to use an OCT grading to identify patients at higher risk of acute coronary events [13]. If this micro-plaque characterization could have an additive value in predicting high-risk vulnerable plaque when compared to a traditional patient's clinical risk profile remains to be proved.

6.6 Near-infrared Spectroscopy (NIRS)

Near-infrared spectroscopy (NIRS) is the last intravascular imaging technique for the study of coronary atherosclerosis approved for clinical use. In this technology, the imaging is obtained analyzing the infrared light reflection by the vessel wall in terms of intensity and wavelength. The NIRS is based on the principle of variable absorption and scattering of near-infrared light by different molecules; this characteristic makes NIRS the only imaging technique able to assess the plaque chemical composition. In other words, while IVUS and OCT can only infer the plaque composition on the basis of signal attenuation (not specific for a single tissue), NIRS can identify plaque components on the basis of its specific spectral signature. In particular, NIRS has high accuracy in the detection of the intra-plaque lipid cores (LCP) and of depleted collagen in fibrous caps [86, 87]. Thus, NIRS provides important information about possible plaque vulnerability.

The results are displayed on a "chemogram" showing the probability of the presence of a lipid-rich plaque: area containing lipid core are represented as yellow and those without lipid core as red. In NIRS validation studies, LCP of interest was defined as a lipid core >200 μm in thickness, >60° in circumferential extent, and with a fibrous cap of thickness <450 μm. The system also reports the lipid-core burden index (LCBI), a quantitative measurement which represents the fraction of yellow pixels whose probability of lipid exceeds 0.6, per 1000 [88]. By convention, the quantitative metric of the lipid core is computed over a 4 mm width windows within explored segments (maxLCBI4mm).

6.6.1 Plaque/Tissue Assessment

NIRS has been extensively tested in an experimental model and also in humans appear as the best invasive imaging modality for the identification of fibro-atheroma [88–90] with a reported sensitivity and specificity >90%. Unfortunately, when used as a single imaging technique NIRS has important limitations: (1) it does not give information about plaque components other than lipid; (2) NIRS does not assess lumen contours or outer vessel dimension preventing plaque burden quantification; (3) it does not localize the lipid components within the plaque and does not give information about the presence of TCFA. This explains why NIRS is not largely used in experimental studies on atherosclerosis and in the clinical area.

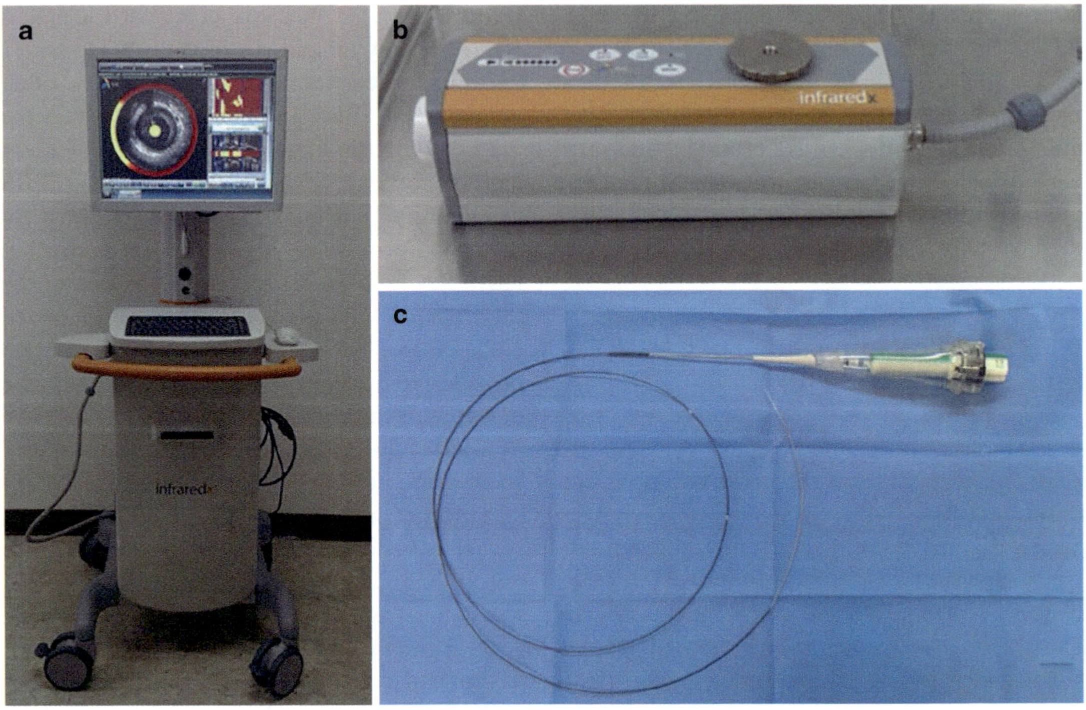

Fig. 6.5 Near-infrared (NIR) spectroscopy system (TVC®, InfraReDx, Burlington, MA, USA) including console (**a**), mechanical rotation pullback device (**b**), and a 3.2F imaging catheter (**c**) containing optical fiber to deliver both NIR light and intravascular ultrasound (IVUS)

To overcome these limitations, efforts were made to develop dual-probe imaging catheters allowing simultaneous assessment of plaque with two complementary imaging modalities [91]. For clinical use, NIRS technology is currently available in combination with IVUS. The NIRS-IVUS system (TVC Insight Coronary Imaging Catheter, InfraRedX, Burlington, MA, USA) includes a scanning NIR laser and a traditional IVUS-sized catheter (Fig. 6.5). The NIRS-IVUS catheter is compatible with a 0.014-inch guidewire and 6F guiding catheter, and both IVUS images and NIRS measurements are co-registered during an automatic pullback acquired at speeds of 0.5, 1.0, or 2.0 mm/s for a maximum imaging length of 15 cm [92]. This hybrid imaging modality combines the resolution and penetration of IVUS with the LCP quantification of NIRS (Fig. 6.6); as a result, the identification of necrotic core or lipid pools is more accurate than with traditional grey-scale IVUS [89].

A combined NIRS-OCT catheter has also been developed and tested in an ex vivo setting. Since the OCT has a spatial resolution capable of detecting inflammatory cells (i.e., macrophages) and fibrous cap thickness, the integration with NIRS could further discriminate the identified LRP on the basis of inflammatory activity [91]. Indeed, in the experimental setting, this prototype showed a detailed and comprehensive imaging assessment of vessel wall morphology and pathophysiology [92].

6.6.2 Fluid-Dynamic Assessment

The destabilization of atherosclerotic plaque is the leading cause of most acute coronary events. Among the local risk factors capable of determining plaque instability, plaque composition, and ESS have central roles. Intra-plaque lipid pool has been strongly associated with plaque vulner-

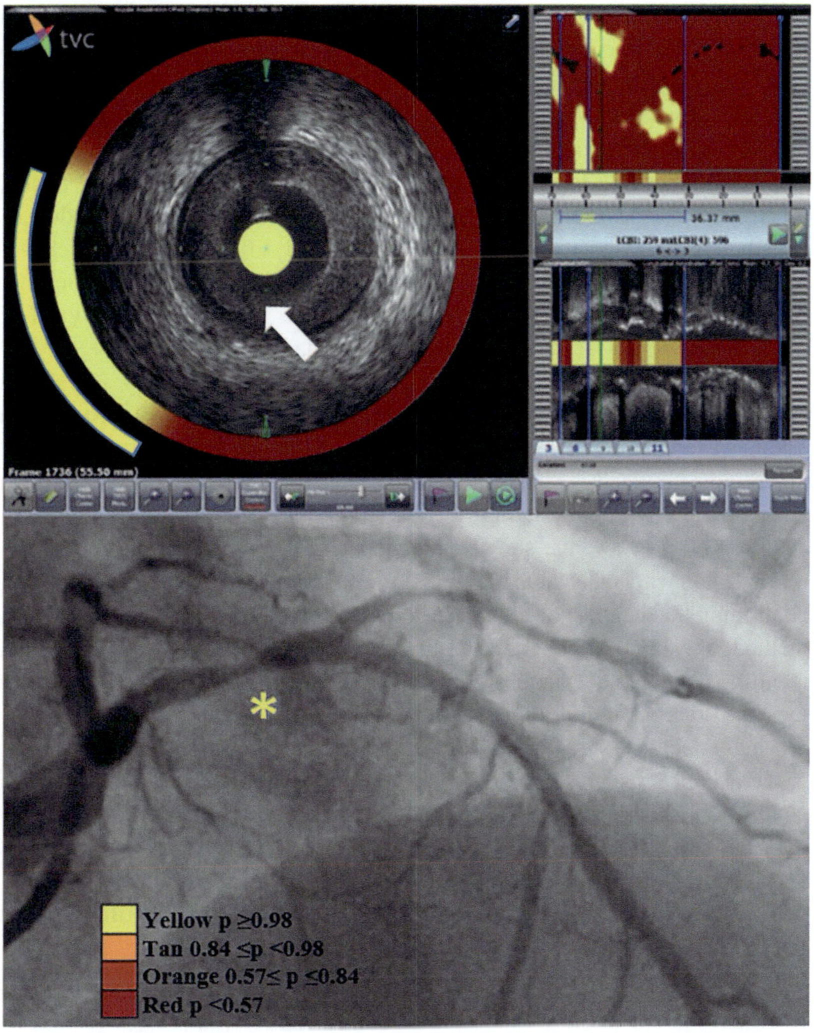

Fig. 6.6 Example of IVUS-NIRS imaging application in a patient with the acute coronary syndrome. Coronary angiography reveals significant stenosis in the proximal left anterior descending artery (*); NIRS shows a large lipid burden within the coronary artery wall (yellow line) localized from 7 to 10 o'clock at cross-sectional reconstruction; intravascular ultrasound (IVUS) shows the presence of plaque rupture (white arrow) at the same location

ability and clinical events [12, 93]. Similarly, a high ESS, the frictional force exerted by the bloodstream on the endothelium, at the level of plaque protruding in the lumen can accelerate the atherosclerosis progression and induce plaque rupture [80, 94].

The co-localization of LCP and ESS, and their synergistic effect on plaque destabilization has been explored and demonstrated in two in vivo studies merging angiography, NIRS, and Doppler wire pressure measurement [95, 96]. According to these studies, LCP co-localizes with exposure to high levels of ESS with a dose-dependent relation. In addition, coronary segments with high ESS showed greater progression of NIRS-derived LCBI and in some cases development of new LCP [95, 96]. Thus, the possibility to co-localize these two parameters could increase our ability to identify the future culprit lesions.

6.6.3 Clinical Implication of CA-NIRS Hybrid Imaging

Histological studies demonstrated as vulnerable lesions have a thin fibrous cap overlying a large necrotic core. Thus, the NIRS, integrated with IVUS or OCT could be the ideal imaging modality to identify plaque prone to rupture. In vivo, this hypothesis has been preliminarily tested in the COLOR registry demonstrating a correlation between vulnerable plaque morphology, assessed by NIRS, and degree of stenosis [97]. The possible clinical implication has then confirmed by the ATHEROREMO-NIRS (The European Collaborative Project on Inflammation and Vascular Wall Remodeling in Atherosclerosis—Near-Infrared Spectroscopy) trial, a sub-study of the ATHEROREMO-IVUS study showing a relationship of LCBI value with the primary clinical end-point both in stable and acute patients [98]. The most recent LRP (Lipid-Rich Plaque) study, a prospective multicentre registry to identify patients and coronary segments at higher risk of major adverse coronary events, showed a higher event rate in lesion with analyzable maxLCBI4mm > 400 confirming the diagnostic value of the NIRS-IVUS methodology [12]. Although the ability of NIRS to identify vulnerable plaques and patients at increased risk of future events has now been convincingly demonstrated, the consequent preventive or therapeutic strategies remain to be determined.

Other relevant implications of a NIRS-based hybrid imaging include the possibility to perform a precise lesion treatment (limited to segments with a high lipid-core burden), and predict the risk of iatrogenic embolization of lipid deposition during revascularization [99].

Finally, the NiRS-IVUS technology could be a tool for monitoring the effect of new pharmacological therapies, such as statins and PCSK9-inhibitors on the lipid burden. Indeed, the YELLOW (Reduction in Yellow Plaque by Aggressive Lipid-Lowering Therapy) trials suggest a significantly higher LCBI4mm reduction in patients undergoing intensive lipid-lowering regimens [100, 101].

6.7 Computed Tomography Coronary Angiography (CTCA)

Computed tomographic coronary angiography (CTCA) represents an attractive noninvasive alternative for the study of coronary atherosclerosis. Several comparative studies showed that CTCA is able to evaluate luminal and outer wall contours of coronary vessels with an accuracy comparable to intravascular imaging techniques [102, 103].

CTCA showed good accuracy in the identification of calcific tissue, but a limited discriminatory capacity in differentiating lipid and fibrotic tissues. A lipid-rich core appears as a low attenuation density area but CTCA resolution is insufficient to identify a TCFA [104, 105].

6.7.1 Plaque/Tissue Assessment

Notwithstanding its limitation in plaque morphology assessment, CTCA would seem able to identify vulnerable lesions; plaque burden, positive remodeling, and napkin ring sign are the elements indicating high-risk plaques prone to progress and cause acute cardiovascular events [106–108]. In particular, the napkin ring—defined as a circular rim of contrast enhancement surrounding the coronary plaque—appears to be the expression of an active inflammation and specific for TFCA [106].

6.7.2 Fluid-Dynamic Assessment

In terms of hybrid imaging, the CTCA allows the reconstruction of the entire coronary tree (Fig. 6.7), complete atherosclerosis burden assessment, and a more accurate 3D vessel reconstruction including also fluid-dynamic parameters (i.e., ESS). Fusion between CTCA and IVUS has been tested and showed advantages in terms of vessel geometry representation, inclusion of side branches (for ESS computing), and accurate rotational alignment with intravascular images [109]. The hybrid reconstruction has been successfully used to compute ESS and to assess its role both in atherosclerotic plaque progression and vessel wall healing post percutaneous coronary revascularization [110]. The main limitation to this approach is that it requires three techniques (CTCA, CA, and IVUS) and similarly to the other reconstruction process is too laborious and time-demanding.

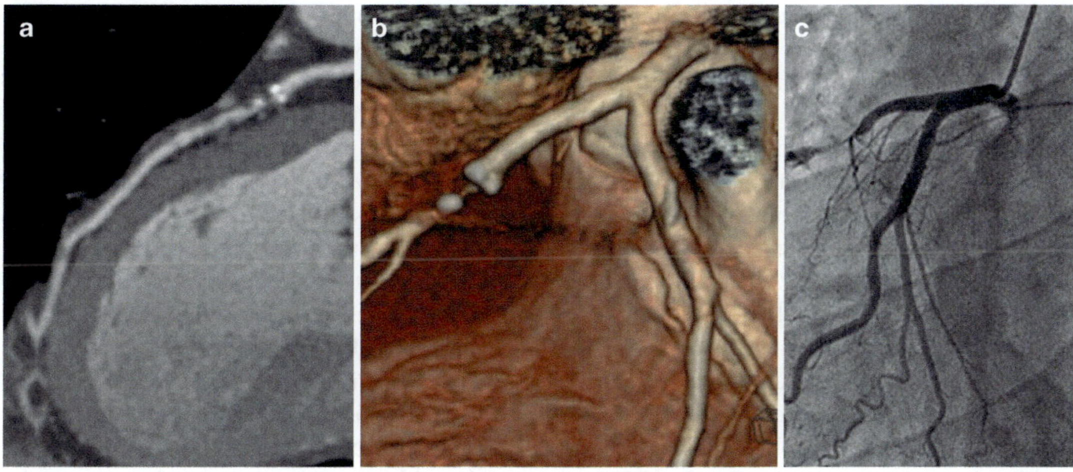

Fig. 6.7 Example of 2D (**a**) and 3D (**b**) vessel reconstruction by CTCA in patient with unstable angina. Coronary angiography (**c**) confirmed the presence of sub-occlusive stenosis of proximal left anterior descending artery

6.7.3 Clinical Implication of CTCA-IVUS-CA Hybrid Imaging

Co-registration of IVUS and CTCA offers the potential for a direct comparison of invasive and noninvasive techniques both in assessing lumen and vessel wall dimensions and in characterizing plaque morphology [102–104]. Notably, CTCA studies showed a high prevalence of high-risk plaques but a prognostic power correlated to total atherosclerotic coronary burden more than to the single complex plaque [111, 112].

Nevertheless, the sensitivity and specificity of these CTCA parameters are variables among the studies and limited data are available on the efficacy of CTCA in detecting vulnerable lesions in patient with established CAD who may benefit from invasive imaging techniques. Thus, if CTCA could be a valid alternative to the invasive imaging techniques for the identification of high-risk plaques, especially in acute patients, remains to be defined.

6.8 The Future of Hydrid Invasive Imaging

Fusion of multiple imaging techniques, taking the best from each and integrating the different information in unique multi-coronary imaging, would represent the natural evolution of invasive hybrid imaging. For example, the fusion of OCT and IVUS could guarantee increased tissue penetration and an accurate plaque components characterization. Table 6.2 summarizes the main advantages and limitations of the existing intravascular imaging methodologies both as a single technique or in hybrid combinations.

Several histology-based studies have demonstrated that combined intravascular imaging provides a more reliable characterization of plaque composition and atherosclerosis evolution [113, 114]. Thus, a hybrid imaging approach could give operators more precise quantitative information (e.g., plaque volume and extension, fibroatheroma vulnerability) useful for treatment guidance.

Different attempts have been made to develop a software system that permits off-line integration of data acquired from different imaging techniques, or dual-probe catheters, able to perform simultaneous multimodality imaging.

All attempts to create user-friendly software have had limited application in research requiring specific acquisition protocols (e.g., biplane angiography), and extensive human interaction in multiple reconstruction steps. Moreover, there are concerns about safety of use of multiple invasive imaging in clinical practice. Indeed, although some reports about the feasibility of combined imaging exist, no clinical advantages have been demonstrated [115].

Regarding simultaneous multimodality imaging, there are many other imaging techniques developed to provide additional information about vessel pathology and biology. These modalities have been combined with IVUS or OCT in dual-probe catheters that are currently under clinical or preclinical evaluation. At present, IVUS-NIRS is the only hybrid imaging catheter approved for clinical use; its role in the detection of unstable plaque and vulnerable patient has been recently demonstrated in the LRP trial [12]. Other possible combinations currently under evaluation are: (1) IVUS-OCT combination (FDA approved); (2) OCT-NIRS; (3) IVUS-near-infrared fluorescence (NIRF); (4) the OCT-NIRF; (5) IVUS-intravascular photoacoustic (IVPA); and (6) the IVUS-time resolved fluorescence spectroscopy catheter.

6.9 Conclusion

In the last two decades, several invasive imaging modalities have been developed to improve the ability in CAD diagnosis and to increase comprehension of atherosclerosis physiopathology. Specific miniaturized catheters have been designed to obtain high-resolution cross-sectional images of vessels and plaques. When compared to CA, these techniques led to a more accurate assessment of atherosclerotic coronary burden in a non-culprit vessel and plaque composition especially in the early stage of disease (e.g., intermediate lesion). This more comprehensive visualization opened new frontiers of research toward the assessment of mechanisms that regulate plaque composition and progression; it includes the study of fluid dynamics and ESS in normal and diseased vessels.

Some of these invasive imaging modalities are currently used in clinical practice, while others remain restricted to research applications. Each technique has unique advantages but also limitations that do not permit a complete visualization of the vessel wall pathology with a single imaging approach. In particular, none of the invasive imaging modalities currently available is able to portray the 3D vessel geometry.

To overcome this drawback, several hybrid attempts, merging data from two or more imaging techniques, have been tested. The creation of a multimodality imaging probe has been proven feasible but is still hampered by technical challenges such as large size of probes, co-registration difficulties, low image quality, and slow image acquisition rates. Presently, the IVUS-NIRS is the only hybrid imaging catheter approved for clinical use but is not able to accurately visualize all plaque characteristics associated with vulnerability phenotype.

Alternatively, the fusion of intravascular imaging and CA or CTCA has enabled the accurate reconstruction of coronary artery geometry and the generation of 3D models allowing the appraisal of blood flow patterns and the definition of the hemodynamic forces at the plaque site. Nevertheless, these hybrid systems are based on complex post-processing analyses requiring time and human-dependent multiple reconstruction steps. Thus, albeit this approach is expected to shed light on pathophysiological mechanisms leading to plaque destabilization, its use is still limited to the research area and needs further validation with histology studies.

In conclusion, hybrid imaging platforms have the potentiality to expand our understanding of atherosclerosis evolution and improving patients' risk stratification. More efforts are required in the upcoming years, in terms of catheter design and co-registration software, to expand clinical use of hybrid imaging for the study of atherosclerosis. Likewise, further studies are required to investigate whether this theoretical progress in the identification of vulnerable plaques will translate into patient outcome improvement.

References

1. Brown BG, Bolson E, Frimer M, Dodge HT. Quantitative coronary arteriography: estimation of dimensions, hemodynamic resistance, and atheroma mass of coronary artery lesions using the arteriogram and digital computation. Circulation. 1977;55:329–37.

2. Burton JR, Teo KK, Buller CE, Plante S, Catellier D, Tymchak W, Taylor D, Dzavik V, Montague TJ. Effects of long term cholesterol lowering on coronary atherosclerosis in patient risk factor subgroups: the Simvastatin/Enalapril Coronary Atherosclerosis Trial (SCAT). Can J Cardiol. 2003;19(5):487–91.
3. Berry C, L'Allier PL, Gregoire J, Lesperance J, Levesque S, Ibrahim R, Tardif JC. Comparison of intravascular ultrasound and quantitative coronary angiography for the assessment of coronary artery disease progression. Circulation. 2007;115(14):1851–7.
4. Mortensen MB, Dzaye O, Steffensen FH, Bøtker HE, Jensen JM, Rønnow Sand NP, Kragholm KH, Sørensen HT, Leipsic J, Mæng M, Blaha MJ, Nørgaard BL. Impact of plaque burden versus stenosis on ischemic events in patients with coronary atherosclerosis. J Am Coll Cardiol. 2020;76(24):2803–13.
5. Task Force Members, Montalescot G, Sechtem U, Achenbach S, Andreotti F, Arden C, Budaj A, Bugiardini R, Crea F, Cuisset T, Di Mario C, Ferreira JR, Gersh BJ, Gitt AK, Hulot JS, Marx N, Opie LH, Pfisterer M, Prescott E, Ruschitzka F, Sabaté M, Senior R, Taggart DP, van der Wall EE, Vrints CJ, ESC Committee for Practice Guidelines, Zamorano JL, Achenbach S, Baumgartner H, Bax JJ, Bueno H, Dean V, Deaton C, Erol C, Fagard R, Ferrari R, Hasdai D, Hoes AW, Kirchhof P, Knuuti J, Kolh P, Lancellotti P, Linhart A, Nihoyannopoulos P, Piepoli MF, Ponikowski P, Sirnes PA, Tamargo JL, Tendera M, Torbicki A, Wijns W, Windecker S, Document Reviewers, Knuuti J, Valgimigli M, Bueno H, Claeys MJ, Donner-Banzhoff N, Erol C, Frank H, Funck-Brentano C, Gaemperli O, Gonzalez-Juanatey JR, Hamilos M, Hasdai D, Husted S, James SK, Kervinen K, Kolh P, Kristensen SD, Lancellotti P, Maggioni AP, Piepoli MF, Pries AR, Romeo F, Rydén L, Simoons ML, Sirnes PA, Steg PG, Timmis A, Wijns W, Windecker S, Yildirir A, Zamorano JL. 2013 ESC guidelines on the management of stable coronary artery disease: the task force on the management of stable coronary artery disease of the European Society of Cardiology. Eur Heart J. 2013;34(38):2949–3003.
6. Tonino PA, Fearon WF, De Bruyne B, Oldroyd KG, Leesar MA, Ver Lee PN, Maccarthy PA, Van't Veer M, Pijls NH. Angiographic versus functional severity of coronary artery stenoses in the FAME study fractional flow reserve versus angiography in multivessel evaluation. J Am Coll Cardiol. 2010;55(25):2816–21.
7. Virani SS, Alonso A, Benjamin EJ, Bittencourt MS, Callaway CW, Carson AP, Chamberlain AM, Chang AR, Cheng S, Delling FN, Djousse L, Elkind MSV, Ferguson JF, Fornage M, Khan SS, Kissela BM, Knutson KL, Kwan TW, Lackland DT, Lewis TT, Lichtman JH, Longenecker CT, Loop MS, Lutsey PL, Martin SS, Matsushita K, Moran AE, Mussolino ME, Perak AM, Rosamond WD, Roth GA, Sampson UKA, Satou GM, Schroeder EB, Shah SH, Shay CM, Spartano NL, Stokes A, Tirschwell DL, VanWagner LB, Tsao CW, American Heart Association Council on Epidemiology and Prevention Statistics Committee and Stroke Statistics Subcommittee. Heart disease and stroke statistics-2020 update: a report from the American Heart Association. Circulation. 2020;141(9):e139–596.
8. Yong AS, Ng AC, Brieger D, Lowe HC, Ng MK, Kritharides L. Threedimensional and two-dimensional quantitative coronary angiography, and their prediction of reduced fractional flow reserve. Eur Heart J. 2011;32:345–53.
9. Bourantas CV, Tweddel AC, Papafaklis MI, Karvelis PS, Fotiadis DI, Katsouras CS, Michalis LK. Comparison of quantitative coronary angiography with intracoronary ultrasound. Can quantitative coronary angiography accurately estimate the severity of a luminal stenosis? Angiology. 2009;60(2):169–79.
10. Tu S, Xu L, Ligthart J, Xu B, Witberg K, Sun Z, Koning G, Reiber JH, Regar E. In vivo comparison of arterial lumen dimensions assessed by co-registered three-dimensional (3D) quantitative coronary angiography, intravascular ultrasound and optical coherence tomography. Int J Cardiovasc Imaging. 2012;28(6):1315–27.
11. Stone GW, Maehara A, Lansky AJ, de Bruyne B, Cristea E, Mintz GS, Mehran R, McPherson J, Farhat N, Marso SP, Parise H, Templin B, White R, Zhang Z, Serruys PW, PROSPECT Investigators. A prospective natural-history study of coronary atherosclerosis. N Engl J Med. 2011;364(3):226–35.
12. Waksman R, Di Mario C, Torguson R, Ali ZA, Singh V, Skinner WH, Artis AK, Cate TT, Powers E, Kim C, Regar E, Wong SC, Lewis S, Wykrzykowska J, Dube S, Kazziha S, van der Ent M, Shah P, Craig PE, Zou Q, Kolm P, Brewer HB, Garcia-Garcia HM, LRP Investigators. Identification of patients and plaques vulnerable to future coronary events with near-infrared spectroscopy intravascular ultrasound imaging: a prospective, cohort study. Lancet. 2019;394(10209):1629–37.
13. Prati F, Romagnoli E, Gatto L, La Manna A, Burzotta F, Ozaki Y, Marco V, Boi A, Fineschi M, Fabbiocchi F, Taglieri N, Niccoli G, Trani C, Versaci F, Calligaris G, Ruscica G, Di Giorgio A, Vergallo R, Albertucci M, Biondi-Zoccai G, Tamburino C, Crea F, Alfonso F, Arbustini E. Relationship between coronary plaque morphology of the left anterior descending artery and 12 months clinical outcome: the CLIMA study. Eur Heart J. 2020;41(3):383–91.
14. Finn AV, Nakano M, Narula J, Kolodgie FD, Virmani R. Concept of vulnerable/unstable plaque. Arterioscler Thromb Vasc Biol. 2010;30(7):1282–92.
15. Falk E, Nakano M, Bentzon JF, Finn AV, Virmani R. Update on acute coronary syndromes: the pathologists' view. Eur Heart J. 2013;34(10):719–28.
16. Janoudi A, Shamoun FE, Kalavakunta JK, Abela GS. Cholesterol crystal induced arterial inflamma-

tion and destabilization of atherosclerotic plaque. Eur Heart J. 2016;37(25):1959–67.
17. Virmani R, Burke AP, Farb A, Kolodgie FD. Pathology of the vulnerable plaque. J Am Coll Cardiol. 2006;47(8 Suppl):C13–8.
18. Chang HJ, Lin FY, Lee SE, Andreini D, Bax J, Cademartiri F, Chinnaiyan K, Chow BJW, Conte E, Cury RC, Feuchtner G, Hadamitzky M, Kim YJ, Leipsic J, Maffei E, Marques H, Plank F, Pontone G, Raff GL, van Rosendael AR, Villines TC, Weirich HG, Al'Aref SJ, Baskaran L, Cho I, Danad I, Han D, Heo R, Lee JH, Rivzi A, Stuijfzand WJ, Gransar H, Lu Y, Sung JM, Park HB, Berman DS, Budoff MJ, Samady H, Shaw LJ, Stone PH, Virmani R, Narula J, Min JK. Coronary atherosclerotic precursors of acute coronary syndromes. J Am Coll Cardiol. 2018;71(22):2511–22.
19. Ozaki Y, Garcia-Garcia HM, Beyene SS, Hideo-Kajita A, Kuku KO, Kolm P, Waksman R. Effect of statin therapy on fibrous cap thickness in coronary plaque on optical coherence tomography—review and meta-analysis. Circ J. 2019;83(7):1480–8.
20. Nair A, Kuban BD, Tuzcu EM, Schoenhagen P, Nissen SE, Vince DG. Coronary plaque classification with intravascular ultrasound radiofrequency data analysis. Circulation. 2002;106(17):2200–6.
21. Yabushita H, Bouma BE, Houser SL, Aretz HT, Jang IK, Schlendorf KH, Kauffman CR, Shishkov M, Kang DH, Halpern EF, Tearney GJ. Characterization of human atherosclerosis by optical coherence tomography. Circulation. 2002;106(13):1640–5.
22. Nudi F, Lotrionte M, Biasucci LM, Peruzzi M, Marullo AGM, Frati G, Valenti V, Giordano A, Biondi-Zoccai G. Comparative safety and effectiveness of coronary computed tomography: systematic review and meta-analysis including 11 randomized controlled trials and 19,957 patients. Int J Cardiol. 2016;222:352–8.
23. D'Ascenzo F, Agostoni P, Abbate A, Castagno D, Lipinski MJ, Vetrovec GW, Frati G, Presutti DG, Quadri G, Moretti C, Gaita F, Zoccai GB. Atherosclerotic coronary plaque regression and the risk of adverse cardiovascular events: a metaregression of randomized clinical trials. Atherosclerosis. 2013;226:178–85.
24. Mintz GS, Nissen SE, Anderson WD, Bailey SR, Erbel R, Fitzgerald PJ, Pinto FJ, Rosenfield K, Siegel RJ, Tuzcu EM, Yock PG. American College of Cardiology Clinical Expert Consensus document on standards for acquisition, measurement and reporting of intravascular ultrasound studies (IVUS). A report of the American College of Cardiology Task Force on clinical expert consensus documents. J Am Coll Cardiol. 2001;37(5):1478–92.
25. Briguori C, Tobis J, Nishida T, Vaghetti M, Albiero R, Di Mario C, Colombo A. Discrepancy between angiography and intravascular ultrasound when analysing small coronary arteries. Eur Heart J. 2002;23(3):247–54.
26. Choi JW, Vardi GM, Meyers SN, Parker MA, Goodreau LM, Davidson CJ. Role of intracoronary ultrasound after high-pressure stent implantation. Am Heart J. 2000;139(4):643–8.
27. Jang JS, Song YJ, Kang W, Jin HY, Seo JS, Yang TH, Kim DK, Cho KI, Kim BH, Park YH, Je HG, Kim DS. Intravascular ultrasound-guided implantation of drug-eluting stents to improve outcome: a meta-analysis. JACC Cardiovasc Interv. 2014;7(3):233–43.
28. Bruining N, Verheye S, Knaapen M, Somers P, Roelandt JR, Regar E, Heller I, de Winter S, Ligthart J, Van Langenhove G, de Feijter PJ, Serruys PW, Hamers R. Three-dimensional and quantitative analysis of atherosclerotic plaque composition by automated differential echogenicity. Catheter Cardiovasc Interv. 2007;70(7):968–78.
29. Hodgson JM, Reddy KG, Suneja R, Nair RN, Lesnefsky EJ, Sheehan HM. Intracoronary ultrasound imaging: correlation of plaque morphology with angiography, clinical syndrome and procedural results in patients undergoing coronary angioplasty. J Am Coll Cardiol. 1993;21(1):35–44.
30. Amano T, Matsubara T, Uetani T, Kato M, Kato B, Yoshida T, Harada K, Kumagai S, Kunimura A, Shinbo Y, Ishii H, Murohara T. Lipid-rich plaques predict non-target-lesion ischemic events in patients undergoing percutaneous coronary intervention. Circ J. 2011;75(1):157–66.
31. Calvert PA, Obaid DR, O'Sullivan M, Shapiro LM, McNab D, Densem CG, Schofield PM, Braganza D, Clarke SC, Ray KK, West NE, Bennett MR. Association between IVUS findings and adverse outcomes in patients with coronary artery disease: the VIVA (VH-IVUS in Vulnerable Atherosclerosis) study. JACC Cardiovasc Imaging. 2011;4(8):894–901.
32. Nair A, Margolis MP, Kuban BD, Vince DG. Automated coronary plaque characterisation with intravascular ultrasound backscatter: ex vivo validation. EuroIntervention. 2007;3(1):113–20.
33. Brugaletta S, Cola C, Martin-Yuste V, Vilahur G, Oriol J, Padro T, Guerra JM, Borras R, Badimon L, Sabate M. Qualitative and quantitative accuracy of ultrasound-based virtual histology for detection of necrotic core in human coronary arteries. Int J Cardiovasc Imaging. 2014;30(3):469–76.
34. Campos CM, Fedewa RJ, Garcia-Garcia HM, Vince DG, Margolis MP, Lemos PA, Stone GW, Serruys PW, Nair A. Ex vivo validation of 45 MHz intravascular ultrasound backscatter tissue characterization. Eur Heart J Cardiovasc Imaging. 2015;16(10):1112–9.
35. Kawasaki M, Takatsu H, Noda T, Ito Y, Kunishima A, Arai M, Nishigaki K, Takemura G, Morita N, Minatoguchi S, Fujiwara H. Noninvasive quantitative tissue characterization and two-dimensional color-coded map of human atherosclerotic lesions using ultrasound integrated backscatter: compari-

son between histology and integrated backscatter images. J Am Coll Cardiol. 2001;38(2):486–92.
36. Sano K, Kawasaki M, Ishihara Y, Okubo M, Tsuchiya K, Nishigaki K, Zhou X, Minatoguchi S, Fujita H, Fujiwara H. Assessment of vulnerable plaques causing acute coronary syndrome using integrated backscatter intravascular ultrasound. J Am Coll Cardiol. 2006;47(4):734–41.
37. Okubo M, Kawasaki M, Ishihara Y, Takeyama U, Yasuda S, Kubota T, Tanaka S, Yamaki T, Ojio S, Nishigaki K, Takemura G, Saio M, Takami T, Fujiwara H, Minatoguchi S. Tissue characterization of coronary plaques: comparison of integrated backscatter intravascular ultrasound with virtual histology intravascular ultrasound. Circ J. 2008;72(10):1631–9.
38. Kawasaki M, Bouma BE, Bressner J, Houser SL, Nadkarni SK, MacNeill BD, Jang IK, Fujiwara H, Tearney GJ. Diagnostic accuracy of optical coherence tomography and integrated backscatter intravascular ultrasound images for tissue characterization of human coronary plaques. J Am Coll Cardiol. 2006;48(1):81–8.
39. Bourantas CV, Papafaklis MI, Athanasiou L, Kalatzis FG, Naka KK, Siogkas PK, Takahashi S, Saito S, Fotiadis DI, Feldman CL, Stone PH, Michalis LK. A new methodology for accurate 3-dimensional coronary artery reconstruction using routine intravascular ultrasound and angiographic data: implications for widespread assessment of endothelial shear stress in humans. EuroIntervention. 2013;9(5):582–93.
40. Stone PH, Maehara A, Coskun AU, Maynard CC, Zaromytidou M, Siasos G, Andreou I, Fotiadis D, Stefanou K, Papafaklis M, Michalis L, Lansky AJ, Mintz GS, Serruys PW, Feldman CL, Stone GW. Role of low endothelial shear stress and plaque characteristics in the prediction of nonculprit major adverse cardiac events: the PROSPECT study. JACC Cardiovasc Imaging. 2018;11(3):462–47.
41. Bourantas CV, Räber L, Sakellarios A, Ueki Y, Zanchin T, Koskinas KC, Yamaji K, Taniwaki M, Heg D, Radu MD, Papafaklis MI, Kalatzis F, Naka KK, Fotiadis DI, Mathur A, Serruys PW, Michalis LK, Garcia-Garcia HM, Karagiannis A, Windecker S. Utility of multimodality intravascular imaging and the local hemodynamic forces to predict atherosclerotic disease progression. JACC Cardiovasc Imaging. 2020;13(4):1021–32.
42. Stone PH, Saito S, Takahashi S, Makita Y, Nakamura S, Kawasaki T, Takahashi A, Katsuki T, Nakamura S, Namiki A, Hirohata A, Matsumura T, Yamazaki S, Yokoi H, Tanaka S, Otsuji S, Yoshimachi F, Honye J, Harwood D, Reitman M, Coskun AU, Papafaklis MI, Feldman CL, PREDICTION Investigators. Prediction of progression of coronary artery disease and clinical outcomes using vascular profiling of endothelial shear stress and arterial plaque characteristics: the PREDICTION study. Circulation. 2012;126(2):172–81.
43. Samady H, Eshtehardi P, McDaniel MC, Suo J, Dhawan SS, Maynard C, Timmins LH, Quyyumi AA, Giddens DP. Coronary artery wall shear stress is associated with progression and transformation of atherosclerotic plaque and arterial remodeling in patients with coronary artery disease. Circulation. 2011;124(7):779–88.
44. Timmins LH, Molony DS, Eshtehardi P, McDaniel MC, Oshinski JN, Giddens DP, Samady H. Oscillatory wall shear stress is a dominant flow characteristic affecting lesion progression patterns and plaque vulnerability in patients with coronary artery disease. J R Soc Interface. 2017;14(127):20160972.
45. Cheng JM, Garcia-Garcia HM, de Boer SP, Kardys I, Heo JH, Akkerhuis KM, Oemrawsingh RM, van Domburg RT, Ligthart J, Witberg KT, Regar E, Serruys PW, van Geuns RJ, Boersma E. In vivo detection of high-risk coronary plaques by radiofrequency intravascular ultrasound and cardiovascular outcome: results of the ATHEROREMO-IVUS study. Eur Heart J. 2014;35(10):639–47.
46. Nissen SE, Tuzcu EM, Schoenhagen P, Brown BG, Ganz P, Vogel RA, Crowe T, Howard G, Cooper CJ, Brodie B, Grines CL, DeMaria AN, REVERSAL Investigators. Effect of intensive compared with moderate lipid-lowering therapy on progression of coronary atherosclerosis: a randomized controlled trial. JAMA. 2004;291(9):1071–80.
47. Nicholls SJ, Ballantyne CM, Barter PJ, Chapman MJ, Erbel RM, Libby P, Raichlen JS, Uno K, Borgman M, Wolski K, Nissen SE. Effect of two intensive statin regimens on progression of coronary disease. N Engl J Med. 2011;365(22):2078–87.
48. Räber L, Taniwaki M, Zaugg S, Kelbæk H, Roffi M, Holmvang L, Noble S, Pedrazzini G, Moschovitis A, Lüscher TF, Matter CM, Serruys PW, Jüni P, Garcia-Garcia HM, Windecker S, IBIS 4 (Integrated Biomarkers and Imaging Study-4) Trial Investigators (NCT00962416). Effect of high-intensity statin therapy on atherosclerosis in non-infarct-related coronary arteries (IBIS-4): a serial intravascular ultrasonography study. Eur Heart J. 2015;36(8):490–500.
49. Sipahi I, Tuzcu EM, Schoenhagen P, Wolski KE, Nicholls SJ, Balog C, Crowe TD, Nissen SE. Effects of normal, pre-hypertensive, and hypertensive blood pressure levels on progression of coronary atherosclerosis. J Am Coll Cardiol. 2006;48(4):833–8.
50. Hong MK, Park DW, Lee CW, Lee SW, Kim YH, Kang DH, Song JK, Kim JJ, Park SW, Park SJ. Effects of statin treatments on coronary plaques assessed by volumetric virtual histology intravascular ultrasound analysis. JACC Cardiovasc Interv. 2009;2(7):679–88.
51. Serruys PW, Garcia-Garcia HM, Buszman P, Erne P, Verheye S, Aschermann M, Duckers H, Bleie O, Dudek D, Botker HE, von Birgelen C, D'Amico D, Hutchinson T, Zambanini A, Mastik F, van Es GA, van der Steen AF, Vince DG, Ganz P, Hamm CW,

Wijns W, Zalewski A, Integrated Biomarker and Imaging Study-2 Investigators. Effects of the direct lipoprotein-associated phospholipase A(2) inhibitor darapladib on human coronary atherosclerotic plaque. Circulation. 2008;118(11):1172–82.
52. Huang D, Swanson EA, Lin CP, Schuman JS, Stinson WG, Chang W, Hee MR, Flotte T, Gregory K, Puliafito CA, Fujimoto JG. Optical coherence tomography. Science. 1991;254(5035):1178–81.
53. Barlis P, Gonzalo N, Di Mario C, Prati F, Buellesfeld L, Rieber J, Dalby MC, Ferrante G, Cera M, Grube E, Serruys PW, Regar E. A multicentre evaluation of the safety of intracoronary optical coherence tomography. EuroIntervention. 2009;5(1):90–5.
54. Takano M, Jang IK, Inami S, Yamamoto M, Murakami D, Okamatsu K, Seimiya K, Ohba T, Mizuno K. In vivo comparison of optical coherence tomography and angioscopy for the evaluation of coronary plaque characteristics. Am J Cardiol. 2008;101(4):471–6.
55. Romagnoli E, Paoletti G, Marco V, Gatto L, Calligaris G, Fabbiocchi F, Fineschi M, Boi A, Albertucci M, Nicholls SJ, Prati F. Comparison between different approaches to evaluate fibrous cap thickness in sequential OCT studies. Minerva Cardioangiol. 2020. https://doi.org/10.23736/S0026-4725.20.05237-8. Epub ahead of print.
56. Tearney GJ, Yabushita H, Houser SL, Aretz HT, Jang IK, Schlendorf KH, Kauffman CR, Shishkov M, Halpern EF, Bouma BE. Quantification of macrophage content in atherosclerotic plaques by optical coherence tomography. Circulation. 2003;107(1):113–9.
57. Tian J, Hou J, Xing L, Kim SJ, Yonetsu T, Kato K, Lee H, Zhang S, Yu B, Jang IK. Significance of intraplaque neovascularisation for vulnerability: optical coherence tomography study. Heart. 2012;98(20):1504–9.
58. Tearney GJ, Regar E, Akasaka T, Adriaenssens T, Barlis P, Bezerra HG, Bouma B, Bruining N, Cho JM, Chowdhary S, Costa MA, de Silva R, Dijkstra J, Di Mario C, Dudek D, Falk E, Feldman MD, Fitzgerald P, Garcia-Garcia HM, Gonzalo N, Granada JF, Guagliumi G, Holm NR, Honda Y, Ikeno F, Kawasaki M, Kochman J, Koltowski L, Kubo T, Kume T, Kyono H, Lam CC, Lamouche G, Lee DP, Leon MB, Maehara A, Manfrini O, Mintz GS, Mizuno K, Morel MA, Nadkarni S, Okura H, Otake H, Pietrasik A, Prati F, Räber L, Radu MD, Rieber J, Riga M, Rollins A, Rosenberg M, Sirbu V, Serruys PW, Shimada K, Shinke T, Shite J, Siegel E, Sonoda S, Suter M, Takarada S, Tanaka A, Terashima M, Thim T, Uemura S, Ughi GJ, van Beusekom HM, van der Steen AF, van Es GA, van Soest G, Virmani R, Waxman S, Weissman NJ, Weisz G, International Working Group for Intravascular Optical Coherence Tomography (IWG-IVOCT). Consensus standards for acquisition, measurement, and reporting of intravascular optical coherence tomography studies: a report from the International Working Group for Intravascular Optical Coherence Tomography Standardization and Validation. J Am Coll Cardiol. 2012;59(12):1058–72.
59. Vergallo R, Crea F. Atherosclerotic plaque healing. N Engl J Med. 2020;383(9):846–57.
60. Kume T, Akasaka T, Kawamoto T, Watanabe N, Toyota E, Neishi Y, Sukmawan R, Sadahira Y, Yoshida K. Assessment of coronary intima-media thickness by optical coherence tomography: comparison with intravascular ultrasound. Circ J. 2005;69(8):903–7.
61. Narula J, Nakano M, Virmani R, Kolodgie FD, Petersen R, Newcomb R, Malik S, Fuster V, Finn AV. Histopathologic characteristics of atherosclerotic coronary disease and implications of the findings for the invasive and noninvasive detection of vulnerable plaques. J Am Coll Cardiol. 2013;61(10):1041–51.
62. Tian J, Ren X, Vergallo R, Xing L, Yu H, Jia H, Soeda T, McNulty I, Hu S, Lee H, Yu B, Jang IK. Distinct morphological features of ruptured culprit plaque for acute coronary events compared to those with silent rupture and thin-cap fibroatheroma: a combined optical coherence tomography and intravascular ultrasound study. J Am Coll Cardiol. 2014;63(21):2209–16.
63. Komukai K, Kubo T, Kitabata H, Matsuo Y, Ozaki Y, Takarada S, Okumoto Y, Shiono Y, Orii M, Shimamura K, Ueno S, Yamano T, Tanimoto T, Ino Y, Yamaguchi T, Kumiko H, Tanaka A, Imanishi T, Akagi H, Akasaka T. Effect of atorvastatin therapy on fibrous cap thickness in coronary atherosclerotic plaque as assessed by optical coherence tomography: the EASY-FIT study. J Am Coll Cardiol. 2014;64(21):2207–17.
64. Rieber J, Meissner O, Babaryka G, Reim S, Oswald M, Koenig A, Schiele TM, Shapiro M, Theisen K, Reiser MF, Klauss V, Hoffmann U. Diagnostic accuracy of optical coherence tomography and intravascular ultrasound for the detection and characterization of atherosclerotic plaque composition in ex-vivo coronary specimens: a comparison with histology. Coron Artery Dis. 2006;17(5):425–30.
65. Manfrini O, Mont E, Leone O, Arbustini E, Eusebi V, Virmani R, Bugiardini R. Sources of error and interpretation of plaque morphology by optical coherence tomography. Am J Cardiol. 2006;98(2):156–9.
66. Xu C, Schmitt JM, Carlier SG, Virmani R. Characterization of atherosclerosis plaques by measuring both backscattering and attenuation coefficients in optical coherence tomography. J Biomed Opt. 2008;13(3):034003.
67. Kume T, Akasaka T, Kawamoto T, Ogasawara Y, Watanabe N, Toyota E, Neishi Y, Sukmawan R, Sadahira Y, Yoshida K. Assessment of coronary arterial thrombus by optical coherence tomography. Am J Cardiol. 2006;97(12):1713–7.
68. Kubo T, Imanishi T, Takarada S, Kuroi A, Ueno S, Yamano T, Tanimoto T, Matsuo Y, Masho T, Kitabata H, Tsuda K, Tomobuchi Y, Akasaka T. Assessment of culprit lesion morphology in acute myocardial

infarction: ability of optical coherence tomography compared with intravascular ultrasound and coronary angioscopy. J Am Coll Cardiol. 2007;50(10):933–9.
69. Jia H, Abtahian F, Aguirre AD, Lee S, Chia S, Lowe H, Kato K, Yonetsu T, Vergallo R, Hu S, Tian J, Lee H, Park SJ, Jang YS, Raffel OC, Mizuno K, Uemura S, Itoh T, Kakuta T, Choi SY, Dauerman HL, Prasad A, Toma C, McNulty I, Zhang S, Yu B, Fuster V, Narula J, Virmani R, Jang IK. In vivo diagnosis of plaque erosion and calcified nodule in patients with acute coronary syndrome by intravascular optical coherence tomography. J Am Coll Cardiol. 2013;62(19):1748–58.
70. Di Vito L, Agozzino M, Marco V, Ricciardi A, Concardi M, Romagnoli E, Gatto L, Calogero G, Tavazzi L, Arbustini E, Prati F. Identification and quantification of macrophage presence in coronary atherosclerotic plaques by optical coherence tomography. Eur Heart J Cardiovasc Imaging. 2015;16(7):807–13.
71. Phipps JE, Vela D, Hoyt T, Halaney DL, Mancuso JJ, Buja LM, Asmis R, Milner TE, Feldman MD. Macrophages and intravascular OCT bright spots: a quantitative study. JACC Cardiovasc Imaging. 2015;8(1):63–72.
72. Nidorf SM, Fiolet A, Abela GS. Viewing atherosclerosis through a crystal lens: How the evolving structure of cholesterol crystals in atherosclerotic plaque alters its stability. J Clin Lipidol. 2020;14(5):619–30.
73. Abela GS, Aziz K, Vedre A, Pathak DR, Talbott JD, Dejong J. Effect of cholesterol crystals on plaques and intima in arteries of patients with acute coronary and cerebrovascular syndromes. Am J Cardiol. 2009;103(7):959–68.
74. Vorpahl M, Nakano M, Virmani R. Small black holes in optical frequency domain imaging matches intravascular neoangiogenesis formation in histology. Eur Heart J. 2010;31:1889.
75. Kume T, Okura H, Yamada R, Koyama T, Fukuhara K, Kawamura A, Imai K, Neishi Y, Uemura S. Detection of plaque neovascularization by optical coherence tomography: ex vivo feasibility study and in vivo observation in patients with angina pectoris. J Invasive Cardiol. 2016;28(1):17–22.
76. Papafaklis MI, Bourantas CV, Yonetsu T, Vergallo R, Kotsia A, Nakatani S, Lakkas LS, Athanasiou LS, Naka KK, Fotiadis DI, Feldman CL, Stone PH, Serruys PW, Jang IK, Michalis LK. Anatomically correct three-dimensional coronary artery reconstruction using frequency domain optical coherence tomographic and angiographic data: head-to-head comparison with intravascular ultrasound for endothelial shear stress assessment in humans. EuroIntervention. 2015;11(4):407–15.
77. Athanasiou LS, Bourantas CV, Siogkas PK, Sakellarios AI, Exarchos TP, Naka KK, Papafaklis MI, Michalis LK, Prati F, Fotiadis DI. 3D reconstruction of coronary arteries using frequency domain optical coherence tomography images and biplane angiography. Conf Proc IEEE Eng Med Biol Soc. 2012;2012:2647–50.
78. Torii R, Stettler R, Räber L, Zhang YJ, Karanasos A, Dijkstra J, Patel K, Crake T, Hamshere S, Garcia-Garcia HM, Tenekecioglu E, Ozkor M, Baumbach A, Windecker S, Serruys PW, Regar E, Mathur A, Bourantas CV. Implications of the local hemodynamic forces on the formation and destabilization of neoatherosclerotic lesions. Int J Cardiol. 2018;272:7–12.
79. Vergallo R, Papafaklis MI, Yonetsu T, Bourantas CV, Andreou I, Wang Z, Fujimoto JG, McNulty I, Lee H, Biasucci LM, Crea F, Feldman CL, Michalis LK, Stone PH, Jang IK. Endothelial shear stress and coronary plaque characteristics in humans: combined frequency-domain optical coherence tomography and computational fluid dynamics study. Circ Cardiovasc Imaging. 2014;7(6):905–11.
80. Slager CJ, Wentzel JJ, Gijsen FJ, Thury A, van der Wal AC, Schaar JA, et al. The role of shear stress in the destabilization of vulnerable plaques and related therapeutic implications. Nat Clin Pract Cardiovasc Med. 2005;2:456–64.
81. Fukumoto Y, Hiro T, Fujii T, Hashimoto G, Fujimura T, Yamada J, et al. Localized elevation of shear stress is related to coronary plaque rupture: a 3-dimensional intravascular ultrasound study with in-vivo color mapping of shear stress distribution. J Am Coll Cardiol. 2008;51:645–50.
82. van Ditzhuijzen NS, Karanasos A, Bruining N, van den Heuvel M, Sorop O, Ligthart J, Witberg K, Garcia-Garcia HM, Zijlstra F, Duncker DJ, van Beusekom HM, Regar E. The impact of Fourier-domain optical coherence tomography catheter induced motion artefacts on quantitative measurements of a PLLA-based bioresorbable scaffold. Int J Cardiovasc Imaging. 2014;30(6):1013–26.
83. Li Y, Gutiérrez Chico JL, Holm NR, Yang W, Hebsgaard L, Christiansen EH, Mæng M, Lassen JF, Yan F, Reiber JH, Tu S. Impact of side branch modeling on computation of endothelial shear stress in coronary artery disease: coronary tree reconstruction by fusion of 3D angiography and OCT. J Am Coll Cardiol. 2015;66(2):125–35.
84. Uemura S, Ishigami K, Soeda T, Okayama S, Sung JH, Nakagawa H, Somekawa S, Takeda Y, Kawata H, Horii M, Saito Y. Thin-cap fibroatheroma and microchannel findings in optical coherence tomography correlate with subsequent progression of coronary atheromatous plaques. Eur Heart J. 2012;33(1):78–85.
85. Xing L, Higuma T, Wang Z, Aguirre AD, Mizuno K, Takano M, Dauerman HL, Park SJ, Jang Y, Kim CJ, Kim SJ, Choi SY, Itoh T, Uemura S, Lowe H, Walters DL, Barlis P, Lee S, Lerman A, Toma C, Tan JWC, Yamamoto E, Bryniarski K, Dai J, Zanchin T, Zhang S, Yu B, Lee H, Fujimoto J, Fuster V, Jang IK. Clinical significance of lipid-rich plaque detected

by optical coherence tomography: a 4-year follow-up study. J Am Coll Cardiol. 2017;69(20):2502–13.
86. Cassis LA, Lodder RA. Near-IR imaging of atheromas in living arterial tissue. Anal Chem. 1993;65(9):1247–56.
87. Gardner CM, Tan H, Hull EL, Lisauskas JB, Sum ST, Meese TM, Jiang C, Madden SP, Caplan JD, Burke AP, Virmani R, Goldstein J, Muller JE. Detection of lipid core coronary plaques in autopsy specimens with a novel catheter-based near-infrared spectroscopy system. JACC Cardiovasc Imaging. 2008;1(5):638–48.
88. Waxman S, Dixon SR, L'Allier P, Moses JW, Petersen JL, Cutlip D, Tardif JC, Nesto RW, Muller JE, Hendricks MJ, Sum ST, Gardner CM, Goldstein JA, Stone GW, Krucoff MW. In vivo validation of a catheter-based near-infrared spectroscopy system for detection of lipid core coronary plaques: initial results of the SPECTACL study. JACC Cardiovasc Imaging. 2009;2(7):858–68.
89. Kang SJ, Mintz GS, Pu J, Sum ST, Madden SP, Burke AP, Xu K, Goldstein JA, Stone GW, Muller JE, Virmani R, Maehara A. Combined IVUS and NIRS detection of fibroatheromas: histopathological validation in human coronary arteries. JACC Cardiovasc Imaging. 2015;8(2):184–94.
90. Inaba S, Mintz GS, Burke AP, Stone GW, Virmani R, Matsumura M, Parvataneni R, Puri R, Nicholls SJ, Maehara A. Intravascular ultrasound and near-infrared spectroscopic characterization of thin-cap fibroatheroma. Am J Cardiol. 2017;119(3):372–8.
91. Bourantas CV, Jaffer FA, Gijsen FJ, van Soest G, Madden SP, Courtney BK, Fard AM, Tenekecioglu E, Zeng Y, van der Steen AFW, Emelianov S, Muller J, Stone PH, Marcu L, Tearney GJ, Serruys PW. Hybrid intravascular imaging: recent advances, technical considerations, and current applications in the study of plaque pathophysiology. Eur Heart J. 2017;38(6):400–12.
92. Kuku KO, Singh M, Ozaki Y, Dan K, Chezar-Azerrad C, Waksman R, Garcia-Garcia HM. Near-infrared spectroscopy intravascular ultrasound imaging: state of the art. Front Cardiovasc Med. 2020;7:107.
93. Schuurman AS, Vroegindewey M, Kardys I, Oemrawsingh RM, Cheng JM, de Boer S, Garcia-Garcia HM, van Geuns RJ, Regar ES, Daemen J, van Mieghem NM, Serruys PW, Boersma E, Akkerhuis KM. Near-infrared spectroscopy-derived lipid core burden index predicts adverse cardiovascular outcome in patients with coronary artery disease during long-term follow-up. Eur Heart J. 2018;39(4):295–302.
94. Brown AJ, Teng Z, Evans PC, Gillard JH, Samady H, Bennett MR. Role of biomechanical forces in the natural history of coronary atherosclerosis. Nat Rev Cardiol. 2016;13(4):210–20.
95. Hartman EMJ, De Nisco G, Kok AM, Hoogendoorn A, Coenen A, Mastik F, Korteland SA, Nieman K, Gijsen FJH, van der Steen AFW, Daemen J, Wentzel JJ. Lipid-rich plaques detected by near-infrared spectroscopy are more frequently exposed to high shear stress. J Cardiovasc Transl Res. 2021;14(3):416–25. https://doi.org/10.1007/s12265-020-10072-x.
96. Shishikura D, Sidharta SL, Honda S, Takata K, Kim SW, Andrews J, Montarello N, Delacroix S, Baillie T, Worthley MI, Psaltis PJ, Nicholls SJ. The relationship between segmental wall shear stress and lipid core plaque derived from near-infrared spectroscopy. Atherosclerosis. 2018;275:68–73.
97. Goldstein JA, Maini B, Dixon SR, Brilakis ES, Grines CL, Rizik DG, Powers ER, Steinberg DH, Shunk KA, Weisz G, Moreno PR, Kini A, Sharma SK, Hendricks MJ, Sum ST, Madden SP, Muller JE, Stone GW, Kern MJ. Detection of lipid-core plaques by intracoronary near-infrared spectroscopy identifies high risk of periprocedural myocardial infarction. Circ Cardiovasc Interv. 2011;4(5):429–37.
98. de Boer S, Baran Y, Garcia-Garcia HM, Eskin I, Lenzen MJ, Kleber ME, Regar E, de Jaegere PJ, Ligthart JM, van Geuns RJ, Lehtimäki T, Laaksonen R, Boersma E, Marz W, Halperin E, Serruys PW, Koenig W. The European Collaborative Project on Inflammation and Vascular Wall Remodeling in Atherosclerosis—Intravascular Ultrasound (ATHEROREMO-IVUS) study. EuroIntervention. 2018;14(2):194–203.
99. Raghunathan D, Abdel-Karim AR, Papayannis AC, daSilva M, Jeroudi OM, Rangan BV, Banerjee S, Brilakis ES. Relation between the presence and extent of coronary lipid core plaques detected by near-infrared spectroscopy with postpercutaneous coronary intervention myocardial infarction. Am J Cardiol. 2011;107(11):1613–8.
100. Kini AS, Baber U, Kovacic JC, Limaye A, Ali ZA, Sweeny J, Maehara A, Mehran R, Dangas G, Mintz GS, Fuster V, Narula J, Sharma SK, Moreno PR. Changes in plaque lipid content after short-term intensive versus standard statin therapy: the YELLOW trial (reduction in yellow plaque by aggressive lipid-lowering therapy). J Am Coll Cardiol. 2013;62(1):21–9.
101. Kini AS, Vengrenyuk Y, Shameer K, Maehara A, Purushothaman M, Yoshimura T, Matsumura M, Aquino M, Haider N, Johnson KW, Readhead B, Kidd BA, Feig JE, Krishnan P, Sweeny J, Milind M, Moreno P, Mehran R, Kovacic JC, Baber U, Dudley JT, Narula J, Sharma S. Intracoronary imaging, cholesterol efflux, and transcriptomes after intensive statin treatment: the YELLOW II study. J Am Coll Cardiol. 2017;69(6):628–40.
102. Boogers MJ, Broersen A, van Velzen JE, de Graaf FR, El-Naggar HM, Kitslaar PH, Dijkstra J, Delgado V, Boersma E, de Roos A, Schuijf JD, Schalij MJ, Reiber JH, Bax JJ, Jukema JW. Automated quantification of coronary plaque with computed tomography: comparison with intravascular ultrasound using a dedicated registration algorithm for fusion-based quantification. Eur Heart J. 2012;33(8):1007–16.
103. Kruk M, Wardziak Ł, Mintz GS, Achenbach S, Pręgowski J, Rużyłło W, Dzielińska Z, Demkow

M, Witkowski A, Kępka C. Accuracy of coronary computed tomography angiography vs intravascular ultrasound for evaluation of vessel area. J Cardiovasc Comput Tomogr. 2014;8(2):141–8.
104. Takahashi S, Kawasaki M, Miyata S, Suzuki K, Yamaura M, Ido T, Aoyama T, Fujiwara H, Minatoguchi S. Feasibility of tissue characterization of coronary plaques using 320-detector row computed tomography: comparison with integrated backscatter intravascular ultrasound. Heart Vessel. 2016;31(1):29–37.
105. Voros S, Rinehart S, Qian Z, Vazquez G, Anderson H, Murrieta L, Wilmer C, Carlson H, Taylor K, Ballard W, Karmpaliotis D, Kalynych A, Brown C 3rd. Prospective validation of standardized, 3-dimensional, quantitative coronary computed tomographic plaque measurements using radiofrequency backscatter intravascular ultrasound as reference standard in intermediate coronary arterial lesions: results from the ATLANTA (assessment of tissue characteristics, lesion morphology, and hemodynamics by angiography with fractional flow reserve, intravascular ultrasound and virtual histology, and noninvasive computed tomography in atherosclerotic plaques) I study. JACC Cardiovasc Interv. 2011;4(2):198–208.
106. Otsuka K, Fukuda S, Tanaka A, Nakanishi K, Taguchi H, Yoshikawa J, Shimada K, Yoshiyama M. Napkin-ring sign on coronary CT angiography for the prediction of acute coronary syndrome. JACC Cardiovasc Imaging. 2013;6(4):448–57.
107. Versteylen MO, Kietselaer BL, Dagnelie PC, Joosen IA, Dedic A, Raaijmakers RH, Wildberger JE, Nieman K, Crijns HJ, Niessen WJ, Daemen MJ, Hofstra L. Additive value of semiautomated quantification of coronary artery disease using cardiac computed tomographic angiography to predict future acute coronary syndrome. J Am Coll Cardiol. 2013;61(22):2296–305.
108. Motoyama S, Ito H, Sarai M, Kondo T, Kawai H, Nagahara Y, Harigaya H, Kan S, Anno H, Takahashi H, Naruse H, Ishii J, Hecht H, Shaw LJ, Ozaki Y, Narula J. Plaque characterization by coronary computed tomography angiography and the likelihood of acute coronary events in mid-term follow-up. J Am Coll Cardiol. 2015;66(4):337–46.
109. van der Giessen AG, Schaap M, Gijsen FJ, Groen HC, van Walsum T, Mollet NR, Dijkstra J, van de Vosse FN, Niessen WJ, de Feyter PJ, van der Steen AF, Wentzel JJ. 3D fusion of intravascular ultrasound and coronary computed tomography for in-vivo wall shear stress analysis: a feasibility study. Int J Cardiovasc Imaging. 2010;26(7):781–96.
110. Hoogendoorn A, Kok AM, Hartman EMJ, de Nisco G, Casadonte L, Chiastra C, Coenen A, Korteland SA, Van der Heiden K, Gijsen FJH, Duncker DJ, van der Steen AFW, Wentzel JJ. Multidirectional wall shear stress promotes advanced coronary plaque development: comparing five shear stress metrics. Cardiovasc Res. 2020;116(6):1136–46.
111. Ferencik M, Mayrhofer T, Bittner DO, Emami H, Puchner SB, Lu MT, Meyersohn NM, Ivanov AV, Adami EC, Patel MR, Mark DB, Udelson JE, Lee KL, Douglas PS, Hoffmann U. Use of high-risk coronary atherosclerotic plaque detection for risk stratification of patients with stable chest pain: a secondary analysis of the PROMISE randomized clinical trial. JAMA Cardiol. 2018;3(2):144–52.
112. Williams MC, Moss AJ, Dweck M, Adamson PD, Alam S, Hunter A, Shah ASV, Pawade T, Weir-McCall JR, Roditi G, van Beek EJR, Newby DE, Nicol ED. Coronary artery plaque characteristics associated with adverse outcomes in the SCOT-HEART study. J Am Coll Cardiol. 2019;73(3):291–301.
113. Brown AJ, Obaid DR, Costopoulos C, Parker RA, Calvert PA, Teng Z, Hoole SP, West NE, Goddard M, Bennett MR. Direct comparison of virtual-histology intravascular ultrasound and optical coherence tomography imaging for identification of thin-cap fibroatheroma. Circ Cardiovasc Imaging. 2015;8(10):e003487.
114. Fujii K, Hao H, Shibuya M, Imanaka T, Fukunaga M, Miki K, Tamaru H, Sawada H, Naito Y, Ohyanagi M, Hirota S, Masuyama T. Accuracy of OCT, grayscale IVUS, and their combination for the diagnosis of coronary TCFA: an ex vivo validation study. JACC Cardiovasc Imaging. 2015;8(4):451–60.
115. Taniwaki M, Radu MD, Garcia-Garcia HM, Heg D, Kelbæk H, Holmvang L, Moschovitis A, Noble S, Pedrazzini G, Saunamäki K, Dijkstra J, Landmesser U, Wenaweser P, Meier B, Stefanini GG, Roffi M, Lüscher TF, Windecker S, Räber L. Long-term safety and feasibility of three-vessel multimodality intravascular imaging in patients with ST-elevation myocardial infarction: the IBIS-4 (integrated biomarker and imaging study) substudy. Int J Cardiovasc Imaging. 2015;31(5):915–26.

Hybrid Cardiac Imaging for the Interventional Cardiologist

7

Niya Mileva, Sakura Nagumo, Jeroen Sonck, and Carlos Collet

7.1 Background

7.1.1 History of CT Development

Since the introduction of computed tomography (CT) more than 40 years ago, considerable progress has been achieved in using CT to evaluate coronary artery stenosis and plaque composition [1, 2]. Non-helical CT, electron beam CT (EBC), and dynamic spatial reconstruction (DSR) technologies provided an important foundation for cardiac imaging [3–5]. Modern era of cardiac CT began in the 1990s with the introduction of single-slice helical CT systems. With the development of 4-slice multislice spiral CT (MSCT) with retrospective electrocardiogram gating, detection of epicardial coronary artery stenosis became possible. However, there were various limitations due to cardiac motion artifacts and calcium blooming in the coronary artery wall [6, 7]. In the 2000s, 16-slice, 64-slice, and 256-slice MSCT scanners were introduced leading to high quantitative and qualitative diagnostic accuracy with reported negative predictive values greater than 97% [1, 8, 9]. Moreover, dual-source computed tomography (DSCT), designed with two X-ray tubes and two corresponding detectors, showed to reduce the time needed by a conventional spiral CT system with increased temporal resolution [10]. DSCT can acquire images of the coronary arteries with reduced motion artifacts in patients with high heart rates and at lower radiation doses compared with previous scanner generations. These technological developments have extended the indication of CT to patients with known coronary disease.

N. Mileva · S. Nagumo · J. Sonck · C. Collet (✉)
Cardiovascular Center Aalst, OLV Hospital, Aalst, Belgium
e-mail: d04sm059@med.showa-u.as.jp

7.1.2 Usefulness of CT for the Diagnosis of CAD

Noninvasive imaging of coronary arteries by coronary CT angiography has increased our understanding of the interactions between lumen, plaque, and physiology at different stages of the atherosclerotic process [11, 12]. Moreover, in patients suspected to have ischemic heart disease, CT can be useful in detecting atherosclerosis in its early phase, to evaluate the presence of obstructive disease and to risk stratify patients based on plaque characteristics [13, 14]. In one randomized clinical trial, the use of coronary CT angiography in patients presenting with chest pain, resulted in reduced incidence of death and myocardial infarction compared to functional noninvasive testing [14]. CCTA is now established in the diagnostic workup of patients suspected to have CAD. Current guidelines emphasize the role of CCTA as a first-line test for patients with symptoms suggestive of obstructive

F. Nudi et al. (eds.), *Hybrid Cardiac Imaging for Clinical Decision-Making*,
https://doi.org/10.1007/978-3-030-99391-7_7

CAD [15]. Nevertheless, CCTA remains a diagnostic tool and its usefulness beyond this phase has not been yet fully explored. This chapter will focus on the implementation of CCTA as a tool to plan and guide coronary interventions in the catheterization laboratory.

7.2 Evaluation of Coronary Arteries Using CT Angiography

After acquisition of the CCTA images, the data are sent to an offline digital workstation for further analysis. A three-dimensional (3D) dataset is formed by integrating separate volume elements called voxels and the raw two-dimensional (2D) CT images. Viewing the axial images enables most of the evaluation of coronary artery disease; however, other reconstructions aid particularly at detailing lesion and plaque characteristics.

For more advanced analysis, semiautomatic extraction of the regions of interest is performed. First, the software segments the heart and coronary vessels. During this process, individual voxels are assigned to certain anatomy or to the background. Following the identification of the heart, the main anatomical structures (i.e., major arteries, veins, atria, ventricles, and myocardium) are segmented. The semiautomatic extraction process may not handle anatomical anomalies or congenital deformities. In the latter case, users can use manual segmentation processing.

The increased spatial and temporal resolution of CCTA enables analysis of the coronary artery tree. The first step of the extraction is to identify the tubular structures in the raw CT data. Then, the coronary tree is traced in the vessel-enhanced data starting at the coronary ostium. The software follows the enhanced structures until the distal vessel or till when the contrast-to-noise ratio reaches a threshold. Most applications also provide automatic vessel labeling and allow for centerline editing and manual vessel tracing if automatic contouring proves to be incorrect.

7.3 CT for Quantitative Plaque Assessment

Once the dataset is segmented and the coronary arteries extracted, a number of tools, such as volume rendering and multiplanar reconstruction (MPR), are useful for visualization. Volume rendering offers a gross overview of the anatomic location of the heart structures. Straight MPR and (rotating) curved MPR provide users a visualization of the entire coronary artery. Straight MPR is particularly suitable for performing quantitative measurements (e.g., cross-sectional area, diameter stenosis and minimal lumen area, lesion and vessel length, etc.). Cross sectional images allow for a detailed luminal and plaque evaluation along the coronary vessel. In addition, Hounsfield unit values of different tissues may permit plaque characterization and identification of lipid-rich and calcified plaques.

7.3.1 Comparison Between CT, Quantitative Coronary Analysis, and Invasive Intravascular Imaging

Visual assessment of coronary stenosis (i.e., percent diameter stenosis) either using invasive coronary angiography or CCTA has been shown to have modest reproducibility [16, 17]. Quantitative coronary analysis (QCA), applying algorithms that detect changes in the brightness function to determine vessel contours, has shown to reduce variability for the assessment of coronary stenosis compared to visual assessment [18, 19].

In vitro, CT-derived QCA analysis has been shown to be accurate and precise for the assessment of coronary stenosis severity [20]. The two most relevant metrics, i.e., minimal lumen diameter (MLD) and reference vessel diameter (RVD) have been shown to have a high degree of agreement with the true luminal dimensions [20]. In a clinical setting, MLD is used to define lesion severity, whereas RVD distal to the lesion is used for percutaneous revascularization planning and selection of stent diameter. In vivo, CT-derived QCA RVD at proximal and distal reference segments have been shown to be in high agreement with luminal dimensions obtained from invasive QCA. Admittedly, QCA, either invasive or noninvasive, has been systematically associated with smaller luminal dimensions compared to intravascular ultrasound (IVUS) [21]. The systematic differences in vessel dimensions between these methods are partially explained by the differences in spatial resolution and the physical properties of the devices. For PCI planning, CT-derived RVD, obtained at healthy coronary segments, can be incorporated into the decision process concerning stent diameter selection. Appropriate stent sizing is of paramount importance to reduce complications associated with PCI [17, 22–24].

The introduction of new CT scanners has enhanced the evaluation of plaque volume and composition [25]. Atherosclerotic plaques can be qualitative and quantitively characterized [26]. The external elastic membrane (EEL) can be outlined allowing assessment of positive remodeling and quantification of plaque burden. Moreover, plaques components can be identified based on the attenuation coefficients expressed in Hounsfield units (HU). Calcified plaques can be easily visualized as "white" hyperechogenic structures with high HU, which permits determining their burden and circumference [27]. It has been proven that a high calcium burden is associated with lower stent expansion and higher rates of adverse events after PCI [28, 29]. Stent expansion, which depends partially on the underlying plaque, is an independent predictor of major adverse events after PCI. Hence, visualization of high calcium burden in the planning phase of coronary procedure may prompt the use of calcium modification techniques (e.g., rotational atherectomy, orbital atherectomy, excimer laser, or intravascular lithoplasty) to facilitate stent expansion [30–32]. On the other hand, CCTA volumetric calcium evaluation was reported to overestimate calcium volume by 60% compared to OCT. Considering this systematic overestimation of calcium plaque by CT, an appropriate interpretation of calcific burden in the noninvasive setting may be possible. On the other side of the spectrum, plaques with low HU, the so-called soft-plaques (i.e., HU < 50) have been identified as independent predictors of acute coronary syndromes, peri-procedural myocardial infarction, and no-reflow phenomenon [13, 33]. Quantitative plaque assessment forms the basis of the three-dimensional plaque reconstructions used during online CT guidance (discussed below). Atherosclerotic plaque components are color-coded based on HU (e.g., white for calcified structures with HU > 320, green for plaque components between 50 and 320 HU, and red for low-attenuation plaques). The results are three-dimensional plaque portrays, a plaque map, that facilitates imaging interpretation, the evaluation of disease extension, volume, and composition. Simultaneous plaque visualization optimizes the analysis of invasive coronary angiography.

Additionally, CCTA overcomes a frequent problem of invasive angiography, i.e., vessel foreshortening and suboptimal length evaluation [17]. Invasive angiographic foreshortening observed in two-dimensional projections impairs accurate evaluation of lesion length [17]. This is a frequent cause of incomplete plaque coverage or geographical miss; these latter issues are associated with adverse events after stent placement. Therefore, improving the accuracy of lesion length measurement may improve patient outcomes in patients undergoing PCI [24]. CT-derived lesion length evaluation incorporates the atherosclerotic extension that is not visible with conventional angiography; thus, this approach mimics the one obtained by intravascular imaging techniques (e.g., IVUS and optical coherence tomography (OCT)). As such, the accurate assessment of plaque extension with CCTA extrapolates the "normal-to-normal" concept described with intravascular imaging [34]. By "landing" the stents on healthy coronary segments, plaque coverage is assured reducing the risk of restenosis and thrombosis. The noninvasive selection of "normal-to-normal" segments is supported by the high diagnostic performance of CT to evaluate normal coronary vessels [35]. Moreover, CT aids in providing the best angiographic projection in the catheterization laboratory thereby minimizing foreshortening and overlapping of the segment of interest. This becomes even more relevant in the evaluation of bifurcation lesions where the visualization of the side-branch ostium is often suboptimal [23].

7.4 CCTA-Guided PCI

7.4.1 Precise PCI and Procedural Planning (P4) Algorithm

The CCTA-guided P4 algorithm is shown in Fig. 7.1. Based on three mainstays namely diagnostic evaluation, catheterization laboratory preparation, and online PCI guidance, the algorithm proposes the incorporation of CT into several phases of coronary evaluation.

7.4.2 Diagnostic Evaluation

The initial part of the algorithm extends the evaluation of the hemodynamic significance of CAD in two domains: (1) Determination of the pattern of CAD (i.e., focal or diffuse) and (2) the prediction of PCI results. Functional evaluation with fractional flow reserve (FFR) derived from CT (FFR_{CT}) characterizes the pathophysiological pattern of CAD noninvasively, this can be visualized either on the color-coded geometry or by a virtual FFR_{CT} pullback curve. The main anatomical and functional patterns of CAD, namely focal or diffuse, can be identified [36]. In cases of the focal functional disease, pressure losses are circumscribed to anatomical stenoses (i.e., lesion-specific ischemia), this vessel phenotype is

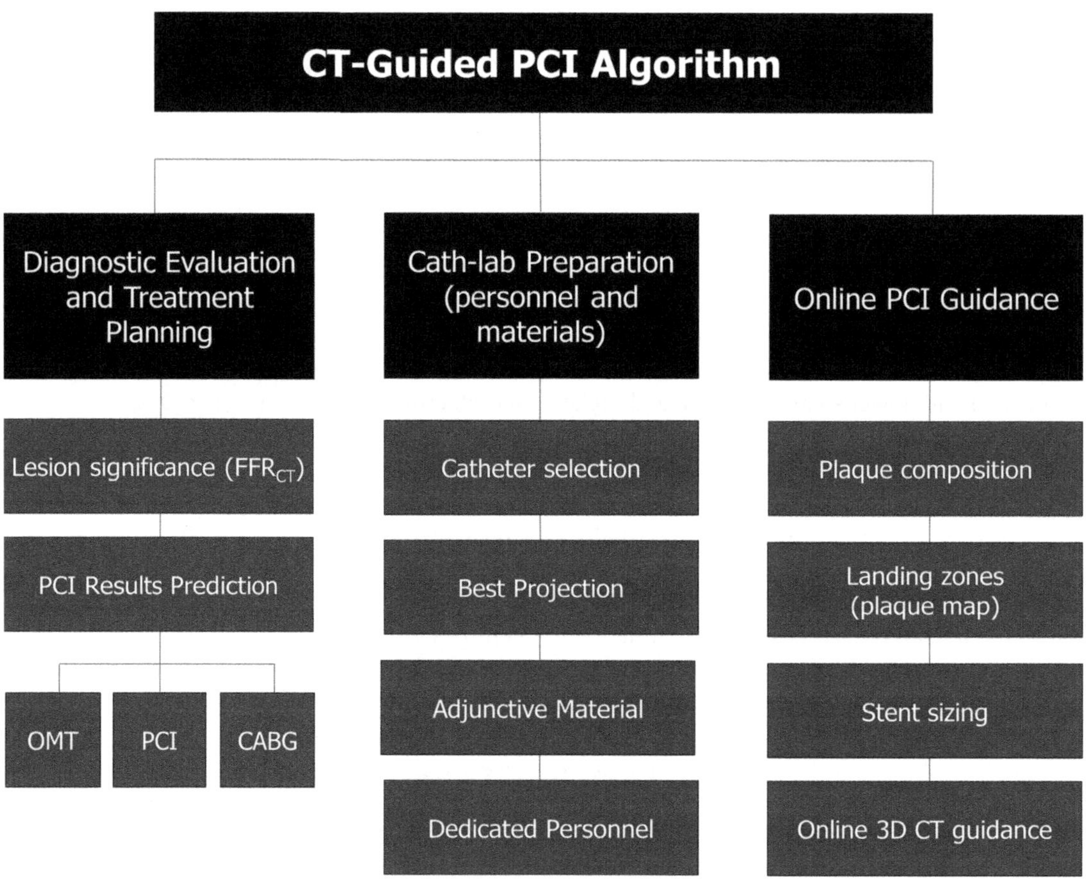

Fig. 7.1 CT-guided Coronary Intervention Algorithm. (Reprinted from article *Collet, C* et al. *Implementing Coronary Computed Tomography Angiography in the Catheterization Laboratory. JACC: Cardiovascular Imaging, 2020* with permission from Elsevier)

favorable for PCI in terms of post-intervention vessel physiology. In contrast, cases of diffuse functional CAD show no focal pressure drops, these vessels often exhibit diffuse atherosclerosis on CCTA, and despite the presence of one or several narrowings, PCI results are suboptimal in terms of post-PCI FFR. Therefore, the evaluation of the anatomic and physiological pattern of CAD aids in predicting the likelihood of functional complete revascularization which is a proxy for relief from angina [36, 37].

The FFR_{CT} planner (HeartFlow Planner, Heartflow, CA, USA) tool is a novel approach to predict the results of PCI in terms of post-PCI FFR. The FFR_{CT} planner tool simulates luminal changes produced by PCI and recalculates coronary pressures using the modified geometry. This may assist to anticipate the benefit of a given PCI strategy. The FFR_{CT} planner depicts the functional extent of CAD and demarcates normal-to-normal segments based on coronary physiology. In combination with anatomical images from CCTA, the anatomical and functional targets for revascularization can be determined. Two case examples of the application of the planner in cases of focal and diffuse CAD are shown in Fig. 7.2. As shown in the case example, PCI restored vessel physiology in focal functional CAD, and this is likely to be translated into a clinical benefit by relief from angina. In contrast, in cases of diffuse functional CAD, suboptimal post-PCI results are plausibly responsible for persistent angina after PCI. Therefore, patient selection for PCI is individualized based on the potential benefit of percutaneous revascularization. The Precise PCI Plan trial (P3 trial) has demonstrated the accuracy and precision of the FFR_{CT} planner-based technology for predicting FFR after PCI [38].

7.4.3 Catheterization Laboratory Preparation

From the evaluation of the position of the coronary ostia to the planning of complex PCI, a noninvasive stratification of the morphological complexity of CAD aids in the organization of the catheterization laboratory. Although relatively uncommon, identification of coronary anomalies informs upon the more adequate type of coronary catheters and cannulation technique. Moreover, CAD in the coronary ostia may change the cannulation strategy avoiding deep vessel catheterization that may conceal an obstructive lesion and flaw invasive FFR measurement. Furthermore, in patients with graft anastomosis in the aorta, CT aids in localizing conduits and expediting cannulation. In these scenarios, a CT-guided approach saves time, contrast, and reduces unnecessary radiation exposure.

Based on CCTA, complex interventions can be better planned in the catheterization laboratory. In case of chronic coronary occlusions, CCTA helps to better identify the distal vessel and route for PCI than invasive angiography and predicts guidewire crossing and procedural success [39]. Beyond chronic total occlusion, other challenging lesion subsets such as left main disease, bifurcations, or severely calcified coronary vessels dedicated devices can be made available to increase the likelihood of success. Moreover, medical centers using CT as the preferred noninvasive test have been shown to have greater PCI to diagnostic catheterization ratio; thereby, transforming the catheterization laboratory into an interventional suite [40].

7.4.4 Online Procedural and PCI Guidance

The 3D reconstruction of the coronary tree during conventional angiography provides a complementary three-dimensional view of the coronary anatomy in the catheterization laboratory. Both lumen and atherosclerotic plaques are reconstructed and projected side by side with the two-dimensional invasive angiography. To facilitate online interpretation, plaques components are color-coded based on their Hounsfield units. The process of coronary vessel reconstruction is shown in Fig. 7.3. During the diagnostic procedure, the right and left coronary arteries are displayed sequentially in coordination with the invasive catheterization. The

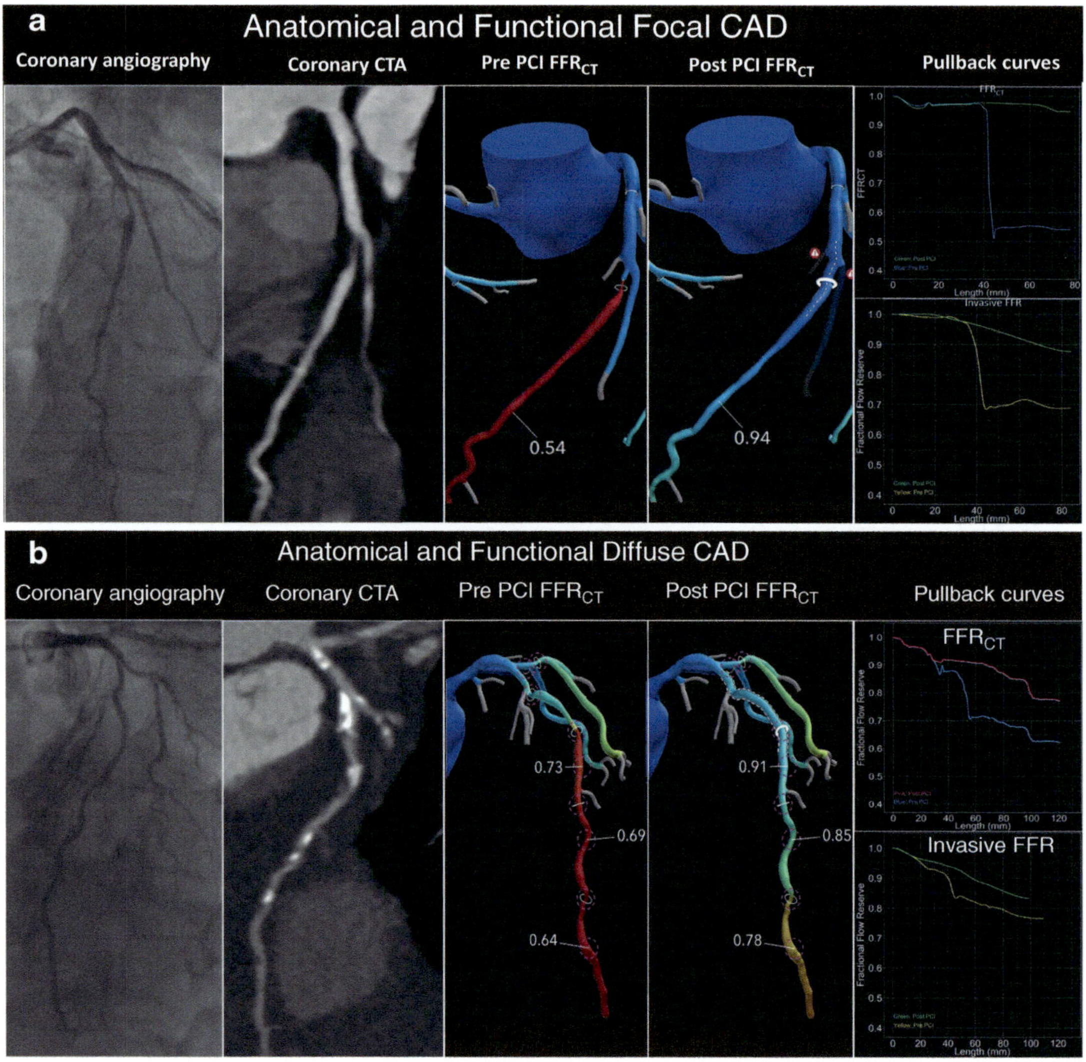

Fig. 7.2 Case examples of focal and diffuse CAD. Panel **a** shows a case with an anatomical and functional focal lesion located in the mid LAD. The virtual pullback curve derived from FFR_{CT} shows a focal pressure drop of approximately 40 FFR_{CT} units related to the lesion. No pressure losses are observed either proximal or distal to the lesion. After virtual PCI, the predicted FFR was 0.94 and invasively measured FFR was 0.90. Panel **b** shows a case of anatomical and functional diffuse CAD in the LAD. The virtual pullback curve derived from FFR_{CT} shows diffuse pressure losses along the vessel length. After virtual PCI, the predicted FFR was 0.78 and invasively measured FFR was 0.82. (Reprinted from article *Collet, C* et al. *Implementing Coronary Computed Tomography Angiography in the Catheterization Laboratory. JACC: Cardiovascular Imaging, 2020* with permission from Elsevier)

movement of the C-arm is tracked in real-time, in order to synchronize the orientation of the three-dimensional coronary tree with the projection of the fluoroscopic C-arm. A manufacturer-independent approach was accomplished by attaching an external sensor, called an inertial measurement unit (IMU), to the C-arm. The IMU continuously communicates the sensor's—and therefore also the C-arm's—orientation with the 3D visualization software (Fig. 7.4). The simultaneous display of the CCTA-derived plaque reconstruction and invasive luminogram optimizes the performance and interpretation of conventional angiography.

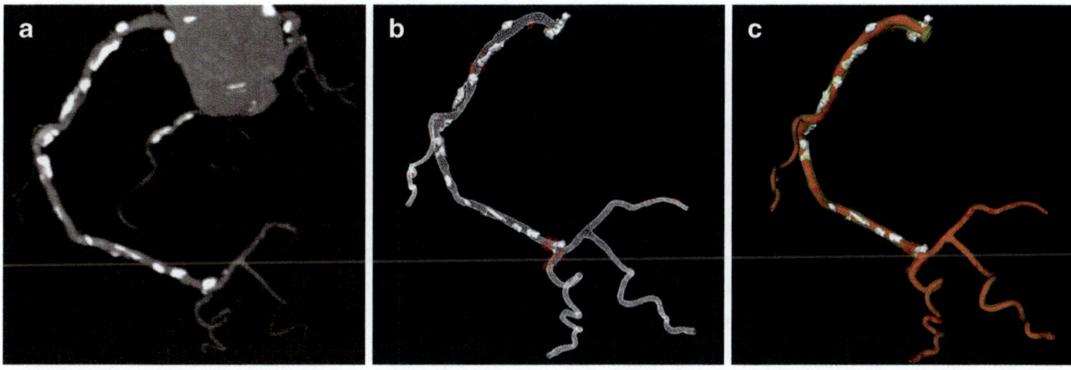

Fig. 7.3 Process of three-dimensional lumen and plaque reconstruction. Panel **a** shows 3D MIP images of a right coronary artery with diffuse calcifications. Panel **b** shows the 3D luminal and plaque reconstruction. And panel **c** shows the color-coded vessel geometry. (Reprinted from article *Collet, C* et al. *Implementing Coronary Computed Tomography Angiography in the Catheterization Laboratory. JACC: Cardiovascular Imaging, 2020* with permission from Elsevier)

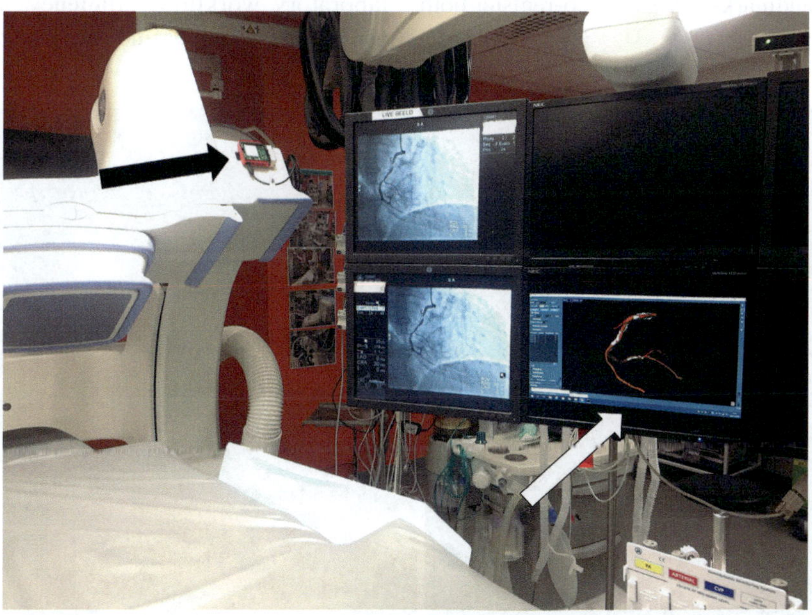

Fig. 7.4 Catheterization laboratory set up for online CT guidance. The cath-lab setup comprises the addition of synchronization hardware between the C-arm and CT software (black arrow) with the projection of the 3D CT-derived geometry projected side by side to the angiographic image (white arrow). (Reprinted from article *Collet, C* et al. *Implementing Coronary Computed Tomography Angiography in the Catheterization Laboratory. JACC: Cardiovascular Imaging, 2020* with permission from Elsevier)

During the procedure, the coronary anatomy derived from CCTA is continuously projected during changes in angiographic projections. At each projection, it is possible to assess the degree of overlapping and foreshortening without additional radiation or contrast. This optimizes lesion visualization and prevents unnecessary angiographic acquisitions. Furthermore, the three-dimensional CCTA model can be used as a 3D roadmap to assist during vessel wiring further reducing the need for additional contrast injection while the wire is advanced.

Guidance of PCI with CCTA is executed following the same principles as with intravascular imaging (e.g., IVUS or OCT) [34]. Preprocedural assessment starts with the evaluation of plaque characteristics, composition, and extension. In presence of severe calcium burden, the operator may be prompted to perform an adequate vessel preparation with pre-dilatation and/or calcium modifying techniques. After stent implantation, post-dilatation with non-compliant balloons may help achieving better stent expansion. Subsequently, lesion length is determined using noninvasive QCA analysis and healthy landing zones proximal and distal to the lesion are identified to ensure complete plaque coverage (Fig. 7.5). The continuous display of CCTA and invasive angiography also allows for the use of anatomical landmarks to visually co-register both modalities.

7.5 Clinical Implications

Coronary CTA is emerging as the preferred method to assess coronary artery disease. Consequently, the number of patients referred for an invasive angiography with a CCTA is expected to increase [41]. In terms of healthcare economics, CCTA is a cost-effective strategy for patients with suspected coronary artery disease [42, 43]. The combined morphological and functional (FFR_{CT}) evaluation of the pattern of coronary artery disease may translate into a better selection of patients for percutaneous revascularization. Likewise, a preprocedural stratification of case complexity may help to better organize timeslots and personnel, and in this way improve the catheterization laboratory workflow, efficiency, and resource utilization. The online procedural and PCI

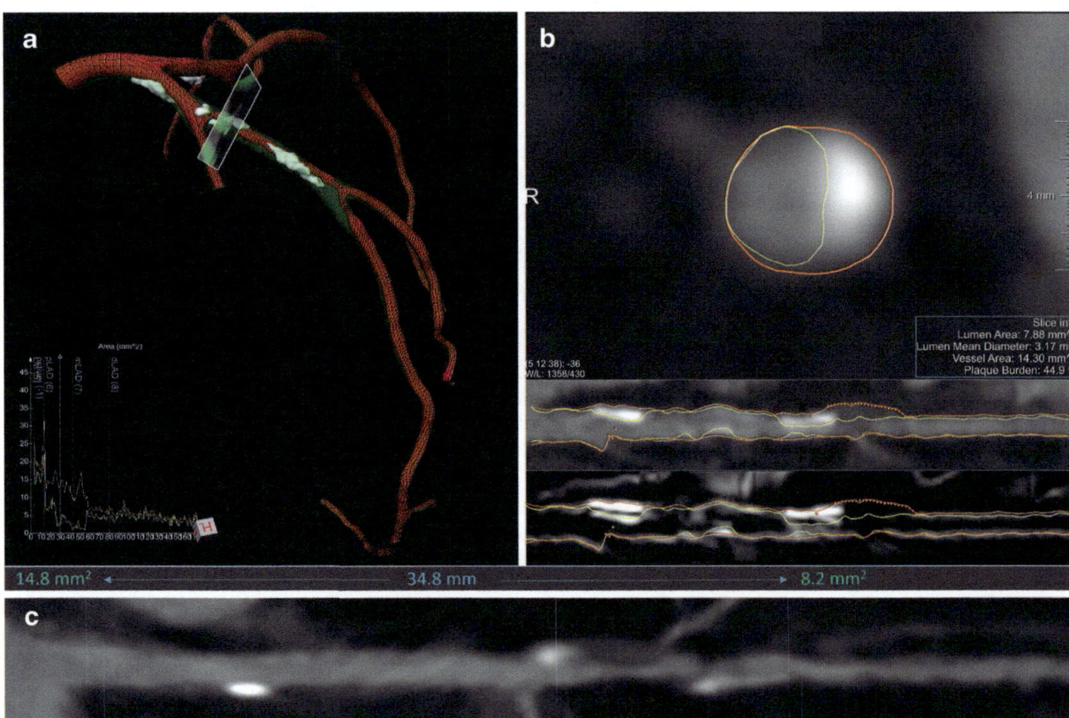

Fig. 7.5 Prototype of measuring tool for online length assessment. Panel **a** shows the 3D reconstruction of a coronary lesion located in the proximal segment of the LAD. Panel **b** shows a tomographic cross-section at the level of the marker. Panel **c** shows a straight MPR reconstruction with the selection of the landing zones and lesion length. (Reprinted from article *Collet, C et al. Implementing Coronary Computed Tomography Angiography in the Catheterization Laboratory. JACC: Cardiovascular Imaging, 2020* with permission from Elsevier)

guidance enhances the evaluation of CAD extent, the identification of optimal landing zones for stents including an improved CAD length assessment and allows for an online 3D visualization of the atherosclerotic process. As such, CCTA provides a "live" IVUS-like imaging of the atherosclerotic plaque. This optimized plaque visualization is likely to be translated into an improved PCI technique with the potential to improve clinical outcomes after PCI. In addition, using CCTA instead of intravascular imaging techniques could reduce a huge burden on healthcare spending.

The integration of CCTA images in the catheterization laboratory is also likely to improve the safety of the procedure in terms of radiation dose and contrast volume. Moreover, the visualization of atherosclerotic disease in apparent "normal" or mild disease angiographic segments might increase the use of invasive functional and imaging assessment (Fig. 7.6). Altogether, the integration of CCTA in the cath-lab has the potential to improve the diagnostic performance of conventional angiography, facilitate coronary revascularization and refine patient management.

7.5.1 Future Perspectives

The integration of noninvasive imaging inside the catheterization laboratory represents a novel approach for the evaluation of CAD. The tools available have been adapted from a diagnostic setting to treatment planning and online guidance of coronary angiography and PCI. Dedicated software must be developed aiming to simplify procedural workflow. Measurement tools that enable online co-registration and simulate cardiac cycle movement can further expand the synergism between CCTA and invasive coronary angiography.

Procedural planning of coronary procedures is likely to become an integral part of the percutaneous treatment of patients with CAD. For this, the evaluation and interpretation of CCTA

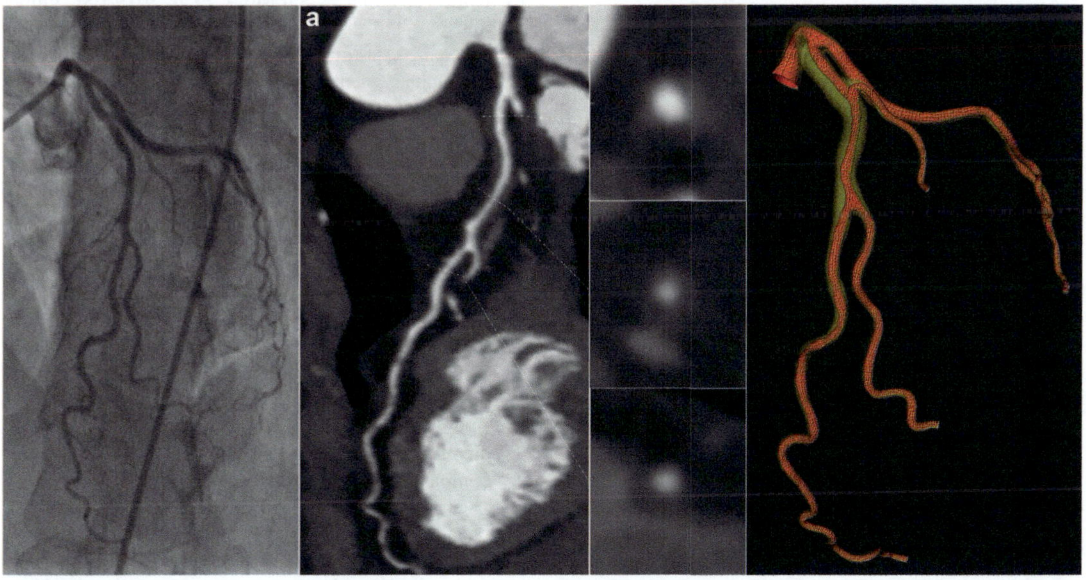

Fig. 7.6 Atherosclerotic disease in apparent "normal" angiographic vessel. Panel **a** shows an MPR image of an LAD with a long noncalcified plaque from the ostial LAD until the takeoff of the second diagonal branch. The cross-sections show noncalcified plaque with positive remodeling. Conventional angiography shows mild disease in the proximal and mid LAD. The co-registration of CCTA and angiography triggered a further invasive functional evaluation of the vessel resulting in an invasive FFR of 0.76. (Reprinted from article *Collet, C* et al. *Implementing Coronary Computed Tomography Angiography in the Catheterization Laboratory. JACC: Cardiovascular Imaging, 2020* with permission from Elsevier)

should become a core competency for an interventional cardiologist. This would require a new training path focused on the guidance of coronary interventions. The randomized Precise Procedural Planning and PCI trial (P4 trial) is currently assessing the effectiveness and safety of CCTA-guided PCI as compared to IVUS-guided PCI (NCT05253677).

7.6 Conclusion

Coronary CTA has become the method of choice for noninvasive evaluation of CAD. Beyond the diagnostic phase, CCTA can be used to improve patient selection for PCI and to plan and guide therapeutic interventions. CCTA adds one dimension to conventional angiography and incorporates the visualization of atherosclerotic plaque in the entire coronary tree. This novel approach has the potential to enhance invasive procedures and improve clinical outcomes. Clinical trials are required to determine the benefits of this approach.

References

1. Schmermund A. The Agatston calcium score: a milestone in the history of cardiac CT. J Cardiovasc Comput Tomogr. 2014;8:414–7.
2. Hurlock GS, Higashino H, Mochizuki T. History of cardiac computed tomography: single to 320-detector row multislice computed tomography. Int J Cardiovasc Imaging. 2009;25(Suppl 1):31–42.
3. Hounsfield GN. Computerized transverse axial scanning (tomography). 1. Description of system. Br J Radiol. 1973;46:1016–22.
4. Sagel SS, Weiss ES, Gillard RG, et al. Gated computed tomography of the human heart. Invest Radiol. 1977;12:563–6.
5. Lipton MJ, Brundage BH, Higgins CB, Boyd DP. CT scanning of the heart. Cardiovasc Clin. 1983;13:385–401.
6. Achenbach S, Giesler T, Ropers D, et al. Detection of coronary artery stenoses by contrast-enhanced, retrospectively electrocardiographically-gated, multislice spiral computed tomography. Circulation. 2001;103:2535–8.
7. Nieman K, Rensing BJ, van Geuns RJ, et al. Usefulness of multislice computed tomography for detecting obstructive coronary artery disease. Am J Cardiol. 2002;89:913–8.
8. Raff GL, Gallagher MJ, O'Neill WW, Goldstein JA. Diagnostic accuracy of noninvasive coronary angiography using 64-slice spiral computed tomography. J Am Coll Cardiol. 2005;46:552–7.
9. Meijboom WB, Van Mieghem CA, van Pelt N, et al. Comprehensive assessment of coronary artery stenoses: computed tomography coronary angiography versus conventional coronary angiography and correlation with fractional flow reserve in patients with stable angina. J Am Coll Cardiol. 2008;52:636–43.
10. Flohr TG, McCollough CH, Bruder H, et al. First performance evaluation of a dual-source CT (DSCT) system. Eur Radiol. 2006;16:256–68.
11. Collet C, Katagiri Y, Miyazaki Y, et al. Impact of coronary remodeling on fractional flow reserve. Circulation. 2018;137:747–9.
12. Norgaard BL, Leipsic J, Gaur S, et al. Diagnostic performance of noninvasive fractional flow reserve derived from coronary computed tomography angiography in suspected coronary artery disease: the NXT trial (Analysis of Coronary Blood Flow Using CT Angiography: Next Steps). J Am Coll Cardiol. 2014;63:1145–55.
13. Motoyama S, Sarai M, Harigaya H, et al. Computed tomographic angiography characteristics of atherosclerotic plaques subsequently resulting in acute coronary syndrome. J Am Coll Cardiol. 2009;54:49–57.
14. Newby DE, Adamson PD, Berry C, et al. Coronary CT angiography and 5-year risk of myocardial infarction. N Engl J Med. 2018;379:924–33.
15. Knuuti J, Wijns W, Saraste A, et al. 2019 ESC guidelines for the diagnosis and management of chronic coronary syndromes: the task force for the diagnosis and management of chronic coronary syndromes of the European Society of Cardiology (ESC). Eur Heart J. 2020;41(3):407–77.
16. de Knegt MC, Linde JJ, Fuchs A, et al. Reproducibility of coronary atherosclerotic plaque characteristics in populations with low, intermediate, and high prevalence of coronary artery disease by multidetector computer tomography: a guide to reliable visual coronary plaque assessments. Int J Cardiovasc Imaging. 2016;32:1555–66.
17. Collet C, Grundeken MJ, Asano T, Onuma Y, Wijns W, Serruys PW. State of the art: coronary angiography. EuroIntervention. 2017;13:634–43.
18. Boogers MJ, Schuijf JD, Kitslaar PH, et al. Automated quantification of stenosis severity on 64-slice CT: a comparison with quantitative coronary angiography. JACC Cardiovasc Imaging. 2010;3:699–709.
19. Papadopoulou SL, Garcia-Garcia HM, Rossi A, et al. Reproducibility of computed tomography angiography data analysis using semiautomated plaque quantification software: implications for the design of longitudinal studies. Int J Cardiovasc Imaging. 2013;29:1095–104.
20. Collet C, Onuma Y, Grundeken MJ, et al. In vitro validation of coronary CT angiography for the evaluation of complex lesions. EuroIntervention. 2018;13:e1823–30.

21. Collet C, Chevalier B, Cequier A, et al. Diagnostic accuracy of coronary CT angiography for the evaluation of bioresorbable vascular scaffolds. JACC Cardiovasc Imaging. 2018;11:722–32.
22. Raber L, Mintz GS, Koskinas KC, et al. Clinical use of intracoronary imaging. Part 1: guidance and optimization of coronary interventions. An expert consensus document of the European Association of Percutaneous Cardiovascular Interventions. Eur Heart J. 2018;39:3281–300.
23. Collet C, Onuma Y, Cavalcante R, et al. Quantitative angiography methods for bifurcation lesions: a consensus statement update from the European Bifurcation Club. EuroIntervention. 2017;13:115–23.
24. Campbell PT, Mahmud E, Marshall JJ. Interoperator and intraoperator (in)accuracy of stent selection based on visual estimation. Catheter Cardiovasc Interv. 2015;86:1177–83.
25. Conte E, Mushtaq S, Pontone G, et al. Plaque quantification by coronary computed tomography angiography using intravascular ultrasound as a reference standard: a comparison between standard and last generation computed tomography scanners. Eur Heart J Cardiovasc Imaging. 2020;21:191–201.
26. van Rosendael AR, Al'Aref SJ, Dwivedi A, et al. Quantitative evaluation of high-risk coronary plaque by coronary CTA and subsequent acute coronary events. JACC Cardiovasc Imaging. 2019;12:1568–71.
27. Dettmer M, Glaser-Gallion N, Stolzmann P, et al. Quantification of coronary artery stenosis with high-resolution CT in comparison with histopathology in an ex vivo study. Eur J Radiol. 2013;82:264–9.
28. Fujino A, Mintz GS, Matsumura M, et al. A new optical coherence tomography-based calcium scoring system to predict stent underexpansion. EuroIntervention. 2018;13:e2182–9.
29. Genereux P, Madhavan MV, Mintz GS, et al. Ischemic outcomes after coronary intervention of calcified vessels in acute coronary syndromes. Pooled analysis from the HORIZONS-AMI (Harmonizing Outcomes With Revascularization and Stents in Acute Myocardial Infarction) and ACUITY (Acute Catheterization and Urgent Intervention Triage Strategy) trials. J Am Coll Cardiol. 2014;63:1845–54.
30. Ali ZA, Brinton TJ, Hill JM, et al. Optical coherence tomography characterization of coronary lithoplasty for treatment of calcified lesions: first description. JACC Cardiovasc Imaging. 2017;10:897–906.
31. Fujino A, Mintz GS, Lee T, et al. Predictors of calcium fracture derived from balloon angioplasty and its effect on stent expansion assessed by optical coherence tomography. JACC Cardiovasc Interv. 2018;11:1015–7.
32. Kobayashi N, Ito Y, Yamawaki M, et al. Optical frequency-domain imaging findings to predict good stent expansion after rotational atherectomy for severely calcified coronary lesions. Int J Cardiovasc Imaging. 2018;34:867–74.
33. Uetani T, Amano T, Kunimura A, et al. The association between plaque characterization by CT angiography and post-procedural myocardial infarction in patients with elective stent implantation. JACC Cardiovasc Imaging. 2010;3:19–28.
34. Maehara A, Matsumura M, Ali ZA, Mintz GS, Stone GW. IVUS-guided versus OCT-guided coronary stent implantation: a critical appraisal. JACC Cardiovasc Imaging. 2017;10:1487–503.
35. Miller JM, Rochitte CE, Dewey M, et al. Diagnostic performance of coronary angiography by 64-row CT. N Engl J Med. 2008;359:2324–36.
36. Collet C, Sonck J, Vandeloo B, et al. Measurement of hyperemic pullback pressure gradients to characterize patterns of coronary atherosclerosis. J Am Coll Cardiol. 2019;74:1772–84.
37. Fournier S, Ciccarelli G, Toth GG, et al. Association of Improvement in fractional flow reserve with outcomes, including symptomatic relief, after percutaneous coronary intervention. JAMA Cardiol. 2019;4:370–4.
38. Mollet NR, Hoye A, Lemos PA, et al. Value of preprocedure multislice computed tomographic coronary angiography to predict the outcome of percutaneous recanalization of chronic total occlusions. Am J Cardiol. 2005;95:240–3.
39. Bradley SM, Spertus JA, Kennedy KF, et al. Patient selection for diagnostic coronary angiography and hospital-level percutaneous coronary intervention appropriateness: insights from the National Cardiovascular Data Registry. JAMA Intern Med. 2014;174:1630–9.
40. Moss AJ, Williams MC, Newby DE, Nicol ED. The updated NICE guidelines: cardiac CT as the first-line test for coronary artery disease. Curr Cardiovasc Imaging Rep. 2017;10:15.
41. Lee SP, Jang EJ, Kim YJ, et al. Cost-effectiveness of coronary CT angiography in patients with chest pain: comparison with myocardial single photon emission tomography. J Cardiovasc Comput Tomogr. 2015;9:428–37.
42. Zeb I, Abbas N, Nasir K, Budoff MJ. Coronary computed tomography as a cost-effective test strategy for coronary artery disease assessment—a systematic review. Atherosclerosis. 2014;234:426–35.
43. Sonck J, Nagumo S, Norgaard B, et al. Clinical Validation of a Virtual Planner for Coronary Interventions Based on Coronary CT Angiography. J Am Coll Cardiol Img. null 2022;0(0). https://doi.org/10.1016/j.jcmg.2022.02.003.

Part II

Hybrid Imaging in Clinical Practice

Systematic Review of Hybrid Cardiac Imaging

8

Susanna Breviario, Davide Tore, Ovidio De Filippo, Gaetano Maria De Ferrari, Paolo Fonio, Fabrizio D'Ascenzo, and Alessandro Depaoli

8.1 The Point of View of the Cardiologists

Hybrid imaging is gaining interest as a relevant field of research and investment in cardiovascular diseases and it is progressively being introduced into routine clinical practice. Indeed, a noninvasive diagnostic test is frequently preferred over an invasive one as the first diagnostic step. Among the formers, hybrid imaging has the unique feature to release anatomical and functional information at the same time. Nowadays, several kinds of hybrid imaging techniques are emerging among them coronary computed tomography angiography (CCTA) generally provides anatomical information while the addition of myocardial perfusion imaging (MPI) allows a contemporary functional evaluation. MPI techniques encompass single photon-emission computed tomography (SPECT), positron emission tomography (PET), and cardiac magnetic resonance (MRI).

In several recent meta-analyses and reviews, hybrid imaging demonstrated improved diagnostic performance compared with stand-alone CCTA or MPI. However, it should be considered that CCTA coupled with SPECT or PET results in increased radiation exposure. On the other side, the increased costs of these methodologies also raised some concerns.

Therefore, this chapter will go through the description of the several methodologies flowing into the common definition of "hybrid imaging." It will provide insights from recent pieces of evidence about hybrid imaging along with its major advantages and drawbacks, to help to address the issue of which clinical scenarios and patients might benefit most from such technologies. Lastly, it will discuss hybrid imaging's future perspectives of development and utilization.

8.1.1 Meta-analysis Results

In recent years, meta-analyses and related reviews have been performed to establish the role and the value of hybrid imaging. Such efforts were prompted by the awareness that anatomic imaging yields the highest sensitivity but performs poorly for specificity, whereas hybrid imaging is supposed to overcome this limitation [1].

In the context of ischemic heart disease, CTA is commonly recommended to rule out obstructive coronary artery disease (CAD) in patients

S. Breviario · O. De Filippo · G. M. De Ferrari
F. D'Ascenzo (✉)
Division of Cardiology, Department of Medical Sciences, University of Turin, Città della Salute e della Scienza, Turin, Italy
e-mail: gaetanomaria.deferrari@unito.it

D. Tore · P. Fonio · A. Depaoli
Division of Radiology, Department of Surgical Sciences, University of Turin, Città della Salute e della Scienza, Turin, Italy
e-mail: paolo.fonio@unito.it

F. Nudi et al. (eds.), *Hybrid Cardiac Imaging for Clinical Decision-Making*,
https://doi.org/10.1007/978-3-030-99391-7_8

deemed at low or intermediate cardiovascular risk [2], due to its high negative predictive value (NPV). This has been confirmed by several meta-analyses [3–5]. Its positive predictive value however was demonstrated to be less relevant. In most cases, this is due to the overestimation of coronary stenosis detected by CTA. Indeed, dense coronary calcifications may deteriorate image quality [6]. CTA proved as the best test for anatomically significant CAD, whereas functional and anatomical-functional (hybrid) tests perform better for the evaluation of functionally significant CAD. In a meta-analysis by Biondi Zoccai et al., noninvasive hybrid imaging tests proved superior to anatomic or stand-alone functional tests to diagnose ischemia-provoking coronary lesions, whereas anatomic imaging performs more accurately to rule out angiographically significant CAD [1].

Recently, novel computed tomography imaging techniques such as stress myocardial computed tomography perfusion (stress-CTP) or noninvasive fractional flow reserve (FFR-CT) have emerged as strategies able to combine both anatomical and functional evaluation, with a positive impact on the diagnosis performance [2]. In a recent meta-analysis, stress-CTP and FFR-CT demonstrated improved diagnostic positive likelihood ratio (PLR) and specificity compared with stand-alone CTA for the detection of hemodynamically relevant coronary stenosis [2]. Myocardial stress-CTP evaluation requires two scans, the first under pharmacologically induced stress, and the other at rest. On the other hand, one of the main strengths of FFR-CT is that this technique requires only a single acquisition, without requiring a stress agent, additional contrast, or additional radiations. Another advantage over stress-CTP is that FFR-CT allows the identification of a specific coronary lesion causing ischemia. However, the performance of such a technique depends on very high image quality. The diagnostic accuracy of FFR-CT varies substantially according to the spectrum of CAD, with high values at advanced stages of the disease, and lower values in the intermediate forms of the disease [2].

Another meta-analysis (Rizvi et al., JACC 2018) concluded that hybrid imaging shows a higher specificity (93%) and positive likelihood ratio (LR+ 12.80) when compared with stand-alone coronary CTA (66% and 3.39; $p < 0.05$) to detect obstructive CAD (Table 8.1).

In particular, while at patient level the hybrid approach showed comparable areas under the curve (AUC) at ROC analysis as compared with stand-alone coronary CTA (0.97 vs 0.93, respectively; $p = 0.132$), on a per-vessel level, hybrid

Table 8.1 Meta-analysis for the diagnostic performance of coronary CTA alone, MPI alone, and cardiac hybrid imaging

	N	Sensitivity (95% CI)	Specificity (95% CI)	PLR (95% CI)	NLR (95% CI)	Diagnostic odds ratio (95% CI)
Per-patient analysis						
Coronary CTA	12	0.90 (0.87–0.92)	0.66 (0.61–0.70)	3.39 (2.22–5.17)	0.06 (0.02–0.23)	53.80 (28.61–101.19)
MPI	9	0.87 (0.83–0.90)	0.83 (0.78–0.87)	5.02 (2.99–8.44)	0.15 (0.09–0.25)	39.55 (15.64–100.02)
Hybrid	12	0.91 (0.88–0.93)	0.93 (0.90–0.95)	12.80 (6.56–24.96)	0.11 (0.07–0.18)	159.00 (57.42–440.25)
Per-vessel analysis						
Coronary CTA	8	0.89 (0.86–0.91)	0.83 (0.81–0.85)	5.75 (4.00–8.26)	0.14 (0.09–0.22)	44.27 (25.39–77.20)
MPI	6	0.78 (0.74–0.81)	0.87 (0.84–0.89)	5.24 (3.52–7.82)	0.25 (0.16–0.39)	22.59 (10.41–49.03)
Hybrid	8	0.84 (0.81–0.87)	0.95 (0.94–0.96)	16.53 (9.14–29.90)	0.14 (0.07–0.26)	137.90 (53.93–352.66)

CI confidence interval, *CTA* computed tomography angiography, *MPI* myocardial perfusion imaging, *PLR* positive likelihood ratio, *NLR* negative likelihood ratio imaging approach showed significantly higher specificity and LR+ (specificity 95% and LR+ 16.53 vs 83% and 5.75 for hybrid imaging and CTA, respectively; $p < 0.0.5$). Moreover, on a per vessel basis, sROC curves showed a significantly higher AUC value for the hybrid approach when compared with stand-alone coronary CTA (0.97 vs 0.93; $p = 0.047$). Particularly, hybrid SPECT/coronary CTA demonstrated the highest sensitivity for assessment of obstructive CAD as compared with PET/coronary CTA ($p < 0.05$). On the contrary, specificity was higher for PET/coronary CTA when compared with SPECT/coronary CTA. Despite these findings, no differences in the SRC curves among the various hybrid imaging techniques were observed [7].

Further studies are required to appropriately compare the individual diagnostic accuracy of different functional and hybrid tests [1].

While CTA estimates the degree of atherosclerotic burden and may reveal some plaques at risk of rupture, it fails to quantify flow-limiting consequences of the luminal stenosis and presents reduced sensitivity in the evaluation of distal coronary segments and side branches [8]. These limits could be offset by MPI information. A functional assessment is particularly required when evaluating intermediate lesions in CTA. To this purpose, at present SPECT represents a well-validated functional test. However, SPECT still suffers from several limitations: it often underestimates the degree of ischemia, particularly in presence of multivessel disease, since the SPECT analysis is either relative (qualitative) or semi-quantitative. Compared with SPECT, PET shows several advantages such as higher image quality, due to higher spatial resolution and reduced attenuation artifacts. The diagnostic accuracy of PET is high. This exam allows identifying multivessel ischemia significantly better when compared with SPECT (74% vs 41%, respectively, Bateman 2006). However, with both methods, the visualization of just small or relative differences in myocardial blood flow (MBF) may lead to the underestimation of CAD. PET allows quantification of the blood flow increasing the diagnostic accuracy of the technique. Another technique able to provide functional data is cardiac magnetic resonance imaging (MRI). MRI can detect myocardial ischemia through pharmacological stress by screening for wall motion abnormalities induced by dobutamine infusion or perfusion abnormalities induced by adenosine [6].

The relationship between the diseased coronary artery and the myocardial perfusion defect can be evaluated on a fusion imaging approach.

In conclusion, the hybrid MPI/CTA imaging techniques can spare unnecessary invasive diagnosis and revascularization in patients with coronary artery lesions but without obvious myocardial ischemia. On the contrary, patients with mild coronary lesion but with severe myocardial ischemia could receive the most adequate treatment by the hybrid approach [8].

8.1.2 Patients Who Might Benefit from Hybrid Imaging

Nowadays, it remains debatable what kind of patients should undergo hybrid imaging examinations for clinical effectiveness and minimization of costs and radiation dose. Patients should be carefully selected when an added value of hybrid imaging may be anticipated. There are several scenarios in which it is recognized that hybrid imaging can provide clinically important information.

Patients with multivessel disease represent a population at increased risk for cardiac events. In this population, a functional test such as SPECT can underestimate the true extent of the disease since this technique emphasizes the territory supplied by the most severe stenosis. A balanced reduction in myocardial hyperemic blood flow may explain the underestimation of clinical cardiovascular risk. By adding an anatomical evaluation, these patients are most likely to benefit from hybrid imaging. Compared to perfusion imaging alone, hybrid imaging may provide an incremental diagnostic value to identify hemodynamically significant coronary lesions [9]. Diagnostic problems for MPI techniques are also found in an increasing number of patients who are affected by obesity. In obese patients, SPECT is prone to false-positive results due to a nonuniform photon attenuation. Regarding this, hybrid imaging could represent a better diagnostic tool [10].

Patients with intermediate pretest likelihood are more likely to yield intermediate or inconclusive results from anatomical studies, as intermediate coronary stenosis was detected by CTA. In this situation, an additional perfusion study may address the hemodynamic significance of these lesions and help to decide whether the patient can be treated medically or needs to be referred for invasive angiography with revascularization.

Side branches are often regarded as prognostically irrelevant but may be associated with significant symptoms. Hybrid imaging allows identifying flow-limiting lesions inside branches for targeted revascularization procedures [9].

Another application of hybrid imaging is the evaluation of chronic total occlusions (CTO). Percutaneous revascularization procedures in patients with CTO are associated with higher rates of complications. Therefore, proof of myocardial ischemia in the area of the occluded vessel is a mandatory prior commitment to any intervention. Hybrid imaging can detect a perfusion defect located in the area of the CTO vessel. The anatomical information provided by CTA are predictors of procedural success and may help to decide between anterograde or retrograde revascularization approaches [9]. Figure 8.1 displays a suggested algorithm to integrate hybrid imaging into routine clinical practice for the diagnosis or follow-up of coronary artery disease both for patients with or without a clinical history of the previous revascularization.

8.1.3 Perspectives on Hybrid Imaging

Over the last 10 years, hybrid imaging has advanced from an intriguing to a useful tool that is finding increasing clinical acceptance. Nowadays, the most popular imaging techniques are SPECT/CT or PET/CT [10].

The current concern about hybrid imaging with SPECT/CT remains the radiation exposure, even if it is expected to decrease in near future with the acquisition of new equipment and protocols. Currently, a newly developed cadmium-zinc-telluride ultrafast semiconductor detector is introduced in the SPECT technique. This system was reported to allow a significant reduction of the scan time and radiotracer dose with high temporal and spatial resolution. It also allows quantitative myocardial blood flow and coronary flow reserve noninvasive evaluation [8].

Moreover, other techniques are now accessible for hybrid imaging, such as cardiac magnetic resonance (CMR). The advantage of CMR is that it does not depend on ionization radiations. On the contrary, its spreading was limited by the fact that perfusion data could only be obtained in three cross-sections of the left ventricle, which is insufficient to extrapolate a 3D volume. However, novel fast perfusion sequences are now available thus allowing to obtain full-coverage volumetric perfusion data of the left ventricle and permitting fusion with 3D volume CTA images [10].

One hybrid imaging technique that is gaining interest is CMR/PET. Since CMR does not currently allow robust coronary angiography, the applications may be different. The experience is nowadays limited only to case-reports, but it could be expected that this combination would be very powerful for viability imaging, in the evaluation of various inflammatory cardiac diseases, and, potentially, in cardiac heart failure [10].

One interesting approach is based on combining functional FFR-CT information with morphological information obtained from CTCA. Preliminary results reveal that FFR-CT may be useful to assess the hemodynamic significance of coronary lesions. These findings need to be confirmed in larger trials. The combination of anatomic imaging (CTA) with a functional evaluation through stress-CTP is another approach that is currently spreading [10] (an example of CTP is provided in Fig. 8.2). Moreover, the latest reports have shown the possibility to calculate noninvasive endothelial shear stress from coronary CTA. The evaluation of endothelial shear stress and wall stress with the aid of hybrid imaging is expected to advance our understanding of the natural history of ischemic cardiac disease [11].

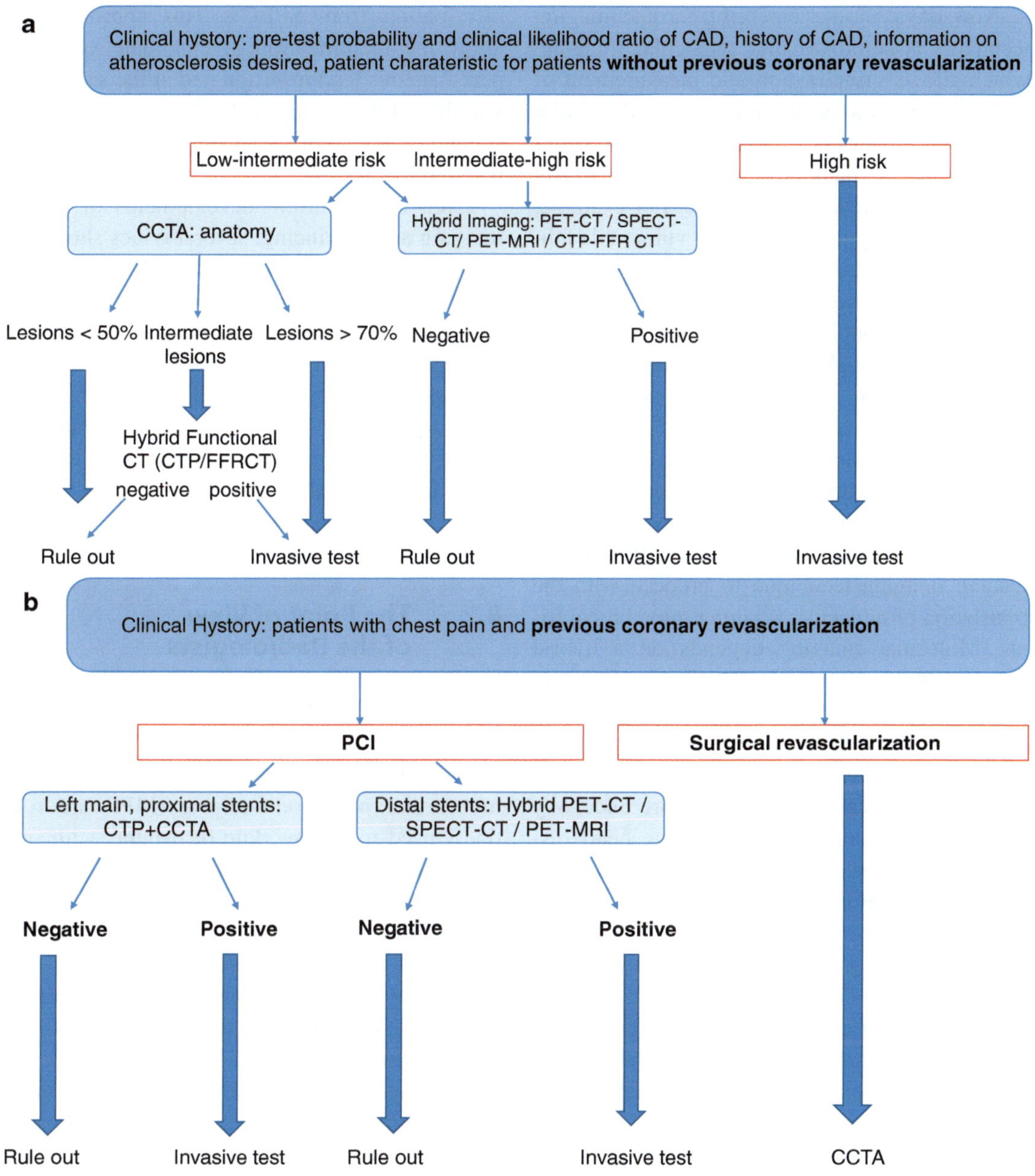

Fig. 8.1 Suggested algorithm to integrate hybrid imaging into routine clinical practice for the detection of coronary artery disease (CAD) according to pretest clinical likelihood of CAD for patients without previous revascularization (**a**) and for those with clinical history of surgical or percutaneous coronary revascularization (**b**). *CCTA* coronary computed tomography angiography, *CTP* computed tomography with perfusion, *FFRCT* fractional flow reserve computed tomography, *PET-CT* positron emission tomography-Computed tomography, *PET-MRI* Positron emission tomography–magnetic resonance imaging

Nowadays, another emerging cardiac imaging technique is cardiovascular molecular imaging, which allows visualization and measurement of biological processes at molecular and cellular levels and provides new targeted probes to better understand the pathophysiological mechanism underlying cardiovascular disease. For example, this kind of imaging can identify vulnerable atherosclerotic plaque before rupture and subsequent MI, biomechanisms that precede left ventricular remodeling and development of heart failure, and, through neuronal imaging, allows to assess the risk of ventricular arrhythmias. Additionally, molecular imaging has great potential to facilitate the development of novel therapies through improved target identification. Regarding its high sensitivity and availability of tracers with a low risk of toxicity, PET is the leading imaging technique to proceed with the translation of molecular imaging into clinical trials. Molecular imaging depends on a hybrid imaging approach, where the nuclear imaging component is used for molecular targeting seen as a hot spot and the anatomical imaging modality is used for localization of the molecular signal [10]. Recently, new developments are underway for PET-based imaging for ischemic heart disease. Among these, the development of new tracers such as 18F-Flurpiridaz has some potential advantages as the one to include high extraction fraction allowing high sensitivity in detecting perfusion defects and longer half-life making it compatible with exercise stress testing. Another new tracer currently under evaluation is 18F-sodium fluoride. Given the potential association of microcalcification with vulnerable plaques, this tracer may identify culprit coronary lesions. Further studies are required to assess the potential of this agent in risk stratification and management of patients with CAD [12].

Another application of hybrid imaging could be the prediction of cardiac resynchronization therapy (CRT) success and the improvement in patient selection. Indeed, CRT nonresponder rates are still high (approximately 30%), particularly in patients with ischemic heart disease. Hybrid imaging may combine venous anatomy evaluation from CT with viability information from SPECT. This approach can allow the identification of candidate veins for percutaneous lead insertion and at the same time viability of this area. It is likely that patients carrying the LV lead in a nonviable territory may not respond to CRT [9].

Even if the current developments of hybrid imaging are convincing, several issues should be addressed for further improvements such as reliability and accuracy of fusion technology, motion compensation (cardiac beating and breathing), tissue deformation with manipulation during procedures, the ability for virtual reality simulation and integration of holographic 4D. The future of fusion imaging combines several imaging tools in a faithful real-time holographic 4D heart model [13].

8.2 The Point of View of the Radiologists

8.2.1 CAC and SPECT

Both calcium score (CAC) and stress-rest SPECT myocardial perfusion imaging (MPI) are routinely used for the workup of patients with suspected coronary artery disease (CAD). CAC may be used in a synergistic fashion with myocardial perfusion imaging (MPI) to improve diagnostic accuracy and clinical decision-making for patients with suspected CAD. An emerging application for CAC is its use as a possible triage test for cardiac stress testing. A meta-analysis demonstrated a low frequency of inducible myocardial ischemia in patients with either zero or very low CAC scores; inducible ischemia was more frequent with increasing CAC scores [14]. A significant variance of incidence of inducible ischemia in patients with intermediate scores was found to be dependent on the diabetic status or metabolic syndrome [15]. Concomitant CAC and SPECT may improve diagnostic accuracy and confidence in SPECT-MPI interpretation. A study compared the interpretation of perfusion images with and without knowledge of the CAC score thus demonstrating that the CAC data allowed to decrease the number of equivocal interpretations

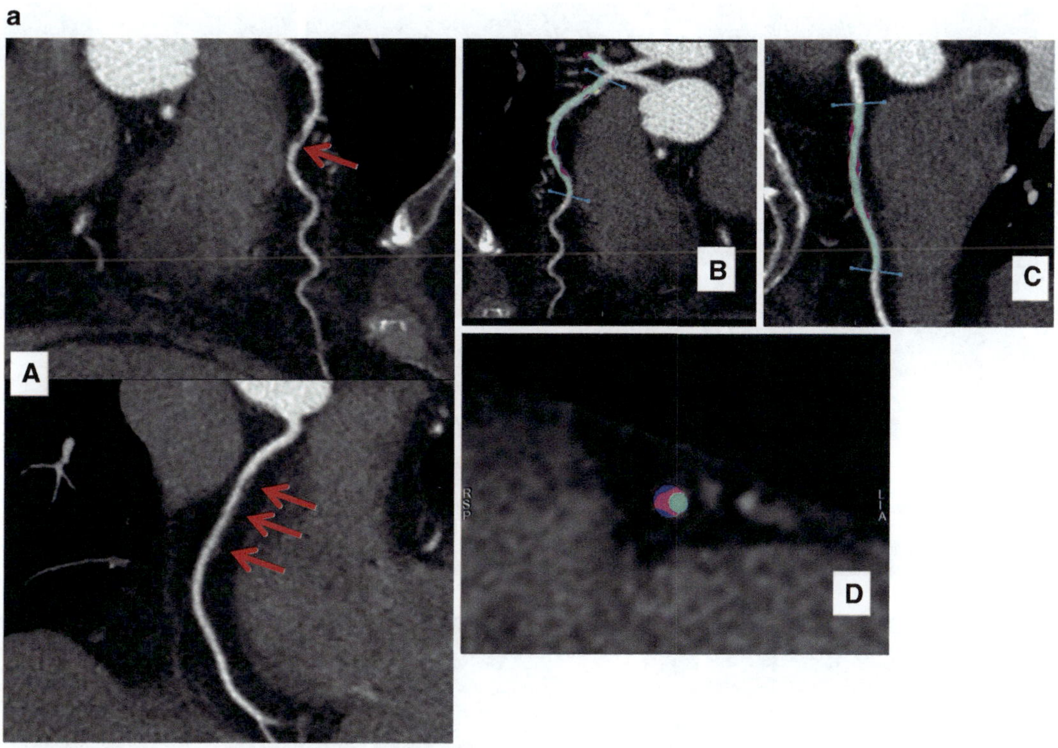

Fig. 8.2 (**a**) Coronary computed tomography angiography with perfusion performed in a patient without a history of previous revascularization, with multiple cardiovascular risk factors (diabetes and hypertension) admitted for worsening dyspnea. Anatomical images (panels A–C): curved planar reformation (CPR) show an intermediate coronary stenosis of the left anterior descending artery (LAD) and diffuse stenotic hypodense plaques of right coronary artery (RCA) (red arrows); panels B and C show vessel and plaque analysis (lipidic plaque high lighted in purple and blue) of LAD and RCA; Panel D shows an axial view of the vessel (LAD) with lipidic plaque highlighted in purple and blue. Perfusion images derived from static CTP (panels E–H): short axis two chamber view show subendocardial perfusion defect in the basal and mid ventricular septum (green arrows), hypodense compared to normally perfused myocardium. Panel H: color map shows perfusion defect in purple/green compared to normal myocardium (orange). Panel I: four chamber long axis image shows subendocardial perfusion defect in the basal and mid ventricular septum (green arrows), hypodense. (**b**) Panela (A–C): volume rendering derived from static stress CTP showing inducible ischemia of basal to mid septum (blue areas) with 3D fusion of the corresponding anatomical coronary tree

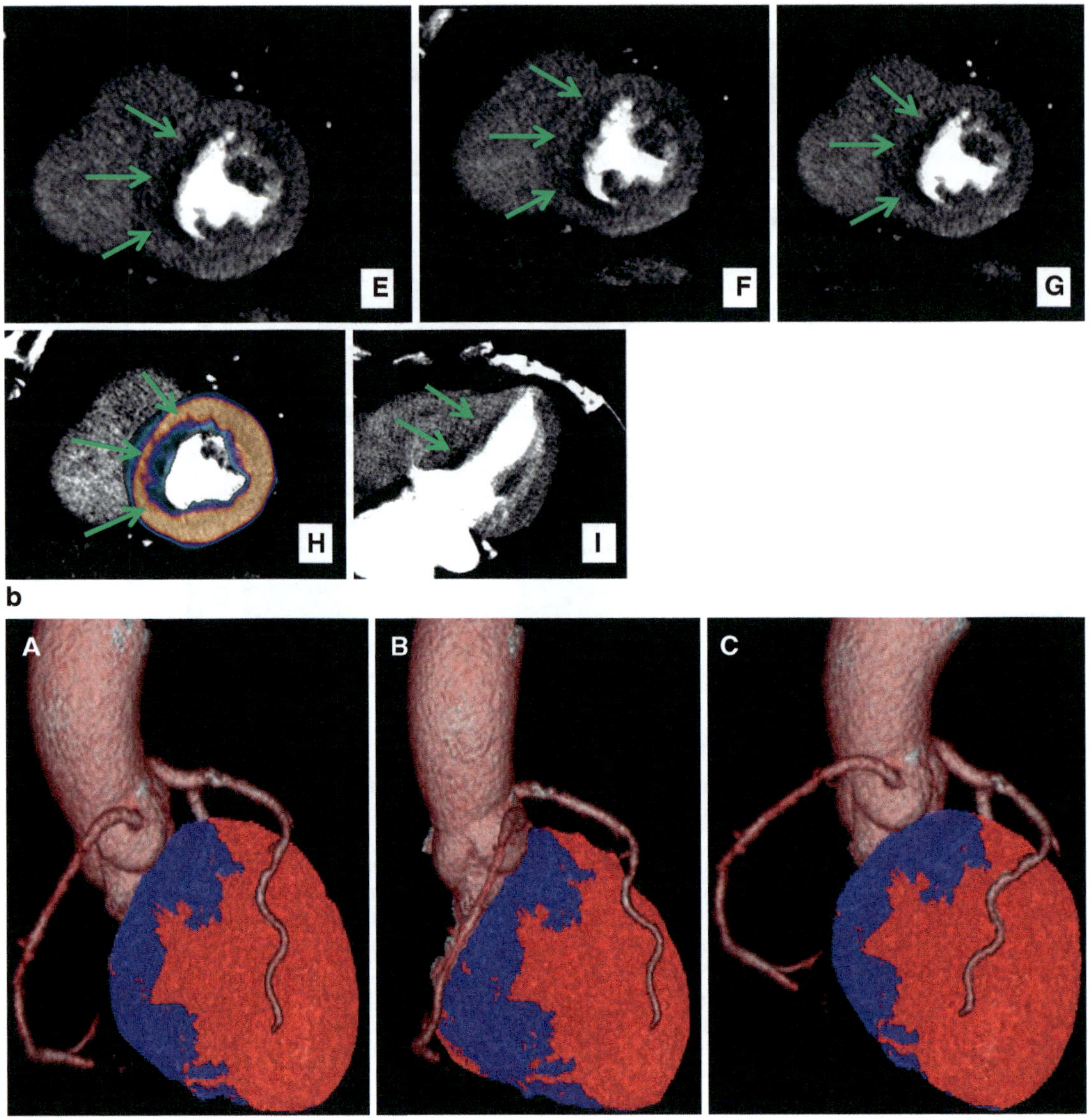

Fig. 8.2 (continued)

from 21 to 9% [16]. Another study showed that CAC imaging could increase the number of stress-only perfusion studies by reducing the need for rest imaging and unnecessary radiation exposure for patients [17]. The synergistic use of CAC and SPECT has been demonstrated to allow a much better long-term risk stratification compared with SPECT-only exams [18, 19]. In current clinical practice with hybrid systems, the CAC scan is generally acquired separately, immediately before the MPI scan [20]. This study protocol with separate CT CAC and attenuation scans results in increased radiation exposure to the patient [21] and lengthens the overall duration of the exam. It should be possible to use the CAC scans also for attenuation correction thus eliminating the need for an additional acquisition on hybrid PET/CT or SPECT/CT scanners. Vendors are currently developing software tools for this purpose.

8.2.2 SPECT and CCTA

CCTA provides high-resolution images of the coronary artery anatomy and allows the assessment of the presence and extent of coronary stenoses even providing prognostic information about the atherosclerotic plaque. There are some limitations to CCTA exams due to beam hardening artifacts from arterial calcifications, coronary stents, and the assessment of luminal stenosis in distal segments of the coronary arteries. Myocardial perfusion imaging (MPI) with SPECT/PET provides functional information on coronary lesions thus allowing prognostic assessment based on the extent and severity of perfusion abnormalities in patients with CAD. Limitations of MPI are due to attenuation, scatter and blur. Hybrid imaging with MPI and CTA provide different and complementary information for the diagnosis and evaluation of CAD, overcoming the limitations of the single modalities.

Hybrid SPECT/CCTA imaging can be obtained with software-based solutions or with hardware-based hybrid scanners. The integration of morphological and functional information provides a detailed view of coronary artery anatomy and myocardial perfusion thus eliminating uncertainties in the relationship between perfusion abnormalities and culprit coronary lesions [22].

Hybrid imaging has an incremental value in the evaluation of functionally relevant coronary artery lesions compared to SPECT or CCTA considered individually, providing higher diagnostic accuracy [23, 24] in the evaluation of patients with suspected CAD. This hybrid imaging technique may reduce the need for unnecessary invasive angiography and revascularization providing morphological and functional information for targeting and treating only clinically significant stenoses. SPECT/CCTA may have a role as a gatekeeper for patients with CAD before invasive diagnostic procedures. Because of the considerable anatomic variability of coronary arteries only half of the population has myocardial perfusion territories corresponding to the 17 segments defined by the American Heart Association [25]. The fusion of morphological and functional imaging permits an unequivocal assessment of the relationship between a diseased coronary artery and perfusion defects providing valuable information to the interventional cardiologist. Moreover, SPECT/CCTA is more accurate than SPECT alone in patients with balanced three-vessel disease that might result in equivocal or false-negative MPI exams while CCTA is very unlikely to miss severe multivessel atherosclerosis [8, 25, 26]. Another possible application for this technique is in the evaluation of treatment outcome in patients with CAD who underwent percutaneous coronary intervention. The reduction of perfusion abnormalities has been related to an increase in left ventricular ejection fraction and improved quality of life [27].

8.2.3 PET/MRI

Hybrid PET/MRI integrating the scanners have been available since 2010 thus allowing to use of the best methods for quantitative stress perfusion (PET) and functional and vitality imaging (MRI) in a single exam [28]. PET/MRI is a promising tool for the evaluation of ischemic heart disease to identify patients who might benefit from revascularization therapy [29]. PET/MRI may provide comprehensive perfusion and myocardial characterization study in a single session integrating a dual tracer protocol such as 13N-NH3 and 18F-FDG combined with late gadolinium enhancement imaging (LGE). PET can reliably identify areas of hibernated or stunned myocardial tissue while LGE can provide a precise assessment of transmural and subendocardial scarring thus providing useful information to guide a possible interventional treatment [30–33]. MRI can also detect small sub-endocardial scars which might be difficult to identify on PET due to its spatial resolution. In order to provide a more accurate risk stratification for major cardiac adverse events, PET can also identify myocardial perfusion-innovation mismatches which are frequently associated with increased mortality because of sudden cardiac arrest with tracers like 15O-water and 11C-meta-hydroxyephedrin3 [29].

A Hybrid PET/MRI study may discriminate between reversible and irreversible myocardial dysfunction in the subacute phase after revascularization in acute coronary syndromes and may have a role in the assessment of myocardial salvage and cardiac remodeling in ACS [34]. Moreover, the MRI part of the exam can rule out coronary artery origin anomalies which is a rare but important incidental finding in about 1% of exams [35, 36]. It is yet to be determined the optimal PET/MRI protocol in order to avoid redundant MRI sequences and/or PET tracer that may be omitted from the protocol. PET/MRI has the potential to be a one-stop-shop approach and for the evaluation of ventricular function and myocardial perfusion; however, there is no scientific evidence to support the value of a combined PET/MRI approach for patients with stable CAD and further research is warranted. A limitation of current PET/MRI studies is the long scan in time which is about 60 min and may not be tolerated by patients with a poor general state.

8.2.4 FFRCT and CTP

CCTA can provide functional data on myocardial tissue perfusion with a post-processing software approach (FFRCT) or with a specific perfusion study protocol.

Fractional flow reserve can be derived from CCTA scan data (FFRCT) using computational fluid dynamics simulation software. There are three principles behind this simulation approach. First, coronary flow at baseline is dependent on myocardial tissue oxygen demand and resting flow can be calculated accounting for myocardial territory-specific ventricular mass. Second, the microcirculatory bed resistance in resting conditions is inversely, not linearly, proportional to the size of the feeding vessel. Third, the microcirculation of the coronary arteries has a predictable response to adenosine [37, 38]. Based on these principles it is possible to simulate coronary blood flow using a 3D model based on patient anatomy. FFRCT is defined as the calculated mean coronary pressure distal to a stenotic lesion divided by the mean estimated blood pressure in the aorta under conditions of maximal hyperemia [39]. To date, one proprietary FFRCT software solution has been approved by FDA and European regulatory authorities for clinical use. The PLATFORM trial evaluated a population of symptomatic patients with suspected CAD with FFRCT or the usual care approach. FFRCT significantly reduced the number of ICAs in patients without obstructive CAD; moreover, the FFRCT approach reduced costs compared with standard care [40]. The PACIFIC FFRCT sub-study compared FFRCT, CCTA, SPECT, and PET for the diagnosis of cardiac ischemia using invasive FFR as a reference standard. FFRCT outperformed CCTA, SPECT, and PET in terms of sensitivity, demonstrated to be more accurate than CCTA and SPECT, and had higher specificity compared with SPECT [41]. The SYNTAX III Revolution study compared the agreement of revascularization strategy based on FFRCT or ICA in patients with three-vessel disease showing a very high concordance in clinical decision-making for both strategies. Moreover, FFRCT permitted to reclassify about 30% of those patients in a lower risk group. These results suggest that deciding between CABG and PCI relying only on noninvasive CCTA and FFRCT is feasible [42]. Myocardial perfusion can be evaluated with CCTA with static or dynamic acquisition protocols in both rest and stress (hyperemia) conditions, similarly to stress cardiac MR and nuclear imaging. Myocardial perfusion defects can be visualized as relatively hypodense areas. Static CTP is obtained with a single acquisition during the first-pass of the contrast medium; consequently, a possible drawback of this protocol is to miss the peak attenuation because only one sample of data is acquired [43]. Static CTP can be performed with two different protocols: rest/stress and stress/rest. A 10–15 min interval between the two acquisitions is needed to allow optimal contrast medium wash-out. In the rest/stress protocol the stress acquisition is performed only in case of evidence of obstructive CAD. Performing stress acquisition first (stress/rest protocol) could mask a fixed perfusion defect secondary to residual contrast contamination in the rest phase, reducing sensitivity for the detection of infarcted areas [43]. Hypoperfusion in stress acquisition with normal perfusion indicates ischemia, hypoperfusion in stress that persists with similar extension in rest is suggestive of myocardial necrosis [44]. Dynamic CTP consists of repeated low-dose acquisitions during intravenous contrast medium injection [45]. The pharmacological stress protocol is similar to static CTP. The images obtained, after motion correction, are used to derive time-attenuation curves (TACs). TACs allow myocardial blood flow (MBF) estimation based on different computational models. Dynamic CTP can quantify MBF (expressed as mL/100 mL/min) for every segment of the myocardium analyzed [46, 47].

CCTA with FFRCT or CTP provides information on coronary anatomy and lumen stenosis, plaque morphology and burden, and also data on myocardial tissue perfusion; examples of native and post-processed CCTA images are shown in Figs. 8.2 and 8.3.

8.2.5 Plaque Imaging

An emerging application for hybrid cardiac imaging with PET/CT is the investigation of vascular plaques. The new hybrid PET/CT scanners, especially with the new resolution-recovery and motion correction techniques, can combine molecular plaque imaging and anatomical information to evaluate coronary lesions. CCTA can identify coronary plaque features associated with increased risk but cannot depict the biological processes implicated in plaque rupture. 18F-FDG is a tracer compound approved for human use extensively used for the detection and staging of tumors and for myocardium vitality imaging [48, 49]. This tracer may have limitations for the study of coronary arteries because of myocardial uptake. Different studies [50–52] highlighted that PET with 18F-sodium-fluoride (18F-NaF) (an inexpensive, widely available, FDA-approved tracer) can identify recently ruptured vulnerable plaque by binding to areas of active microcalcification, which is a well-established histological

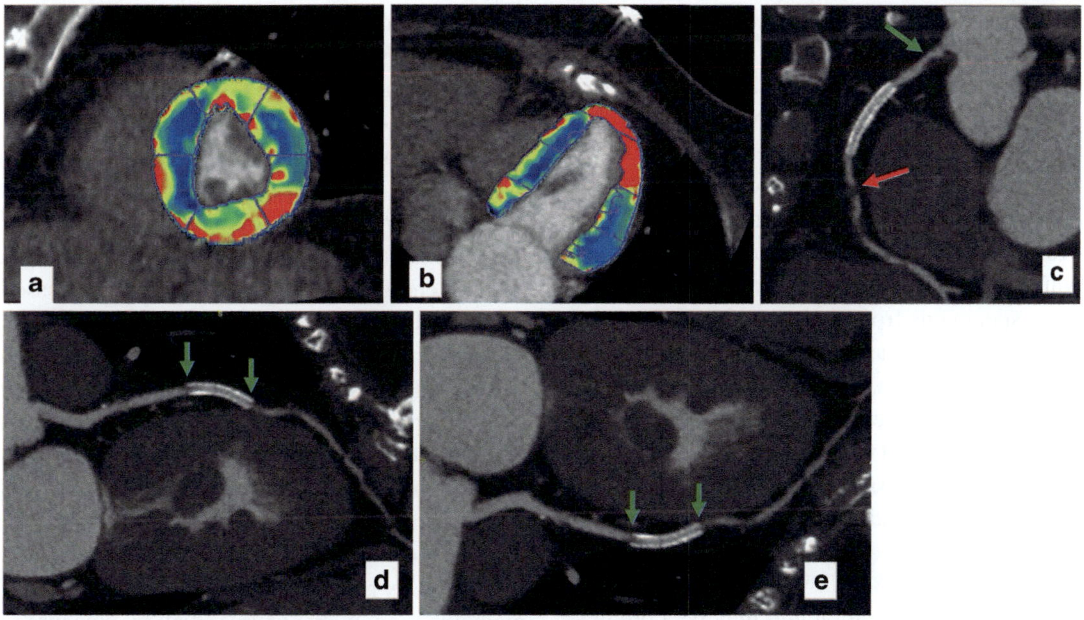

Fig. 8.3 perfusion maps of myocardial blood flow (panels **a** and **b**) derived from dynamic stress CTP performed in the same patient of Fig. 8.2 who underwent stenting of RCA and LAD with new symptom onset. Panel **a** short axis, panel **b** long axis, inducible ischemic territory shown in blue (basal to apical septal wall and basal to mid anterolateral wall). Anatomical images from rest CCTA (panel **c**–**e**): curved planar reformation (CPR). Panel **c**: RCA stenting, severe stenosis of proximal RCA (green arrow) and occlusion of distal RCA (red arrow). Panel **d**–**e**: proximal and distal intra stent restenosis of LAD (green arrows)

marker of high-risk disease. Hybrid imaging with high-resolution CCTA allows to correctly localize the tracer uptake in the coronary arteries for 18F-FDG and for 18F-NaF. Only a few studies regarding PET/CT with the 18F-FDG tracer for the evaluation of CAD have been reported to date. Increased 18F-FDG signal along the course of coronary arteries in patients with known CAD has been reported but without confirmation that atherosclerotic plaques existed at the sites of increased uptake [53]. A Higher 18F-FDG signal at culprit plaque sites has been demonstrated in patients with acute coronary syndromes [54]. Another study demonstrated increased 18F-FDG uptake in culprit sites in patients with acute myocardial infarction but failed to detect increased signal in nearly half of those patients, highlighting the challenging nature of in vivo coronary artery plaque metabolic imaging [55]. These results indicate that the detection of inflammation in the coronary arteries by hybrid PET/CTA imaging with 18F-FDG remains controversial.

It has been suggested that 18F-NaF can potentially provide information about the formation and progression of atherosclerotic plaque and vascular plaque biology [56, 57]. Dweck et al. have used a hybrid PET/CT scanner to study coronary arterial uptake of 18F-NaF and 18F-FDG as markers of active plaque calcification and inflammation [50]; increased coronary 18F-NaF activity had higher rates of prior cardiovascular events and angina. Joshi et al. compared 18F-NaF uptake with histology in carotid endarterectomy specimens from patients with symptomatic carotid artery disease and with IVUS in patients with stable angina. The highest coronary 18F-NaF uptake was seen in culprit plaques; 18F-NaF uptake occurred at the site of all carotid plaque ruptures and was associated with histological evidence of active calcification, macrophage infiltration, apoptosis, and necrosis [58]. Dweck et al. confirmed that 18F-NaF uptake can identify active tissue calcification and may be a predictor of disease progression in patients with calcific aortic stenosis [59]. 18F-NaF PET/CT is a promising application for hybrid PET/CT imaging for the identification of vulnerable plaques in the coronary arteries and in other vessels.

8.2.6 Radiation Dose Considerations

All medical exams involving ionizing radiations must be performed respecting the principles of justification and optimization [60, 61]. It is generally accepted that no diagnostic exposure is justified without a valid clinical indication and that the possible clinical benefit for the patient should outweigh the risk associated with radiation exposure. Moreover, exams should be performed respecting the ALARA/ALARP principles (as low as reasonably achievable/as low as reasonably practicable), that is to say with the lowest dose compatible with sufficient diagnostic image quality. The introduction of hybrid imaging techniques, in particular those combining PET or SPECT with CT, has raised concerns regarding patient radiation protection. Hybrid imaging modalities bring multiple challenges for radiation dose recording and monitoring and protection strategies.

Radiation dose in cardiac CT exams is related to radiation tube settings (kV and mA), cardiac gating modality (retrospective or prospective), use of iterative reconstruction algorithms, exposure length, and duration of the acquisition which are influenced by both scanner hardware specifications (number of detectors row, z-axis coverage, gantry rotation speed, etc.) and clinical parameters of the patient (such as heart rate and arrhythmias). The SI unit of exposure is air kerma (kinetic energy released in the matter), expressed in units of dose (gray [Gy]), where 1 Gy equals 1 J/kg. In CT exams dose is evaluated with CTDIvol (exposure on a single slice, mGy) and dose length product (DLP), which is the product of CTDIvol and total scan length (measured in mGy × cm) [62]. The effective dose is obtained by multiplying DLP by a conversion factor (mSv × mGy^{-1} × cm^{-1}) depending on the patient age and the region examined [63]. In nuclear medicine modalities, where radiation exposure to the patient is due to the radioactive decay of radiopharmaceutical agents, exposure is quantified using the administered activity relative to the concentration of the tracer (megabecquerels [MBq]) and is influenced by the physical properties of the radiopharmaceutical and its pharmacokinetics [64]. These different exposure metrics are measured in different units (i.e., Sv and Becquerels) so the individual radiation burden from each modality in hybrid imaging must be reported separately. A solution could be to convert the different exposure metrics into a common measure to quantify effective dose. Estimated doses from hybrid imaging procedures are more prone to error compared with radiologic or nuclear medicine exams considered individually because they are affected by all factors that may influence dose in the single modalities. Radiation doses from CT, PET, and SPECT exams, considered individually, may be relatively high among all medical imaging procedures, and consequently, when combined, might result in very high doses of radiation to the patient, compared with other imaging modalities. Many hybrid cardiac imaging protocols have been used in literature resulting in a great variety of radiation doses [65] (summarized in Table 8.2). Exposure information and subsequent dose estimates should be incorporated into imaging devices in order to record and monitor doses over time. However, critical information necessary to estimate dose from nuclear medicine procedures is not currently part of the standard DICOM header (i.e., administered activity, radiopharmaceutical administered, etc.)

This should require a joint effort of international medical societies to develop a consensus on what information should be recorded and how does should be estimated and manufacturers have to implement this information in the DICOM header [66].

In order to minimize risk from radiation exposure, only those patients who can really benefit from undergoing a hybrid imaging examination should be referred for such exams (i.e., the principle of justification) and the minimum amount of radiation should be administered to acquire diagnostic information (i.e., the principle of optimization).

Even if optimization strategies may significantly reduce exposure and dose, hybrid imaging

Table 8.2 Burden of radiation

Source	Typical ED (mSv)
Nonmedical exposures	
Backscatter for airport screening	0.0008
One-way flight, Helsinki to New York	0.05
Miner or nuclear industry worker (annual)	2
Background radiation to public (annual, worldwide)	2.4
Average annual limit, radiation workers	20
Lifetime occupational limit (Germany)	400
Noncardiac medical imaging	
Chest x-ray, posteroanterior	0.02
Chest x-ray, posteroanterior and lateral	0.1
Mammogram	0.7
Head CT	2
Abdominal CT	10
Nuclear cardiology	
Low dose 99mTc stress-only (450 MBq)	3
One day rest/stress or stress/rest 99mTc (450/1350 MBq)	13
Two day 99mTc (750/750 MBq)	11
201Tl rest-redistribution (92 MBq)	11
Dual isotope (US protocol) (120 MBq Tl/1110 MBq 99mTc)	22
18F Fluorodeoxglucose (275 MBq)	5
82Rb rest/stress (1665/1665 MBq)	2
13 N-ammonia rest/stress (555/555 MBq)	2
15O-water rest/stress (500/500 MBq)	1
153Gd line source attenuation correction	0.001
Cardiac CT	
Attenuation correction	
CT attenuation correction scan	<1
Calcium scoring	
Electron beam CT	1
Multidetector-row CT	3
Coronary CT angiography	
Prospectively triggered, 100 kVp	2
Prospectively triggered, 120 kVp	3
Retrospectively gated ESTCM, 120 kVp	14
Retrospectively gated, 120 kVp	20
Cardiac catheterization	
Diagnostic catheterization	7
Percutaneous coronary intervention	20

Adapted from Einstein AJ, Knuuti J, Eur Heart J, 33, 573–578, 2012 should be used only in patients for whom the diagnostic utility is expected to be high and when indicated by evidence-based clinical practice guidelines.

When using hybrid imaging equipment, routine acquisition of both functional and anatomical information may be unwarranted unless there is strong clinical justification for both. Hybrid technology offers the opportunity for "test layering," avoiding unnecessary radiation exposure.

8.3 Conclusions

Hybrid imaging represents a new frontier in the field of cardiovascular diagnostic and is progressively gaining interest as it allows a reliable diagnosis of many different cardiac diseases, mainly avoiding the necessity of an invasive test as the first step. Choose a single imaging test (anatomic or functional) to detect a certain disease is often hard for clinicians because every test carries several limits. Hybrid imaging appears as an optimal choice in many cases, as it allows the fusion of anatomical and functional elements in a single test, along with their strengths and weaknesses. Nowadays, these techniques are not yet widespread because of their high costs and the limited availability of types of machinery. However, hybrid imaging development is going fast and probably this kind of imaging will represent the first diagnostic step in many different cardiovascular diseases in the near future.

References

1. Biondi-Zoccai G, Versaci F, Iskandrian AE, Schillaci O, Nudi A, Frati G, et al. Umbrella review and multivariate meta-analysis of diagnostic test accuracy on hybrid noninvasive imaging for coronary artery disease. J Nucl Cardiol. 2020;27(5):1744–55.
2. Hamon M, Geindreau D, Guittet L, Bauters C, Hamon M. Additional diagnostic value of new CT imaging techniques for the functional assessment of coronary artery disease: a meta-analysis. Eur Radiol. 2019;29(6):3044–61.
3. Hamon M, Biondi-Zoccai GGL, Malagutti P, Agostoni P, Morello R, Valgimigli M, et al. Diagnostic performance of multislice spiral computed tomography of coronary arteries as compared with conventional invasive coronary angiography: a meta-analysis. J Am Coll Cardiol. 2006;48:1896–910.
4. Haase R, Schlattmann P, Gueret P, Andreini D, Pontone G, Alkadhi H, et al. Diagnosis of obstructive coronary artery disease using computed tomography angiography in patients with stable chest pain depending on clinical probability and in clinically important subgroups: meta-analysis of individual patient data. BMJ. 2019;365:l1945.
5. Schlattmann P, Schuetz GM, Dewey M. Influence of coronary artery disease prevalence on predictive values of coronary CT angiography: a meta-regression analysis. Eur Radiol. 2011;21(9):1904–13.
6. Kajander S. CT and PET/CT hybrid imaging of coronary artery disease. 2010.
7. Rizvi A, Han D, Danad I, Hartaigh BÓ, Lee JH, Gransar H, et al. Diagnostic performance of hybrid cardiac imaging methods for assessment of obstructive coronary artery disease compared with stand-alone coronary computed tomography angiography a meta-analysis. JACC Cardiovasc Imaging. 2018;11(4):589–99.
8. Qiu L, Tan H, Cheng D, Shi H, et al. The incremental clinical value of cardiac hybrid SPECT/CTA imaging in coronary artery disease. Nucl Med Commun. 2018;39(6):469–78.
9. Gaemperli O, Bengel FM, Kaufmann PA. Cardiac hybrid imaging. Eur Heart J. 2011;32(17):2100–8.
10. Gaemperli O, Saraste A, Knuuti J. Cardiac hybrid imaging. Eur Heart J Cardiovasc Imaging. 2012;13:51–60.
11. Giannopoulos AA, Gaemperli O. Hybrid imaging in ischemic heart disease. Rev Esp Cardiol. 2018;71(5):382–90.
12. Chen K, Miller EJ, Sadeghi MM. PET-based imaging of ischemic heart disease. PET Clin. 2019;14(2):211–21.
13. Veulemans V, Hellhammer K, Polzin A, Bönner F, Zeus T, Kelm M. Current and future aspects of multimodal and fusion imaging in structural and coronary heart disease. Clin Res Cardiol. 2018;107(Suppl 2):49–54.
14. Bavishi C, Argulian E, Chaterjee S, Rozanski A. Coronary artery calcium score and the frequency of stress-induced myocardial ischemia during myocardial perfusion imaging. JACC Cardiovasc Imaging. 2016;9(5):580–9.
15. Wong ND, Rozanski A, Gransar H, Miranda-Peats R, Kang X, Hayes S, et al. Metabolic syndrome and diabetes are associated with an increased likelihood of inducible myocardial ischemia among patients with subclinical atherosclerosis. Diabetes Care. 2005;28:1445–50.
16. Mouden M, Ottervanger JP, Timmer JR, et al. The influence of coronary calcium score on the interpretation of myocardial perfusion imaging. J Nucl Cardiol. 2014;21:368–7.
17. Uretsky S, Cohen R, Argulian E, et al. Combining stress-only myocardial perfusion imaging with coronary calcium scanning as a new paradigm for ini-

tial patient workup: an exploratory analysis. J Nucl Cardiol. 2015;22:89–97.
18. Chang SM, Nabi F, Xu J, et al. The coronary artery calcium score and stress myocardial perfusion imaging provide independent and complementary prediction of cardiac risk. J Am Coll Cardiol. 2009;54(20):1872–82.
19. Engbers E, Timmer JR, Ottervanger JP, Mouden M, et al. Prognostic value of coronary artery calcium scoring in addition to SPECT myocardial perfusion imaging in symptomatic patients. Circ Cardiovasc Imaging. 2016;9(5):e003966.
20. Di Carli MF, Dorbala S, Hachamovitch R. Integrated cardiac PET-CT for the diagnosis and management of CAD. J Nucl Cardiol. 2006;132:139–44.
21. Kim KP, Einstein AJ, Berrington de Gonzalez A. Coronary artery calcification screening: estimated radiation dose and cancer risk. Arch Intern Med. 2009;16913:1188.
22. Gaemperli OST, Kaufmann PA. SPECT-CT fusion imaging integrating anatomy and perfusion. Eur Heart J. 2007;28:145.
23. Sato A, Nozato T, Hikita H, Yoshida M, Narita S, Fukunaga T, et al. Incremental value of combining 64-slice computed tomography angiography with stress nuclear myocardial perfusion imaging to improve noninvasive detection of coronary artery disease. J Nucl Cardiol. 2010;17:19–26.
24. Kadokami T, Ando S, Momii H, Yoshida M, Narita S, Fukunaga T, et al. Diagnostic performance of cardiac fusion images from myocardial perfusion imaging and multislice computed tomography coronary angiography for assessment of hemodynamically significant coronary artery lesions: an observational study. Nucl Med Commun. 2012;33:60–8.
25. Pereztol-Valdes O, Candell-Riera J, Santana-Boado C, Angel J, Aguadé-Bruix S, Castell-Conesa J, et al. Correspondence between left ventricular 17 myocardial segments and coronary arteries. Eur Heart J. 2005;26:2637–43.
26. Javadi MS, Lautamaki R, Merrill J, Voicu C, Epley W, McBride G, et al. Definition of vascular territories on myocardial perfusion images by integration with true coronary anatomy: a hybrid PET/CT analysis. J Nucl Med. 2010;51:198–203.
27. Sun D, Wang J, Tian Y, et al. Multimodality imaging evaluation of functional and clinical benefits of percutaneous coronary intervention in patients with chronic total occlusion lesion. Theranostics. 2012;2:788–800.
28. Nensa F, Bamberg F, Rischpler C, et al. Hybrid cardiac imaging using PET/MRI: a joint position statement by the European Society of Cardiovascular Radiology (ESCR) and the European Association of Nuclear Medicine (EANM). Eur Radiol. 2018;28(10):4086–101.
29. Harms HJ, Lubberink M, de Haan S, et al. Use of a single 11C-meta-Hydroxyephedrine scan for assessing flow-innervation mismatches in patients with ischemic cardiomyopathy. J Nucl Med. 2015;56:1706–11.
30. Nordenskjöld AM, Hammar P, Ahlström H, et al. Unrecognized myocardial infarction assessed by cardiac magnetic resonance imaging-prognostic implications. PLoS One. 2016;11:1–12.
31. Krumm P, Zitzelsberger T, Weinmann M, et al. Cardiac MRI left ventricular global function index and quantitative late gadolinium enhancement in unrecognized myocardial infarction. Eur J Radiol. 2017;92:11–6.
32. Fukushima K, Javadi MS, et al. Prediction of short-term cardiovascular events using quantification of global myocardial flow reserve in patients referred for clinical 82Rb PET perfusion imaging. J Nucl Med. 2011;52:726–32.
33. Klumpp B, Seeger A, Bretschneider C, et al. Is myocardial stress perfusion MR-imaging suitable to predict the long term clinical outcome after revascularization? Eur J Radiol. 2013;82:1776–82.
34. Masci PG, Bogaert J. Post myocardial infarction of the left ventricle: the course ahead seen by cardiac MRI. Cardiovasc Diagn Ther. 2012;2:113–27.
35. Prakken NH, Cramer MJ, Olimulder MA, et al. Screening for proximal coronary artery anomalies with 3-dimensional MR coronary angiography. Int J Cardiovasc Imaging. 2010;26:701–10.
36. Mangold S, Kramer U, Franzen E, et al. Detection of cardiovascular disease in elite athletes using cardiac magnetic resonance imaging. Rofo. 2013;185:1167–74.
37. West GB, Brown JH, Enquist BJ. A general model for the origin of allometric scaling laws in biology. Science. 1997;276(5309):122–6.
38. Steele BN, Olufsen MS, Taylor CA. Fractal network model for simulating abdominal and lower extremity blood flow during resting and exercise conditions. Comput Methods Biomech Biomed Engin. 2007;10(1):39–51.
39. Serruys PW, Girasis C, Papadopoulou SL, et al. Non-invasive fractional flow reserve: scientific basis, methods and perspectives. EuroIntervention. 2012;8(4):511–9.
40. Douglas PS, Pontone G, Hlatky MA, et al. Clinical outcomes of fractional flow reserve by computed tomographic angiography-guided diagnostic strategies vs. usual care in patients with suspected coronary artery disease: the prospective longitudinal trial of FFR (CT): outcome and resource impacts study. Eur Heart J. 2015;36(47):3359–67.
41. Driessen RS, Danad I, Stuijfzand WJ, et al. Comparison of coronary computed tomography angiography, fractional flow reserve, and perfusion imaging for ischemia diagnosis. J Am Coll Cardiol. 2019;73(2):161–73.
42. Collet C, Onuma Y, Andreini D, et al. Coronary computed tomography angiography for heart team decision-making in multivessel coronary artery disease. Eur Heart J. 2018;39:3689–98.
43. Rossi A, Merkus D, Klotz E, et al. Stress myocardial perfusion: imaging with multidetector CT. Radiology. 2014;270:25–46.

44. Mehra VC, Valdiviezo C, Arbab-Zadeh A, et al. A stepwise approach to the visual interpretation of CT-based myocardial perfusion. J Cardiovasc Comput Tomogr. 2011;5:357–69.
45. Danad I, Szymonifka J, Schulman-Marcus J, Min JK. Static and dynamic assessment of myocardial perfusion by computed tomography. Eur Heart J Cardiovasc Imaging. 2016;8:836–44.
46. Ho KT, Chua KC, Klotz E, Panknin C. Stress and rest dynamic myocardial perfusion imaging by evaluation of complete time–attenuation curves with dual-source CT. JACC Cardiovasc Imaging. 2010;3:811–20.
47. Bamberg F, Marcus RP, Becker A, Hildebrandt K, Bauner K, Schwarz F, Greif M, von Ziegler F, Bischoff B, Becker HC, Johnson TR, Reiser MF, Nikolaou K, Theisen D. Dynamic myocardial CT perfusion imaging for evaluation of myocardial ischemia as determined by MR imaging. JACC Cardiovasc Imaging. 2014;7(3):267–77.
48. Tillisch J, Brunken R, Marshall R, et al. Reversibility of cardiac wall-motion abnormalities predicted by positron tomography. N Engl J Med. 1986;314:884–8.
49. Maddahi J, Schelbert H, Brunken R, et al. Role of thallium-201 and PET imaging in evaluation of myocardial viability and management of patients with coronary artery disease and left ventricular dysfunction. J Nucl Med. 1994;354:707–15.
50. Dweck MR, Chow MW, Joshi NV, et al. Coronary arterial 18F-sodium fluoride uptake: a novel marker of plaque biology. J Am Coll Cardiol. 2012;59(17):1539–48.
51. Irkle A, Vesey AT, Lewis DY, et al. Identifying active vascular microcalcification by (18)F-sodium fluoride positron emission tomography. Nat Commun. 2015;6:7495.
52. Joshi NV, Vesey AT, Williams MC, et al. 18F-fluoride positron emission tomography for identification of ruptured and high-risk coronary atherosclerotic plaques: a prospective clinical trial. Lancet. 2014;383(9918):705–13.
53. Wykrzykowska J, Lehman S, Williams G, Parker JA, et al. Imaging of inflamed and vulnerable plaque in coronary arteries with 18F-FDG PET/CT in patients with suppression of myocardial uptake using a low-carbohydrate, high-fat preparation. J Nucl Med. 2009;504:563–8.
54. Rogers IS, Nasir K, Figueroa AL, et al. Feasibility of FDG imaging of the coronary arteries: comparison between acute coronary syndrome and stable angina. JACC Cardiovasc Imaging. 2010;34:388–97.
55. Cheng VY, Slomka PJ, Le Meunier L, et al. Coronary arterial 18F- FDG uptake by fusion of PET and coronary CT angiography at sites of percutaneous stenting for acute myocardial infarction and stable coronary artery disease. J Nucl Med. 2012;534:575–83.
56. Derlin T, Richter U, Bannas P, et al. Feasibility of 18F-sodium fluoride PET/CT for imaging of atherosclerotic plaque. J Nucl Med. 2010;516:862–5.
57. Derlin T, Toth Z, Papp L, et al. Correlation of inflammation assessed by 18F-FDG PET, active mineral deposition assessed by 18F-fluoride PET, and vascular calcification in atherosclerotic plaque: a dual-tracer PET/CT study. J Nucl Med. 2011;527:1020–7.
58. Joshi NV, Vesey AT, Williams MC, et al. F-fluoride positron emission tomography for identification of ruptured and high-risk coronary atherosclerotic plaques: a prospective clinical trial. Lancet. 2013;383:705–13.
59. Dweck MR, Jenkins WS, Vesey AT, et al. 18F-NaF Uptake is a marker of active calcification and disease progression in patients with aortic stenosis. Circ Cardiovasc Imaging. 2014;7(2):371–8.
60. Medical Exposure Directive (MED) 97/43/Euratom (CEC 1997).
61. International Commission on Radiological Protection: radiation protection: radiological protection and safety in medicine. ICRP publication no. 73. Elsevier Science; 1996.
62. Managing patient dose in multi-detector computed tomography (MDCT). ICRP publication 102. Ann IRCP 2007;37(1):1–79.
63. Matsubara K, Koshida K, Noto K, et al. Relationship between specific organ doses and volumetric CT dose indices in multidetector CT studies. J Med Imaging Radiat Oncol. 2011;55(5):493–7.
64. International Commission on Radiological Protection (ICRP). Radiation dose to patients from radiopharmaceuticals. ICRP publication 53. Ann ICRP. 1988;18(1–4):1–388.
65. Einstein AJ, Knuuti J. Cardiac imaging: does radiation matter? Eur Heart J. 2012;33:573–8.
66. Mercuri M, Rehani MM, Einstein AJ. Tracking patient radiation exposure: challenges to integrating nuclear medicine with other modalities. J Nucl Cardiol. 2012;19(5):895–900.

Hybrid Cardiac Viability Assessment

9

Kenji Fukushima and Michinobu Nagao

9.1 Introduction

Management of patients with symptomatic left ventricular dysfunction is a common issue in leading countries due to high morbidity and mortality. Particularly, in the era of a super-aging society, etiologic diagnosis using noninvasive imaging technique is more crucial more than ever due to the global emergence of heart failure [1]. When the patients are diagnosed as having obstructive coronary artery disease after myocardial infarction (MI), noninvasive imaging is highly valuable in determining whether revascularization is appropriate in addition to optimal medical therapy, and as widely known, myocardial viability testing is an established approach as well as the evaluation of coronary anatomical burden [2]. Myocardial viability is mostly defined as "dysfunctional myocardium which has potential for functional recovery after revascularization," and is termed "stunning" and "hibernation" in clinical practice [3, 4]. Myocardial stunning is recognized as a condition of reversible cardiac dysfunction induced by ischaemic burden, and it is considered that the resting myocardial blood flow is preserved. The term "myocardial hibernation" is used to indicate chronic cardiac dysfunction due to persistent hypoxia and reduced blood flow during both rest and exertion. It is hypothesized that myocardial oxygen consumption is regionally downregulated to protect against cell necrosis [3, 5]. Considering that dysfunctional myocardium is mostly caused by chronic obstructive disease after MI, it has been mainly discussed for "hibernating myocardium" in clinical practice. Since the functional recovery by revascularization in patients after MI was initially reported in 1971, accumulated evidence over the decades suggested the clinical value of prospective identification of selected candidates who would benefit from coronary revascularization [6–9]. However, the accurate identification and differentiation of "hibernation" and "stunning" is still challenging because the true pathophysiology of the transition from acute ischemic insult to irreversible fibrosis under chronic status after MI remains uncertain, while acute stunning is a well-defined phenomenon and investigated in animal models [10, 11]. Moreover, in a clinical setting, these phenomena may frequently coexist in an infarct myocardium. Nevertheless, the detection of viable myocardium is an essential strategy for patients after myocardial infarction, particularly in those with symptomatic LV dysfunction. In

K. Fukushima (✉)
Department of Nuclear Medicine, and Cardiology, Saitama Medical University International Medical Center, Saitama, Japan
e-mail: kfukush4@saitama-med.ac.jp

M. Nagao
Department of Diagnostic Imaging and Nuclear Medicine, Tokyo Women's Medical University, Tokyo, Japan
e-mail: nagao.michinobu@twmu.ac.jp

F. Nudi et al. (eds.), *Hybrid Cardiac Imaging for Clinical Decision-Making*,
https://doi.org/10.1007/978-3-030-99391-7_9

this chapter, we summarize various noninvasive imaging modalities briefly, and discuss the clinical availability and usefulness of hybrid assessment for the detection of viable myocardium.

9.2 Current Consensus for Myocardial Viability Testing

Table 9.1 shows the noninvasive imaging modalities currently available in routine clinical practice. As shown in the table, multiple techniques can be used to detect viable myocardium, and each has different imaging targets (i.e., residual perfusion, metabolism, contractile reserve, and extent of irreversible fibrosis). Each imaging modality demonstrates various findings of viable myocardium as manifestation of pathological change after myocardial infarction (e.g., wall thickness, contractile reserve, perfusion-metabolism mismatch, delayed perfusion, and extent of fibrosis). Mostly, echocardiography or magnetic resonance imaging demonstrates structural abnormality such as remodeling or deformation, and nuclear imaging is employed to visualize the metabolic or membrane dysfunction of injured but surviving cells. To date, there is still no gold standard imaging technique, and as listed in the table, each modality has its own advantages and disadvantages. Ideally, the patients should undergo all available imaging modalities to precisely determine the benefit of revascularization. However, the availability of each imaging technique is occasionally limited due to high cost, local expertise, and institutional availability. Table 9.2 shows the list of studies for comparison or hybrid analysis. Among numerous studies, it is obvious that combined analyses or comparative studies mostly included nuclear imaging and echocardiography or cardiac magnetic resonance imaging (CMR). This trend is quite convincing

Table 9.1 Non-invasive imaging for viability testing

Modalities	Physiological basis	Imaging procedure/protocol	Study duration	Evaluation	Clinical evidence	Disadvantage, contraindication
SPECT	Viable tissue	Vasodilator stress/rest	5–24 h	Defect size, reversibility, uptake	++	Radiation exposure, vasodilator stress, low emission energy (TL)
		Rest/24 h redistribution/ reinjection				
PET	Viable tissue	Vasodilator rest/ stress	1–2 h	Defect size, uptake	++	Radiation exposure
		Glucose loading, insulin clamp				
Cardiac magnetic resonance	Scar tissue	Cine, T2weighted, strain, delayed enhancement	1 h	Wall motion, thickness, transmurality of delayed enhancement	++	Device implant, contrast media
CT	Scar tissue	Contrast-enhanced, delayed enhancement	10–20 min	Wall thickness, hypoenhanced, transmurality of delayed enhancement	–	Radiation exposure, contrast media
Dobutamine stress echo	Contractility reserve	Dobutamine stress	10–20 min	Contractile response	++	Dobutamine stress
Contrast echo	Viable tissue	Microvascular perfusion	30 min		+	

Table 9.2 Hybrid analysis or comparison by multi-modality imaging

Modality	First author	Year	Journal	Modalities	Feature	Pts
Echo and Nuclear	Marzullo [12]	1993	Am J Cardiol	DSE, Tc, TL		14
	Baer [13]	1995	Circulation	DSE, FDG		42
	Arnese [14]	1995	Circulation	DSE vs. TL		43
	Mariani [15]	1995	Am J Cardi Imaging	DSE, Tc, and FDG		16
	Vanoverschelde [16]	1996	J Am Coll Cardiol	DSE vs. TL	Exercise-TL	73
	Nagueh [17]	1997	J Am Coll Cardiol	MCE vs. DSE vs. TL		18
	Qureshi [18]	1997	Circulation	DSE and TL		44
	Pagano [19]	1999	Heart	DSE and FDG		35
	Pasquet [20]	1999	Am J Cardiol	DSE and Rb		66
	Rambaldi [21]	1999	Am J Cardiol	DSE and Tc/FDG	FDG-SPECT	110
	Cornel [22]	1999	J Nucl Cardiol	DSE vs. TL, FDG		40
	Cwajg [23]	2000	J Am Coll Cardiol	DES vs. TL	EDD	44
	Anseslmi [24]	2000	Int J Cardiol	DES vs. TL		19
	Ozdemir [25]	2000	Acta Cardiol	DSE and TL		17
	Yong [26]	2001	Circulation	Echo and TL	LV inflow	40
	Yuan [27]	2001	Echocardiography	DSE vs. FDG	Doppler Echo	30
	Yoshinaga [28]	2001	J Nucl Med	Tc vs. DSE and FDG	Dobutamine Tc	23
	Yasugi [29]	2002	Circ J	DSE vs. TL/BMIPP		35
	Leoncini [30]	2010	Am J Cardiol	DSE, Tc	Dobutamine Tc	37
	Barrington [31]	2004	Eur J Nucl Med Mol Imaging	DSE vs. FDG/NH3, or TL and Tc		47
	Schinkel [32]	2004	Am J Med	DSE and Tc		198
	Tani [33]	2004	Circ J	DSE vs. FDG, TL, and BMIPP		30
	Ling [34]	2006	Am Heart J	Echo and TL	nitroglycerin-dobutamine	32
	Hickman [35]	2007	Int J Cardiol	MCE vs. Tc		56
	Dwivedi [36]	2009	Am J Cardiol	MCE and Tc		99
	He [37]	2009	Clin Nucl Med	TL vs. Echo		38
	Mollema [38]	2010	Circ Cardiovasc Imaging	Strain and Tc	Global strain	147
	Gong [39]	2013	Int J Cardiovasc Imaging	Strain, DSE and Tc		42
	Al Moudi [40]	2014	J Geriatr Cardiol	FDG vs DSE and Tc		30
	Ismail [41]	2015	Minerva Cardioangiol	DOB-Strain and Tc	Dobutamine Strain	60
	Sharma [42]	2018	J Echo	Strain, DSE, and FDG		57
	Orloff [43]	2018	Echocardiography	Strain vs. Tc		47
	Liu [44]	2019	Medicine (Baltimore)	Strain, MIBI, FDG	Strain	40
	Verma [45]	2019	Open Access Maced J Med Sci	MCE, DSE vs. Tc		50
	Nelson [46]	2004	J Am Coll Cardiol	DSE, TL	RD-TL	60
	LaGanna [47]	2000	Eur Heart J	DSE, TL	RD-TL	28

(continued)

Table 9.2 (continued)

Modality	First author	Year	Journal	Modalities	Feature	Pts
CMR and Nuclear	Baer [48]	1994	Eur Heart J	CMR, Tc		55
	Baer [13]	1995	Circulation	CMR, FDG	Dobutamine CMR	35
	Klein [49]	2002	Circulation	CMR-LGE, FDG, NH3		31
	Gunning [50]	2002	J Am Coll Cardiol	CMR, Tc, TL	Dobutamine CMR	23
	Knuesel [51]	2003	Circulation	CMR, FDG		19
	Kitagawa [52]	2003	Radiology	CMR, TL		22
	Kuhl [53]	2003	J Am Coll Cardiol	CMR, FDG		26
	Lee [54]	2003	Radiology	CMR, Tc		20
	Schmidt [55]	2004	Magn Reson Imaging	CMR, FDG	Dobutamine CMR	40
	Gulberlet [56]	2005	Eur Radiol	CMR vs. TL		20
	Misko [57]	2006	J Cardiovasc Magn Reson	CMR and		18
	Solar [58]	2006	Int Heart J	CMR-LGE vs. TL		32
	Wang [59]	2006	Chin Med Sci J	CMR-LGE vs. Tc and FDG		7
	Wu [60]	2007	Int J Cardiovasc Imaging	CMR-LGE vs. TL and FDG		116
	Roes [61]	2009	Eur J Nucl Med Mol Imaging	CMR vs. Tc and FDG		60
	Liu [44]	2009	Nucl Med Commun	CMR-LGE vs. Tc and FDG		34
	Rischphler [62]	2015	Eur Heart J Cardiovasc Imaging	CMR vs. FDG	Hybrid PETMR	28
	Hunold [63]	2018	World J Cardiol	CMR-LGE and FDG		105
	Timmer [64]	2018	J Nucl Cardiol	CMR-LGE vs. 15O		28
	Kiko [65]	2020	J Nucl Cardiol	CMR-LGE and FDG	Hybrid PETMR, CTO	28
	Beitzke [66]	2020	Acta Radiol	CMR-LGE, NH3/FDG		39
	Wu [67]	2007	J Nucl Med	CMR-LGE, FDG, TL		41
CMR and CT	Habis [68]	2007	J Am Coll Cardiol	CT-DE vs DSE		36
	Sato [69]	2008	Eur Heart J	CT-DE vs TL		52
	Shapiro [70]	2010	J Cardiovasc Comput Tomogr	CMR-LGE vs. CT-PD		17
	Goetti [71]	2011	Eur Radiol	CMR-LGE vs. CT-DE	high-pitch CT	24
Echo and CMR	Mghaieth [72]	2020	Medicine (Baltimore)	Strain Echo and LGE-CMR		31
	Lipiec [73]	2011	Kardiol Pol	Strain Echo and LGE-CMR		40
Echo, CMR, and Nuclear	Baer [74]	1996	Am J Cardiol	DSE, CMR, FDG	Dobutamine Transesophageal	43

Echo echocardiography, *LVEF* left ventricular ejection fraction, *OMT* optimal medical treatment, *PCI* percutaneous coronary intervention, *CABG* coronary artery bypass grafting, *Echo* echocardiography, *MCE* myocardial contrast echocardiography, *DSE* dobutamine stress echocardiography, *FDG* 18F fluorodeoxyglucose, *NH3* 13N ammonia, *TL* 201Thallium, *MIBI* 99mTc sestamibi, *Tc* technitium, *CTO* chronic total occlusion, *CMR* cardiovascular magnetic resonance imaging, *LGE* late gadlinium enhancement because there are substantial needs for combined assessment by these different imaging targets [75–78]. Several authors performed a direct comparison of dobutamine stress echocardiography (DSE) and myocardial perfusion single photon emission computed tomography (SPECT), and Bax et al. reported the agreement between SPECT and DSE was 72% [79]. However, nearly half of the myocardial segments without a perfusion defect did not show contractile reserve. This can be one possible reason why the combined analysis or hybrid assessment significantly increases diagnostic accuracy by compensating for insufficient accuracy in the single modality [62, 80–82]. As shown in Table 9.2, the most employed combination was dobutamine stress echo and nuclear cardiology. In the initial pooled analysis of 37 studies, Bax et al. reported an overall sensitivity of 84%, and specificity of 81% for predicting functional recovery, and ^{201}thallium (TL) showed higher sensitivity and lower specificity compared to DSE [83]. Schinkel et al. also summarized several studies that compared DSE and TL in patients with acute myocardial infarction and reported DSE showed higher specificity than that of TL [84]. The combination of DSE and ^{99m}Tc (Tc) agents was also investigated. A meta-analysis showed diagnostic accuracy is comparable between TL and Tc agents (the sensitivity were 87% and 83%; the specificity were 56% and 57% for TL and Tc, respectively), while the uptake and retention of Tc agents are different from that of TL [85]. In a direct comparison between perfusion SPECT tracers, Cuccolo et al. reported that the optimal threshold cutoffs for the prediction of viability were 58% and 55% uptake for TL and Tc agents, respectively [86]. Kauffman et al. reported the worth of TL and Tc agents for viability testing is comparable [87]. After introducing ^{18}F-fluorodeoxyglucose positron emission tomography (FDG-PET) for viability study, many studies consisted of two or more combined studies with perfusion PET or SPECT tracers, and they focused on "perfusion-metabolism mismatch," namely "reduced perfusion but residual metabolism" [88–93]. Combined assessment using echocardiography and myocardial glucose metabolism have also been studied [13, 19, 27].

In a meta-analysis focused on FDG and DSE, Allman et al. enrolled 3088 patients 25 months follow up, and reported that the revascularization to viable myocardium had reduced nearly 80% in annual mortality rate (3.2% vs. 16% for revascularization vs. medical therapy) [94]. Among a subset of the studies compared two or more imaging techniques, the pooled analysis showed that DSE had a significantly higher positive predictive value (84% vs. 75%) and a lower negative predictive value compared to PET and SPECT (69 vs 80%) [85]. In multiple meta-analyses including various imaging techniques, Schinkel et al. compared FDG and DSE for available imaging modalities and concluded that FDG was the most sensitive (80–85%), and DSE was the most specific (85–90%) in predicting functional recovery after revascularization [85]. Tables 9.2 and 9.3 also showed comparison studies and combined analysis of multimodality imaging including vasodilator-enhanced technique. In the 1990s, most comparative studies focused on the comparison of DSE and rest MPI or FDG imaging for viability testing [13, 14, 18, 21, 23, 138–146]. Leoncini et al. have introduced dobutamine stress into ^{99m}Tc sestamibi gated SPECT and compared to DSE [147]. Other than dobutamine, several vasodilators (i.e., nitrate, dipyridamole) have been used to enhance residual viability, and a few studies have tested the combination [146, 148]. The viability testing with nitrate in nuclear cardiology was firstly reported by He and Bisi et al., and nitrate significantly enhanced the viable segments compared to conventional SPECT alone [149, 150]. Slart et al. reported that the administration of nitrate has significantly increased for myocardial blood flow in viable myocardium and improved the diagnostic accuracy when FDG was used as gold standard (sensitivity 80% and specificity 100%) [128]. These investigations suggested that the combined analysis or adding dobutamine stress may enhance the diagnostic value of non-invasive, rest imaging study. However, there is a significant limitation in evaluating wall kinetics when infarct myocardium shows a severe defect compared to CMR as a standard [151]. More recently, CMR has been frequently employed to test the feasibil-

Table 9.3 Hybrid analysis of different technique in single modality

Modality	First author	Year	Journal	Modalities	Feature	Pts
Echo	deFilippi [95]	1995	Circulation	MCE vs. DSE		35
	Iwakura [96]	2010	Circ J	Strain and DSE	Automation	23
CMR	Yun [97]	2014	Int J Cardiovasc Imaging	LGE and WHCA		70
	Gerbaud [98]	2010	Am J Cardiol	DOB, LGE, MVO		69
Nuclear	Tamaki [99]	1991	J Nucl Med	TL vs. FDG	RI-TL	18
	Altehoefer [88]	1994	J Nucl Med	FDG, Tc		111
	Altehoefer [89]	1994	Eur J Nucl Med	Tc and FDG		46
	Lucignani [90]	1992	Eur J Nucl Med	Tc and FDG		14
	Gropler [100]	1992	J Am Coll Cardiol	Acetate and 15O		16
	Dondi [101]	1993	Eur J Nucl Med	Tc vs. TL		30
	Yoshida [93]	1993	J Am Coll Cardiol	Rb vs. FDG		35
	Gropler [100]	1992	J Am Coll Cardiol	Acetate and FDG		34
	Udelson [102]	1994	Circulation	TL vs. Tc		31
	Kawamoto [103]	1994	Ann Nucl Med	BMIPP vs. TL and FDG		22
	Altehoefer [89]	1994	Eur J Nucl Med	TL vs. FDG		111
	vom Dahl [92]	1994	Circulation	NH3 and FDG		37
	Tamaki [91]	1995	Circulation	NH3 and FDG		61
	vom Dahl [104]	1996	J Am Coll Cardiol	Tc and FDG		193
	Gerber [105]	1996	Circulation	NH3 and FDG		39
	Wolpers [106]	1997	Circulation	Acetate and FDG		30
	vom Dahl [107]	1997	J Nucl Med	FDG and Tc		161
	Cornel [108]	1997	Int J Card Imaging	TL	DOB, RD, RI-TL	26
	Flotats [109]	1997	Eur J Nucl Med	Tc vs. TL	Nitrate Tc	15
	Gerber [110]	1998	J Nucl Med	NH3, 15O		30
	Cuocolo [86]	2000	J Nucl Cardiol	TL and Tc		43
	Fukuchi [111]	2000	J Nucl Med	FDG and Tc		18
	Matsuno [112]	2001	Nucl Med Commun	Tc vs. TL		79
	Yoshinaga [28]	2002	Eur J Nucl Med Mol Imaging	Tc vs. FDG	DOB-Tc	23
	Acampa [113]	2002	J Nucl Cardiol	Tc vs. Tc and TL		17
	Maruyama [114]	2002	Ann Nucl Med	Tc vs. FDG		33
	De Boer [115]	2003	Nucl Med Commun	FDG and Tc		19
	Yoshinaga [116]	2004	J Nucl Med	Acetate and FDG		20
	Giorgetti [117]	2004	J Nucl Cardiol	Tc vs. FDG	Nitrate	23
	Orea [118]	2004	Rev Invest Clin	Tc vs. TL	GIK	72
	Slart [119]	2004	J Nucl Cardiol	Tc vs. FDG	Attenuation correction	33

Table 9.3 (continued)

Modality	First author	Year	Journal	Modalities	Feature	Pts
	Toyama [120]	2004	Ann Nucl Med	TL vs. PYP and FDG	GIK	21
	Yamakawa [121]	2004	Ann Nucl Med	FDG and Tc	Gated FDG	48
	Matsunari [122]	2005	Eur J Nucl Med Mol Imaging	FDG/NH3 and Tc		33
	Desideri [123]	2005	J Am Coll Cardiol	NH3 and FDG		261
	Schinkel [124]	2005	AmJ Cardiol	Tc vs. FDG		
	Wu [125]	2005	J Nucl Cardiol	FDG and Tc vs. TL	FDG-SPECT	42
	Alexanderson [126]	2006	Arch Cardiol Mex	TL vs. FDG		23
	Roelants [127]	2006	Nucl Med Commun	Tc vs. NH3/FDG	Attenuation correction	30
	Slart [128]	2006	J Nucl Med	NH3 vs. FDG	Nitrate	25
	Gunel [129]	2009	Ann Nucl Med	Tc vs. TL	Isosorbide dinitrate, exercise	26
	Raja [130]	2012	J Nucl Cardiol	Tc and FDG	Nitrate	54
	Uebleis [131]	2013	Int J Cardiovasc Imaging	Tc and FDG		224
	Dong [132]	2018	Ann Nucl Med	Tc and FDG	CTO	104
	Moody [133]	2019	J Nucl Cardiol	Rb vs. FDG		120
	Zhang [134]	2020	J Nucl Cardiol	FDG and Tc	Wall thicknenning	83
	Sun [135]	2020	J Nucl Cardiol	FDG and Tc	CTO	164
	Duncan [136]	2000	Am J Cardiol	Tc vs TL	Gated Tc	30
	Narula [137]	2000	J Am Coll Cardiol	Tc, TL	DOB-Tc	54
	Kauffmann [87]	1996	J Am Coll Cardiol	Tc, TL		20

LVEF left ventricular ejection fraction, *OMT* optimal medical treatment, *PCI* percutaneous coronary intervention, *CABG* coronary artery bypass grafting, *Echo* echocardiography, *MCE* myocardial contrast echocardiography, *DSE* dobutamine stress echocardiography, *FDG* 18F fluorodeoxyglucose, *NH3* 13N ammonia, *TL* 201Thallium, *MIBI* 99mTc sestamibi, *Tc* technitium, *CTO* chronic total occlusion, *CMR* cardiovascular magnetic resonance imaging, *LGE* late gadolinium enhancement, *WHCA* whole heart coronary MRA, *MVO* microvascular obstruction

ity of viability imaging. CMR has distinctive advantages including excellent soft tissue contrast without using a contrast media, and functional assessment with good penetration at which echocardiography may occasionally fail [152]. Comparison or combined analysis of CMR and nuclear cardiology have increased in the 2000s, and several studies have assessed wall thickness, motion, the extent of fibrosis, and metabolism simultaneously [44, 49, 60, 61, 66]. Moreover, Baer et al. firstly introduced dobutamine stress CMR and compared FDG [13]. From this point of view, the hybrid PETMR system is the ideal technology which has a capability of combing the molecular and functional information simultaneously [62, 65, 66].

Table 9.4 shows randomized clinical trials. The PARR-2 (Positron emission tomography And Recovery following Revascularization phase 2) trial was a multicenter randomized clinical study which enrolled 430 patients with left ventricular ejection fraction (LVEF) <35% to determine the usefulness of FDG guided revascularization compared to standard care without FDG [158]. In a short-time period (1 year), a statistical trend towards to a lower rate of cardiovascular events (cardiac death, MI, and hospitalization) was not observed. However, in a

Table 9.4 Systematic review, meta-analysis, and multiinstitutional studies

	Author or study	Year	Journal	Modality	Studies	Patients
Systematic-reviews/meta-analysis	Schinkel [85]	2007	J Nucl Med	CMR, DSE, TL, Tc, DSE, and FDG	NA	NA
	Bax [83]	1997	J Am Coll Cardiol	TL, FDG, Tc, DSE	37	NA
	Romeo [153]	2012	JACC Cardiovasc Imaging	CMR, LGE, DOB	24	698
	Allman [94]	2002	J Am Coll Cardiol	TL, FDG, and DSE	24	3088
	Orlandini [154]	2015	Int J Cardiol	DSE, FDG, TL, and Tc	36	4328
	Tsai [155]	2014	Nucl Med Commun	FDG, Tc, and TL	8	310
	Inaba [156]	2010	J Nucl Cardiol	FDG, Stress echo, Tc, TL	29	4167
	Bourque [157]	2003	Am Heart J		4	1244
Randomized or Multicenter	PARR-2 [158]	2007	J Am Coll Cardiol	FDG		218
	Ottawa-FIVE [159]	2010	J Nucl Med	FDG		56
	STICH [160]	2011	N Engl J Med	DSE		1212
	CHRISTMASS [161]	2003	Lancet	Echo		305
	OAT-NUC [162]	2011	Am Heart J	SPECT		124
	Gebaud [98]	2010	Am J Cardiol	CMR, LGE, DOB, MVO		69
	HEART [163]	2010	Eur J Heart Fail	Echo, Nuclear		138
Ongoing	HYBRIDHEART					NA
	IMAGE-HF					NA
	VIAMI					NA

LVEF left ventricular ejection fraction, *OMT* optimal medical treatment, *PCI* percutaneous coronary intervention, *CABG* coronary artery bypass grafting, *Echo* echocardiography, *MCE* myocardial contrast echocardiography, *DSE* dobutamine stress echocardiography, *FDG* 18F fluorodeoxyglucose, *NH3* 13N ammonia, *TL* 201Thallium, *MIBI* 99mTc sestamibi, *Tc* technitium, *CTO* chronic total occlusion, *CMR* cardiovascular magnetic resonance imaging, *LGE* late gadolinium enhancement, *WHCA* whole heart coronary MRA, *MVO* microvascular obstruction

post hoc analysis including 75% of the patients who adhered to the PET recommendation, a significant reduction in adverse outcomes was observed in the PET guided group, indicating the imaging guided decision-making and follow up has a positive impact on the patients. A PARR-2 substudy was followed to determine the thresholds of FDG parameters and revealed that a perfusion-metabolism mismatch >7% showed significantly reduced primary events [164]. Substudy of PARR-2, Ottawa-FIVE showed significant benefits in the FDG guided revascularization when FDG is easily accessible and the expertized image interpretation is guaranteed (events 19% in the PET arm versus 41% in the standard care) [159]. This evidence suggests that it requires physicians or surgeons adhered to imaging and the assessment by experienced image interpreters. Similar findings were also reported from several other investigations [34, 165–167], and this indicates that the detection of "residual metabolic activity in infarct myocardium" is crucial to determine whether to perform revascularization or not. Summarizing the above, it is emphasized that transmural fibrosis with a low level of residual glucose metabolism and a dyskinetic thinned wall is unlikely to show functional recovery by revascularization.

The STICH (the Surgical Treatment for Ischemic Heart Failure) trial and STICHES (STICH extension study) showed a strong impact on the current belief on the usefulness of myocardial viability testing [160]. The study randomized 1212 patients after MI with LVEF 35% or lower to optimal medical therapy (OMT) and OMT plus coronary artery bypass grafting (CABG). A 10-year follow-up revealed that CABG improved all mortality, but myocardial viability testing did not contribute to distinguish candidates who would benefit from revascularization [168, 169]. Furthermore, LVEF improvement was also observed in the OMT group, and interestingly, reducing mortality was not associated with LVEF improvement. From the result of the study, the authors emphasized the risk of misleading in employing single viability testing due to its variability and the difficulty of determining the optimal cut-off. In STICH trials, the authors also noted that the current definition "functional recovery improve prognosis" which has been accepted as truth for decades should be reconsidered [170–173]. In a long-term follow-up, the merit of surgical intervention still seems controversial. The STICH and STICHES extension has shown that invasive revascularization had significantly improved patients' outcomes including death and hospitalization compared to conservative therapy [174]. However, surgical revascularization did not improve cardiac function. Also, it should be noted that the STICH trials did not enroll the candidate with renal insufficiency, while PARR-2 study included more patients with chronic kidney disease.

The latest trend for the investigation of viability testing has become more diverse. Wu et al. focused on the patients that were 50 years old or younger and found that younger patients have more chance to recover with revascularization [175]. The pathophysiology in transition or recovery of myocardial ischemia should be influenced by more complex and diverse causes (i.e., age, sex, neurohormonal factors), while most investigations had focused on functional recovery or mortality. To unravel the complexity of interaction by various factors, the usefulness of multimodality imaging technique should be continuously investigated.

9.3 Echocardiography

In a clinical setting, echocardiography is widely available due to its portability, less invasiveness, and cost-effectiveness. Initially, the usefulness of measuring end-diastolic thickness was tested, and the thicknesses of over 6 mm have been recognized as a sign of functional recovery after revascularization [13]. Currently, contractile reserve under pharmacological stress is the most common criterion and has been extensively studied. Usually, dipyridamole, atropine, and dobutamine are listed as stress agents, and dobutamine is mainly used throughout the world. Standard protocol is based on the studies for detecting myocardial ischemia. The most frequently employed technique is low-high dose (5–10 μg/kg/min up to over 15 μg/kg/min) to evaluate biphasic response of wall motion in infarct territory, while nonviable myocardium does not show this response. A meta-analysis included 32 studies of 1090 patients reported mean sensitivity and specificity of 82% and 79% [83]. Other investigations reported combined use of dipyridamole and dobutamine improved the accuracy for predicting wall motion recovery after revascularization [146, 148]. Contraindications of dobutamine stress are (1) inducible ventricular arrhythmia, (2) left ventricular outflow obstruction, (3) severe hypertension, and (4) aortic aneurysm [176]. Myocardial contrast echocardiography (MCE) is an imaging technique that utilizes air-filled microbubbles (approximate mean size 3 μm) which emulate red blood cells to evaluate myocardial microvascular perfusion. Although it has not been clinically widely used, MCE has established its predictive value of functional recovery [177]. MCE is used to evaluate the spatial extent of viable tissue post MI [178, 179]. DeFillipi et al. compared MCE and DSE for 35 patients with LV dysfunction after MI, and had good concordance but DSE had better specificity and positive predictive value [95]. Recently, detection of myocardial deformation using strain analysis by two- or three-dimensional speckle tracking technique has been widely studied [39, 180, 181].

9.4 Single Photon Emission Computed Tomography

Scintigraphic imaging with SPECT has been the most common technique in detecting viability due to its accessibility in nuclear cardiology clinics. ^{201}Thallium chloride (TL) is a potassium analog which is transported by Na+/K+ ATPase channel reflecting cell membrane integrity, namely detecting survived cells with preserved intra-extra cellular potassium gradient. TL also has the advantage of demonstrating a high first pass extraction fraction (approximately 80%), and the redistribution phenomenon as reversible ischemia [182]. Various imaging protocols have been validated and tested including delayed rest-18–24 h redistribution, and redistribution—reinjection techniques. Several investigations showed that the TL reinjection technique demonstrated additive value for detecting defect reversibility [183–185]. Viability testing with the delayed rest-redistribution TL image has initially presented the usefulness of detecting reversible myocardium in apparently fixed perfusion defect undergoing routine stress-rest protocols [186–188]. From a number of studies, findings indicating viability are as follows: (1) Tracer uptake is maintained at more than 50% in delayed or reinjection images. (2) Redistribution phenomenon in delayed or/and reinjection image (10% recovery of %uptake is mostly used). The accuracy of myocardial viability testing by TL revealed high sensitivity but low specificity [83, 85]. Although TL has been used widely for viability testing, considerable limitations are discussed, such as lower emission showing a false defect, relatively longer protocols, and radiation exposure. Particularly, TL can produce the highest effective dose, and minimization of radiation exposure is desired [189].

^{99m}Tc agents (^{99m}Tc tetrofosmin and sestamibi) are commonly used myocardial flow tracers. The physiologic property of those tracers is lipophilic cationic which is rapidly taken into myocardial cell via passive diffusion and stabilized in the mitochondria. The protocol is mostly based on routine stress—rest study and occasionally rest only [190–192]. From the accumulated evidence, the diagnostic accuracy is almost similar to that of TL, despite a significant difference in the physiologic property including redistribution and washout [87, 101, 193, 194]. In routine clinical practice, it is desirable to perform additional imaging study for viability testing when the patients show a fixed defect with LV dysfunction. For instance, in addition to routine SPECT protocols such as stress-rest, or rest only scan, the patient can undergo viability testing such as delayed redistribution or rest-reinjection TL protocol subsequently. The use of single or combination of pharmacological agents (i.e., dobutamine, nitrate, and dipyridamole) has been studied and shown to improve the detectability of myocardial viability [195–197]. ^{123}I-BMIPP (BMIPP) is a free fatty acid analog which simulates myocardial fatty acid metabolism, and is currently clinically unavailable except in Japan. BMIPP is frequently used for ischemic heart disease including acute coronary syndrome. BMIPP also can demonstrate diagnostic ability for myocardial viability showing discordant uptake less than a perfusion image, and this is recognized as perfusion fatty acid metabolism mismatch [29, 198–200]. BMIPP can contribute as an additive value to detect viable myocardium over by perfusion tracer only. Other than the above, cardiac sympathetic imaging using ^{123}I-(MIBG) is currently under investigation for viability testing (IMAGE-HF) [201].

9.5 Positron Emission Tomography

Compared to SPECT, PET image offers a far better spatial resolution and improvements to the time-consuming issue. Among various tracers including flow tracers (^{15}O-H_2O, ^{13}N-ammonia, ^{82}Rb, etc.) and metabolic agents (^{18}F-fluorodeoxyglucose = FDG, ^{11}C-acetate, etc.), most clinical evidence was investigated using

FDG [107, 202–204]. The accumulated evidence of viability testing by using FDG was mostly from comparing with SPECT or PET perfusion tracers to detect a discrepant uptake so-called perfusion and glucose metabolism mismatch. However, unlike flow tracers, cardiac FDG uptake is strongly affected by metabolic circumstances. High insulin and glucose with low fatty acid levels are strictly required to maximize cardiac glucose uptake. The usual protocols are oral glucose loading for non-diabetic, and insulin-euglycemic clamp for diabetic patients. Insulin-euglycemic clamp protocols are relatively time-consuming due to strict monitoring of blood glucose levels and dose adjustment of insulin I.V. until the administration of FDG [205–210]. Possible assessment by the combination of flow tracer and FDG can be summarized as follows: reduced wall motion with preserved both flow and FDG uptake is stunned, reduced wall motion and regional flow but preserved FDG uptake is hibernating (this status can be categorized as perfusion—glucose metabolism mismatch), and reduced wall motion with perfusion and FDG defect (matched defect, and FDG %uptake less than 50) is considered to be a nonviable scar. Disadvantages of nuclear cardiology are as follows; radiation exposure (still higher than cardiac CT), relatively longer duration of exams, and high cost.

9.6 Cardiac Magnetic Resonance

Cardiac magnetic resonance (CMR) imaging represents cardiac morphology and wall characteristics with a high spatial resolution for either ischemic or nonischemic myocardial disease. Unlike other modalities, the main advantage of CMR is the direct visualization of wall contractility and magnitude of damage, and late gadolinium enhancement (LGE) is the most powerful visualization technique of myocardial fibrosis [211]. Myocardial viability can be determined using visual or quantitative grading of transmural extent of LGE in the myocardial wall, and identifying the residual-epicardial rim can be visualized simultaneously as a sign of viability (magnitude of LGE extent <50%). CMR scan in conjunction with dobutamine has been validated, and the initial experiences were established to predict significant coronary artery stenosis [212]. Subsequently, dobutamine stress CMR was validated to evaluate myocardial viability in a similar procedure to echocardiography (i.e., contractile reserve, wall thickness) in addition to identifying scar tissue [13, 213]. Detection of myocardial viability is usually interpreted as follows: end-diastolic wall thickness >5.5 mm in resting cine-MRI or show contractile reserve under dobutamine stress, and a dysfunctional wall with a sub-endocardial extent by delayed enhancement [64, 153, 214, 215]. In addition to demonstrating wall kinetics and infarct transmurality with high spatial resolution, CMR can contribute using different magnetic resonance techniques such as strain encoded magnetic resonance (SENC) or tagging cine [216, 217]. Several studies reported the ability of SENC for the detection of myocardial viability, and showed high sensitivity (82–100%) and wide range of specificity (47–94%) [218]. Disadvantages of CMR are a contraindication of contrast media including chronic renal disease, relatively longer duration, and claustrophobic conditions in enclosed space. Although the implantable electronical device is contraindicated for CMR, recent technological development of MRI-conditional devices which ensure the patients' safety. However, it should be noted that the frequent metal artifacts cause insufficient diagnosis [219].

9.7 Hybrid Assessment of Myocardial Viability for Clinical Cases Using Different Imaging Techniques

As is widely known, a myocardial perfusion SPECT image can underestimate myocardial viability, especially in the infero-posterior region due to lower emission, and PET images provide a more accurate diagnosis to identify viable myocardium. Additionally, combined myocardial perfusion imaging and FDG can visualize hibernating and viable myocardium as a perfusion-glucose metabolism mismatch.

Case 1

A 70-year-old man with a recent myocardial infarction. He complained of shortness of breath on slight exertion. He had a history of diabetes and dyslipidemia. Dipyridamole stress-rest myocardial perfusion SPECT showed a severe defect in the anterior wall (Fig. 9.1 left). FDG-PET revealed decreased uptake in anterior wall. However, %uptake was over 50 in the basal ant and septal area, which showed typical "perfusion-glucose metabolism mismatch" and residual glucose metabolism was indicated (Fig. 9.1 middle). ECG-gated FDG-PET showed LVEF of 37%. This case was referred for revascularization.

Case 2

A 60-year-old man who was suspected of old anterior infarction underwent myocardial perfusion imaging. He was in preoperative status for knee replacement surgery and had a history of active bronchial asthma. Rest TL-BMIPP cardiac dual SPECT was performed and revealed an anterior perfusion defect, and BMIPP showed a more severe defect, which showed "perfusion—fatty acid metabolism mismatch." The infarct myocardium was expected as viable (Fig. 9.2 middle). CMR study was performed post-operation and showed reduced wall motion in the anterior with a significant extent of late gadolinium enhancement. However, a non-enhanced viable rim was observed in the anterior wall. The transmural extent was approximately 50% in the apex and less than 50% in the anteroseptal wall (Fig. 9.2 right).

Case 3

A 65-year-old man with multivessel disease was referred for noninvasive imaging. Coronary angiography showed total occlusion in the right coronary artery, distal left circumflex, and severe stenosis in the proximal left anterior descending artery (LAD). Stress-rest MPI showed a severe anterior defect, and partially reversible ischemia in the anteroseptal wall (Fig. 9.3 left). FDG-PET revealed a severe defect in the anterior wall, and functional recovery with revascularization was hardly expected. However, maintained glucose metabolism was observed in the anteroseptal wall (Fig. 9.3 middle). Similar to FDG, CMR showed a significant transmural extent of delayed enhancement in

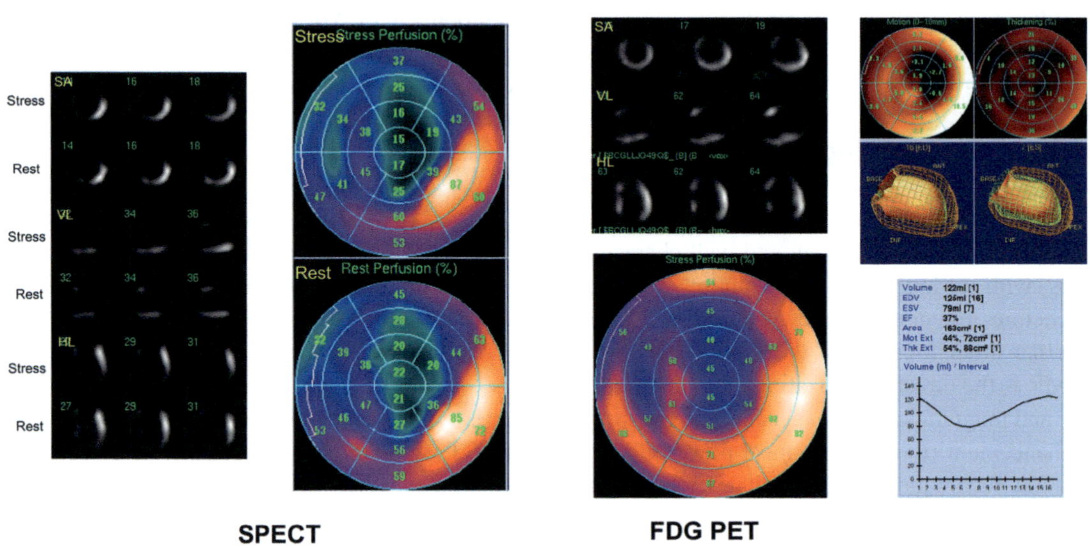

Fig. 9.1 Representative case of myocardial perfusion glucose metabolism mismatch is shown. Pharmacological stress-rest perfusion SPECT demonstrated a significant defect in left anterior descending artery (LAD) territory %uptake lower than 40% which indicated poor viability. However, myocardial FDG-PET by insulin-clamp protocol revealed residual uptake in the anterior wall and %uptake was around 45–50%, and this finding indicated myocardial hibernation. ECG-gated FDG-PET showed significantly reduced LVEF (37%)

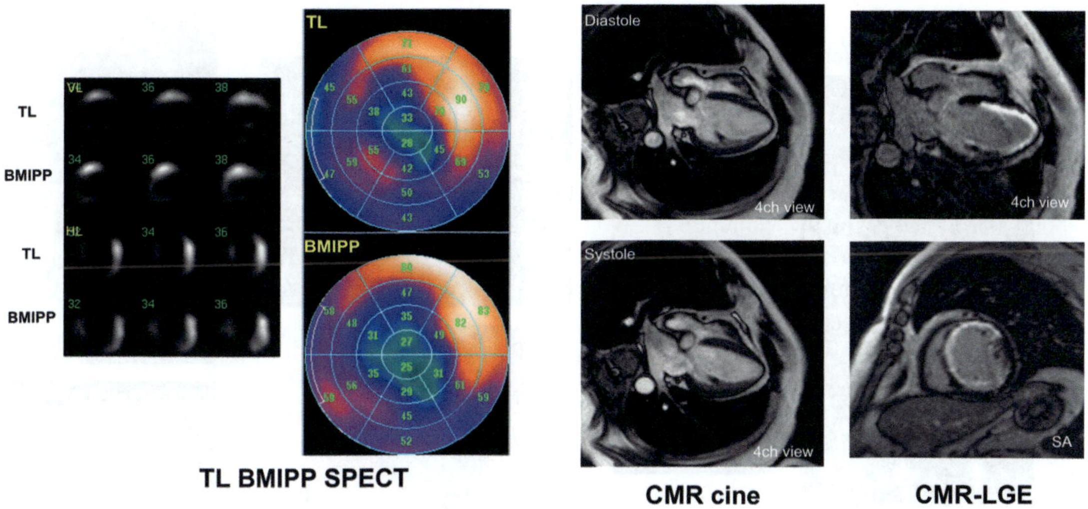

Fig. 9.2 Case of ^{201}TL and ^{123}I-BMIPP dual SPECT and cardiac MRI (CMR) in a patient with anterior and inferior myocardial infarction (MI) is shown. ^{201}TL (left upper panel) showed significantly reduced uptake in antero-apical and inferior region and ^{123}I-BMIPP (left lower panel) shows a discordant severe defect in the wider area, which indicated myocardial viability as "perfusion fatty acid metabolism mismatch." CMR showed preserved wall thickness in anterior and inferior walls despite significant systolic dysfunction (right middle panel), and the delayed enhancement demonstrated non-transmural hyperenhancement in the area of anterior and inferior wall (right panel)

the antero-apical wall, and a non-transmural pattern was identified in the anteroseptal wall, which indicated maintained viability (Fig. 9.3 right). Both viable and nonviable myocardium were distribution of culprit lesion in LAD. In a clinical practice, this heterogeneity of defects can be frequently experienced, and viable and nonviable myocardium may coexist in the cilprit territory.

Case 4

A 67-year-old woman with recent MI underwent stress-rest myocardial SPECT. SPECT showed a significant inferior defect and partially reversible (Fig. 9.4 left). As expected, FDG-PET revealed preserved uptake in the infarct lesion (Fig. 9.4 middle). Coronary angiography revealed total occlusion in the right coronary artery, and revascularization was performed. Two years later, the perfusion defect in the inferior wall had significantly recovered and %uptake in the revascularized area improved from 30–40% to 40–50%. Cardiac function also significantly improved (LVEF 28% → 41%). Follow up scan is useful to monitor the recovery after revascularization.

Case 5

A 65-year-old man who underwent emergency coronary stenting in RCA was referred for examination due to persistent cardiac dysfunction. He had a history of old MI and PCI to LAD. ^{99m}Tc tetrofosmin stress-rest myocardial perfusion SPECT showed an anterior and infero-posterior defect where myocardial %uptake was less than 40%. FDG revealed significantly reduced myocardial glucose metabolism which indicated scar tissue. He has already been post status of revascularizations, and a follow-up angiography revealed no significant restenosis or new lesion. Six years later, follow-up SPECT showed a similar extent of perfusion defect. However, LV dysfunction became worse, indicating the progression of myocardial remodeling (LVEF 35% → 23% and LVEDV 160 mL → 230 mL) (Fig. 9.5).

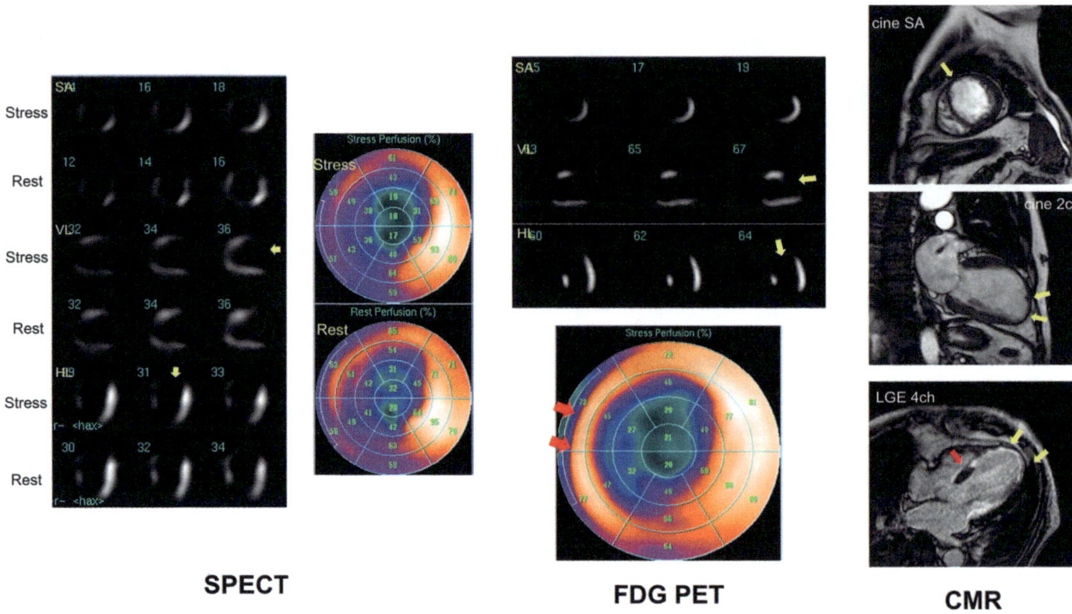

Fig. 9.3 Hybrid analysis of myocardial perfusion, glucose metabolism, and fibrosis in a patient with anterior myocardial infarction is shown. Stress-rest myocardial perfusion ^{201}TL SPECT demonstrated a significant defect in anterior, and redistribution in anteroseptal wall (left panel). FDG-PET revealed preserved glucose metabolism in atero-basal area while persistent defect was observed in distal LAD territory. Myocardial viability was expected in antero-basal area, but less likely in distal LAD territory (middle panel). Cardiac MRI demonstrated remarkably thinned wall with transmural enhancement in LAD territory, while the basal anteroseptal wall was non-transmural fibrosis with preserved wall thickness (right panel)

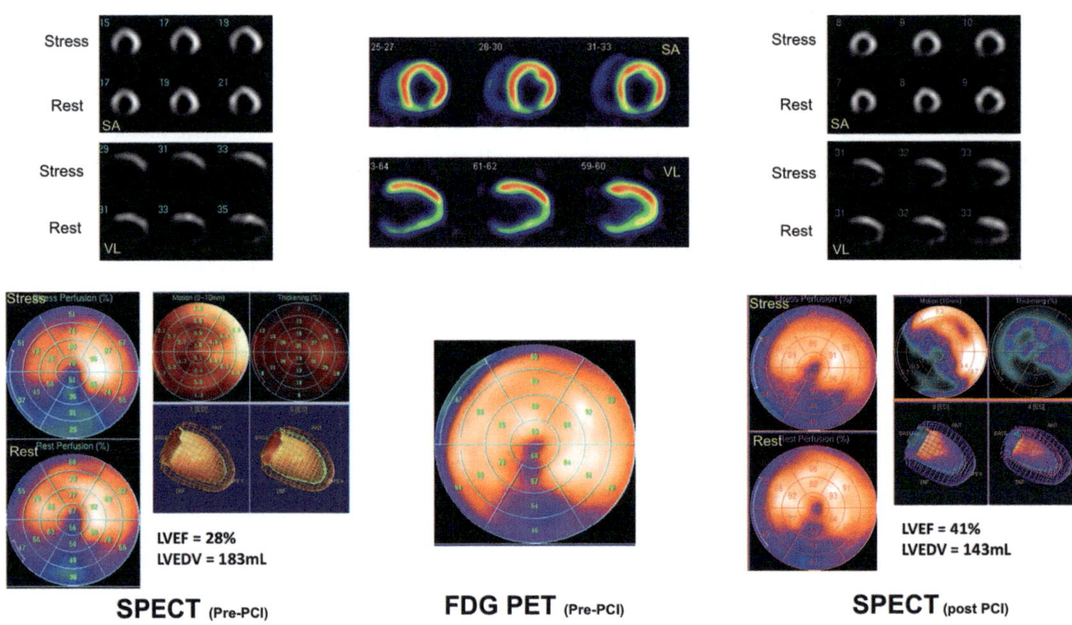

Fig. 9.4 Typical case of preserved myocardial glucose metabolism with perfusion defect in patients with inferior MI. ^{99m}Tc tetrofosmin myocardial perfusion SPECT imaging showed significant inferior defect with reduced cardiac function (LVEF 28%, EDV 183 mL). FDG-PET study showed approximately 50% of uptake in the inferior area which indicated preserved myocardial viability. The patient underwent percutaneous coronary intervention (PCI) in the right coronary artery. Two years after PCI, myocardial uptake and cardiac function significantly recovered (LVEF 41%, EDV 116 mL)

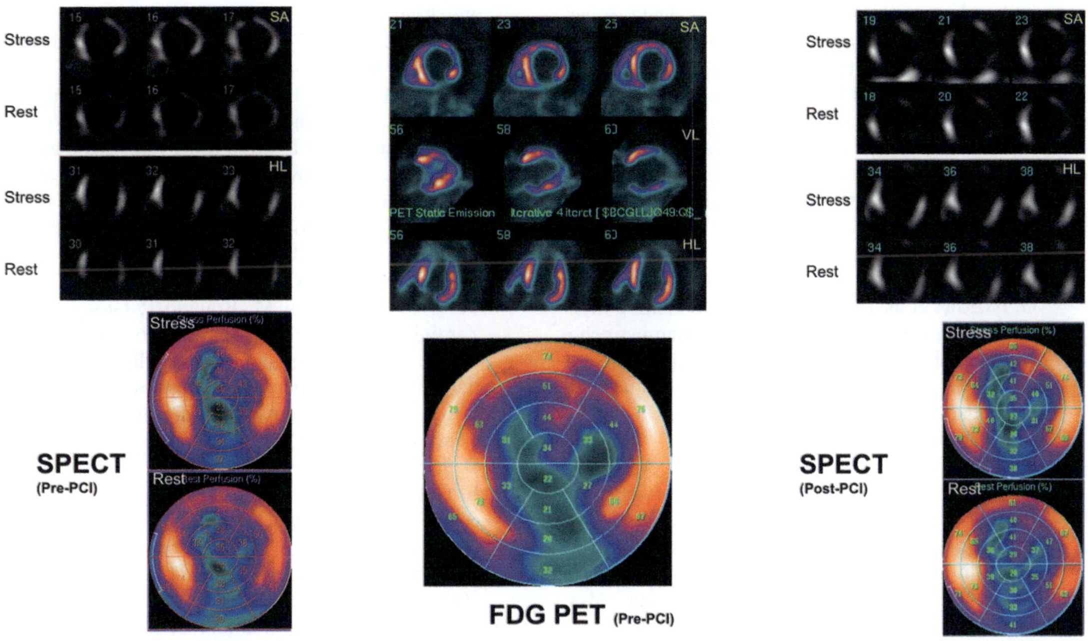

Fig. 9.5 A case of ischaemic cardiomyopathy after MI in multivessel territory is shown. A 65-year-old male was post status of PCI to LAD and RCA prior viability testing. ^{99m}Tc tetrofosmin stress-rest myocardial perfusion SPECT showed anterior and infero-posterior defects where myocardial %uptake was less than 40% (left panel). FDG-PET demonstrated significantly reduced myocardial glucose metabolism which indicated irreversible scarr (middle panel). During follow-up, neither in-stent restenosis nor new lesion was documented. Six years later, follow-up SPECT showed a similar extent of perfusion defect, and LV dysfunction has become worse (LVEF 15%–12%, EDV 316 mL–413 mL)

References

1. Roger VL. Heart failure epidemic: it's complicated. Circulation. 2018;138:25–8.
2. Bax JJ, Delgado V. Myocardial viability as integral part of the diagnostic and therapeutic approach to ischemic heart failure. J Nucl Cardiol. 2015;22:229–45.
3. Camici PG, Prasad SK, Rimoldi OE. Stunning, hibernation, and assessment of myocardial viability. Circulation. 2008;117:103–14.
4. Ammirati E, Rimoldi OE, Camici PG. Myocardial viability in ischemic left ventricular dysfunction. N Engl J Med. 2011;365:471; author reply 472–473.
5. Kloner RA, Bolli R, Marban E, Reinlib L, Braunwald E. Medical and cellular implications of stunning, hibernation, and preconditioning: an NHLBI workshop. Circulation. 1998;97:1848–67.
6. Rees G, Bristow JD, Kremkau EL, Green GS, Herr RH, Griswold HE, Starr A. Influence of aortocoronary bypass surgery on left ventricular performance. N Engl J Med. 1971;284:1116–20.
7. Chatterjee K, Swan HJ, Parmley WW, Sustaita H, Marcus HS, Matloff J. Influence of direct myocardial revascularization on left ventricular asynergy and function in patients with coronary heart disease. With and without previous myocardial infarction. Circulation. 1973;47:276–86.
8. Diamond GA. Hibernating myocardium. Am Heart J. 1989;118:1361.
9. Rahimtoola SH. The hibernating myocardium. Am Heart J. 1989;117:211–21.
10. Braunwald E, Kloner RA. The stunned myocardium: prolonged, postischemic ventricular dysfunction. Circulation. 1982;66:1146–9.
11. Matsuzaki M, Gallagher KP, Kemper WS, White F, Ross J Jr. Sustained regional dysfunction produced by prolonged coronary stenosis: gradual recovery after reperfusion. Circulation. 1983;68:170–82.
12. Marzullo P, Parodi O, Picano E, Sambuceti G, Reisenhofer B, Gimelli A, Distante A, L'Abbate A. Imaging of myocardial viability: a head-to-head comparison among nuclear, echocardiographic, and angiographic techniques. Am J Card Imaging. 1993;7:143–51.
13. Baer FM, Voth E, Schneider CA, Theissen P, Schicha H, Sechtem U. Comparison of low-dose dobutamine-gradient-echo magnetic resonance imaging and positron emission tomography with [18F]fluorodeoxyglucose in patients with chronic coronary artery disease. A functional and morpho-

logical approach to the detection of residual myocardial viability. Circulation. 1995;91:1006–15.
14. Arnese M, Cornel JH, Salustri A, Maat A, Elhendy A, Reijs AE, Ten Cate FJ, Keane D, Balk AH, Roelandt JR, et al. Prediction of improvement of regional left ventricular function after surgical revascularization. A comparison of low-dose dobutamine echocardiography with 201Tl single-photon emission computed tomography. Circulation. 1995;91:2748–52.
15. Mariani MA, Palagi C, Donatelli F, Mengozzi G, Biadi O, Vanoli G, Landoni C, Paolini G, Lucignani G, Fazio F, et al. Identification of hibernating myocardium: a comparison between dobutamine echocardiography and study of perfusion and metabolism in patients with severe left ventricular dysfunction. Am J Card Imaging. 1995;9:1–8.
16. Vanoverschelde JL, D'Hondt AM, Marwick T, Gerber BL, De Kock M, Dion R, Wijns W, Melin JA. Head-to-head comparison of exercise-redistribution-reinjection thallium single-photon emission computed tomography and low dose dobutamine echocardiography for prediction of reversibility of chronic left ventricular ischemic dysfunction. J Am Coll Cardiol. 1996;28:432–42.
17. Nagueh SF, Vaduganathan P, Ali N, Blaustein A, Verani MS, Winters WL Jr, Zoghbi WA. Identification of hibernating myocardium: comparative accuracy of myocardial contrast echocardiography, rest-redistribution thallium-201 tomography and dobutamine echocardiography. J Am Coll Cardiol. 1997;29:985–93.
18. Qureshi U, Nagueh SF, Afridi I, Vaduganathan P, Blaustein A, Verani MS, Winters WL Jr, Zoghbi WA. Dobutamine echocardiography and quantitative rest-redistribution 201Tl tomography in myocardial hibernation. Relation of contractile reserve to 201Tl uptake and comparative prediction of recovery of function. Circulation. 1997;95:626–35.
19. Pagano D, Lewis ME, Townend JN, Davies P, Camici PG, Bonser RS. Coronary revascularisation for postischaemic heart failure: how myocardial viability affects survival. Heart. 1999;82:684–8.
20. Pasquet A, Williams MJ, Secknus MA, Zuchowski C, Lytle BW, Marwick TH. Correlation of preoperative myocardial function, perfusion, and metabolism with postoperative function at rest and stress after bypass surgery in severe left ventricular dysfunction. Am J Cardiol. 1999;84:58–64.
21. Rambaldi R, Poldermans D, Bax JJ, Boersma E, Valkema R, Elhendy A, Vletter WB, Fioretti PM, Roelandt JR, Krenning EP. Dobutamine stress echocardiography and technetium-99m-tetrofosmin/fluorine 18-fluorodeoxyglucose single-photon emission computed tomography and influence of resting ejection fraction to assess myocardial viability in patients with severe left ventricular dysfunction and healed myocardial infarction. Am J Cardiol. 1999;84:130–4.
22. Cornel JH, Bax JJ, Elhendy A, Visser FC, Boersma E, Poldermans D, Sloof GW, Fioretti PM. Agreement and disagreement between "metabolic viability" and "contractile reserve" in akinetic myocardium. J Nucl Cardiol. 1999;6:383–8.
23. Cwajg JM, Cwajg E, Nagueh SF, He ZX, Qureshi U, Olmos LI, Quinones MA, Verani MS, Winters WL, Zoghbi WA. End-diastolic wall thickness as a predictor of recovery of function in myocardial hibernation: relation to rest-redistribution T1-201 tomography and dobutamine stress echocardiography. J Am Coll Cardiol. 2000;35:1152–61.
24. Anselmi M, Golia G, Maines M, Marino P, Goj C, Turri M, Cavaggioni M, Braggio P, Giorgetti PG, Zardini P. Comparison between low-dose dobutamine echocardiography and thallium-201 scintigraphy in the detection of myocardial viability in patients with recent myocardial infarction. Int J Cardiol. 2000;73:213–23.
25. Ozdemir M, Berk F, Boyaci B, Diker E, Kural T, Ibis E, Goksel S. Comparison of low-dose dobutamine echocardiography and thallium-201 reinjection for the determination of myocardial viability in the early post myocardial infarction period. Acta Cardiol. 2000;55:289–94.
26. Yong Y, Nagueh SF, Shimoni S, Shan K, He ZX, Reardon MJ, Letsou GV, Howell JF, Verani MS, Quinones MA, Zoghbi WA. Deceleration time in ischemic cardiomyopathy: relation to echocardiographic and scintigraphic indices of myocardial viability and functional recovery after revascularization. Circulation. 2001;103:1232–7.
27. Yuan D, Kuhl H, Nowak B, Kleinhans E, Kaiser HJ, Franke A, Bull U, Hanrath P, Hoffmann R. Pulsed tissue Doppler imaging to assess myocardial viability by quantification of regional myocardial functional reserve. Echocardiography. 2001;18:657–64.
28. Yoshinaga K, Morita K, Yamada S, Komuro K, Katoh C, Ito Y, Kuge Y, Kohya T, Kitabatake A, Tamaki N. Low-dose dobutamine electrocardiograph-gated myocardial SPECT for identifying viable myocardium: comparison with dobutamine stress echocardiography and PET. J Nucl Med. 2001;42:838–44.
29. Yasugi N, Koyanagi S, Ohzono K, Sakai K, Matsumoto T, Sako S, Homma T, Azakami S, Hiroki T. Comparative study of dobutamine stress echocardiography and dual single-photon emission computed tomography (thallium-201 and I-123 BMIPP) for assessing myocardial viability after acute myocardial infarction. Circ J. 2002;66:1132–8.
30. Leoncini M, Sciagra R, Maioli M, Bellandi F, Marcucci G, Sestini S, Chiocchini S, Dabizzi RP. Usefulness of dobutamine Tc-99m sestamibi-gated single-photon emission computed tomography for prediction of left ventricular ejection fraction outcome after coronary revascularization for ischemic cardiomyopathy. Am J Cardiol. 2002;89:817–21.
31. Barrington SF, Chambers J, Hallett WA, O'Doherty MJ, Roxburgh JC, Nunan TO. Comparison of sestamibi, thallium, echocardiography and PET for the detection of hibernating myocardium. Eur J Nucl Med Mol Imaging. 2004;31:355–61.

32. Schinkel AF, Bax JJ, Elhendy A, van Domburg RT, Valkema R, Vourvouri E, Bountioukos M, Rizzello V, Biagini E, Agricola E, Krenning EP, Simoons ML, Poldermans D. Long-term prognostic value of dobutamine stress echocardiography compared with myocardial perfusion scanning in patients unable to perform exercise tests. Am J Med. 2004;117:1–9.
33. Tani T, Teragaki M, Watanabe H, Muro T, Yamagishi H, Akioka K, Takeuchi K, Yoshikawa J. Prediction of functional recovery in patients with myocardial infarction after revascularization—comparison of low-dose dobutamine stress echocardiography with fluorine-18 fluorodeoxyglucose positron emission tomography. Jpn Circ J. 2001;65:177–81.
34. Ling LH, Christian TF, Mulvagh SL, Klarich KW, Hauser MF, Nishimura RA, Pellikka PA. Determining myocardial viability in chronic ischemic left ventricular dysfunction: a prospective comparison of rest-redistribution thallium 201 single-photon emission computed tomography, nitroglycerin-dobutamine echocardiography, and intracoronary myocardial contrast echocardiography. Am Heart J. 2006;151:882–9.
35. Hickman M, Janardhanan R, Dwivedi G, Burden L, Senior R. Clinical significance of perfusion techniques utilising different physiological mechanisms to detect myocardial viability: a comparative study with myocardial contrast echocardiography and single photon emission computed tomography. Int J Cardiol. 2007;114:139–40.
36. Dwivedi G, Janardhanan R, Hayat SA, Lim TK, Senior R. Comparison between myocardial contrast echocardiography and (99m)technetium sestamibi single photon emission computed tomography determined myocardial viability in predicting hard cardiac events following acute myocardial infarction. Am J Cardiol. 2009;104:1184–8.
37. He YM, Yang XJ, Wu YW, Zhang B. Twenty-four-hour thallium-201 imaging enhances the detection of myocardial ischemia and viability after myocardial infarction: a comparison study with echocardiography follow-up. Clin Nucl Med. 2009;34:65–9.
38. Mollema SA, Delgado V, Bertini M, Antoni ML, Boersma E, Holman ER, Stokkel MP, van der Wall EE, Schalij MJ, Bax JJ. Viability assessment with global left ventricular longitudinal strain predicts recovery of left ventricular function after acute myocardial infarction. Circ Cardiovasc Imaging. 2010;3:15–23.
39. Gong L, Li D, Chen J, Wang X, Xu T, Li W, Ren S, Wang C. Assessment of myocardial viability in patients with acute myocardial infarction by two-dimensional speckle tracking echocardiography combined with low-dose dobutamine stress echocardiography. Int J Cardiovasc Imaging. 2013;29:1017–28.
40. Al Moudi M, Sun ZH. Diagnostic value of (18) F-FDG PET in the assessment of myocardial viability in coronary artery disease: a comparative study with (99m)Tc SPECT and echocardiography. J Geriatr Cardiol. 2014;11:229–36.
41. Ismail M, Khalid S, Eldemerdash S, Elmallal W, Bahy H, Nammas W. The percent change of strain and strain rate under dobutamine stress echocardiography predicts viability following myocardial infarction. Minerva Cardioangiol. 2015;63:483–93.
42. Sharma A, Sood A, Mittal BR, Vijayvergiya R. Assessment of myocardial viability using echocardiographic strain imaging in patients with ST-elevation myocardial infarction: comparison with cardiac PET imaging. J Echocardiogr. 2020;18(4):240–52.
43. Orloff E, Fournier P, Bouisset F, Moine T, Cournot M, Elbaz M, Carrie D, Galinier M, Lairez O, Cognet T. Myocardial multilayer strain does not provide additional value for detection of myocardial viability assessed by SPECT imaging over and beyond standard strain. Echocardiography. 2018;35:1300–9.
44. Liu Q, Zhao S, Yan C, Lu M, Jiang S, Zhang Y, Li S, Liu Y, Yang M, He Z. Myocardial viability in chronic ischemic heart disease: comparison of delayed-enhancement magnetic resonance imaging with 99mTc-sestamibi and 18F-fluorodeoxyglucose single-photon emission computed tomography. Nucl Med Commun. 2009;30:610–6.
45. Verma B, Singh A. Comparison of contrast enhanced low-dose dobutamine stress echocardiography with 99mTc-sestamibi single-photon emission computed tomography in assessment of myocardial viability. Open Access Maced J Med Sci. 2019;7:1287–92.
46. Nelson C, McCrohon J, Khafagi F, Rose S, Leano R, Marwick TH. Impact of scar thickness on the assessment of viability using dobutamine echocardiography and thallium single-photon emission computed tomography: a comparison with contrast-enhanced magnetic resonance imaging. J Am Coll Cardiol. 2004;43:1248–56.
47. La Canna G, Rahimtoola SH, Visioli O, Giubbini R, Alfieri O, Zognio M, Milan E, Ceconi C, Gargano M, Lo Russo R, Ferrari R. Sensitivity, specificity, and predictive accuracies of non-invasive tests, singly and in combination, for diagnosis of hibernating myocardium. Eur Heart J. 2000;21:1358–67.
48. Baer FM, Smolarz K, Theissen P, Voth E, Schicha H, Sechtem U. Regional 99mTc-methoxyisobutyl-isonitrile-uptake at rest in patients with myocardial infarcts: comparison with morphological and functional parameters obtained from gradient-echo magnetic resonance imaging. Eur Heart J. 1994;15:97–107.
49. Klein C, Nekolla SG, Bengel FM, Momose M, Sammer A, Haas F, Schnackenburg B, Delius W, Mudra H, Wolfram D, Schwaiger M. Assessment of myocardial viability with contrast-enhanced magnetic resonance imaging: comparison with positron emission tomography. Circulation. 2002;105:162–7.
50. Gunning MG, Anagnostopoulos C, Davies G, Knight CJ, Pennell DJ, Fox KM, Pepper J, Underwood SR. Simultaneous assessment of myocardial viability and function for the detection of hibernating myocardium using ECG-gated 99Tcm-tetrofosmin emission tomography: a comparison with 201Tl

emission tomography combined with cine magnetic resonance imaging. Nucl Med Commun. 1999;20:209–14.
51. Knuesel PR, Nanz D, Wyss C, Buechi M, Kaufmann PA, von Schulthess GK, Luscher TF, Schwitter J. Characterization of dysfunctional myocardium by positron emission tomography and magnetic resonance: relation to functional outcome after revascularization. Circulation. 2003;108:1095–100.
52. Kitagawa K, Sakuma H, Hirano T, Okamoto S, Makino K, Takeda K. Acute myocardial infarction: myocardial viability assessment in patients early thereafter comparison of contrast-enhanced MR imaging with resting (201)Tl SPECT. Single photon emission computed tomography. Radiology. 2003;226:138–44.
53. Kuhl HP, Beek AM, van der Weerdt AP, Hofman MB, Visser CA, Lammertsma AA, Heussen N, Visser FC, van Rossum AC. Myocardial viability in chronic ischemic heart disease: comparison of contrast-enhanced magnetic resonance imaging with (18)F-fluorodeoxyglucose positron emission tomography. J Am Coll Cardiol. 2003;41:1341–8.
54. Lee VS, Resnick D, Tiu SS, Sanger JJ, Nazzaro CA, Israel GM, Simonetti OP. MR imaging evaluation of myocardial viability in the setting of equivocal SPECT results with (99m)Tc sestamibi. Radiology. 2004;230:191–7.
55. Schmidt M, Voth E, Schneider CA, Theissen P, Wagner R, Baer FM, Schicha H. F-18-FDG uptake is a reliable predictory of functional recovery of akinetic but viable infarct regions as defined by magnetic resonance imaging before and after revascularization. Magn Reson Imaging. 2004;22:229–36.
56. Gutberlet M, Frohlich M, Mehl S, Amthauer H, Hausmann H, Meyer R, Siniawski H, Ruf J, Plotkin M, Denecke T, Schnackenburg B, Hetzer R, Felix R. Myocardial viability assessment in patients with highly impaired left ventricular function: comparison of delayed enhancement, dobutamine stress MRI, end-diastolic wall thickness, and TI201-SPECT with functional recovery after revascularization. Eur Radiol. 2005;15:872–80.
57. Misko J, Dziuk M, Skrobowska E, Szalus N, Pietrzykowski J, Warczynska A. Co-registration of cardiac MRI and rest gated SPECT in the assessment of myocardial perfusion, function and viability. J Cardiovasc Magn Reson. 2006;8:389–97.
58. Solar M, Zizka J, Dolezal J, Klzo L, Tintera J, Vizda J, Ceral J. Contrast-enhanced magnetic resonance and thallium scintigraphy in the detection of myocardial viability: a prospective comparative study. Int Heart J. 2006;47:521–32.
59. Wang YN, Jin ZY, Zhang ZH, Kong LY, Chen LB, Zhou L, Sun HY, Zhang H, Miao Q. Assessment of myocardial viability with contrast-enhanced magnetic resonance imaging and comparison with single-photon emission computed tomography. Chin Med Sci J. 2006;21:239–44.
60. Wu YW, Tadamura E, Kanao S, Yamamuro M, Marui A, Komeda M, Toma M, Kimura T, Togashi K. Myocardial viability by contrast-enhanced cardiovascular magnetic resonance in patients with coronary artery disease: comparison with gated single-photon emission tomography and FDG position emission tomography. Int J Cardiovasc Imaging. 2007;23:757–65.
61. Roes SD, Kaandorp TA, Marsan NA, Westenberg JJ, Dibbets-Schneider P, Stokkel MP, Lamb HJ, van der Wall EE, de Roos A, Bax JJ. Agreement and disagreement between contrast-enhanced magnetic resonance imaging and nuclear imaging for assessment of myocardial viability. Eur J Nucl Med Mol Imaging. 2009;36:594–601.
62. Rischpler C, Langwieser N, Souvatzoglou M, Batrice A, van Marwick S, Snajberk J, Ibrahim T, Laugwitz KL, Nekolla SG, Schwaiger M. PET/MRI early after myocardial infarction: evaluation of viability with late gadolinium enhancement transmurality vs. 18F-FDG uptake. Eur Heart J Cardiovasc Imaging. 2015;16:661–9.
63. Hunold P, Jakob H, Erbel R, Barkhausen J, Heilmaier C. Accuracy of myocardial viability imaging by cardiac MRI and PET depending on left ventricular function. World J Cardiol. 2018;10:110–8.
64. Timmer SAJ, Teunissen PFA, Danad I, Robbers L, Raijmakers P, Nijveldt R, van Rossum AC, Lammertsma AA, van Royen N, Knaapen P. In vivo assessment of myocardial viability after acute myocardial infarction: a head-to-head comparison of the perfusable tissue index by PET and delayed contrast-enhanced CMR. J Nucl Cardiol. 2017;24:657–67.
65. Kiko T, Yokokawa T, Misaka T, Masuda A, Yoshihisa A, Yamaki T, Kunii H, Nakazato K, Takeishi Y. Myocardial viability with chronic total occlusion assessed by hybrid positron emission tomography/magnetic resonance imaging. J Nucl Cardiol. 2021;28(5):2335–42.
66. Beitzke D, Rasul S, Lassen ML, Pichler V, Senn D, Stelzmuller ME, Nolz R, Loewe C, Hacker M. Assessment of myocardial viability in ischemic heart disease by PET/MRI: comparison of left ventricular perfusion, hibernation, and scar burden. Acad Radiol. 2020;27:188–97.
67. Wu YW, Tadamura E, Yamamuro M, Kanao S, Marui A, Tanabara K, Komeda M, Togashi K. Comparison of contrast-enhanced MRI with (18) F-FDG PET/201Tl SPECT in dysfunctional myocardium: relation to early functional outcome after surgical revascularization in chronic ischemic heart disease. J Nucl Med. 2007;48:1096–103.
68. Habis M, Capderou A, Ghostine S, Daoud B, Caussin C, Riou JY, Brenot P, Angel CY, Lancelin B, Paul JF. Acute myocardial infarction early viability assessment by 64-slice computed tomography immediately after coronary angiography: comparison with low-dose dobutamine echocardiography. J Am Coll Cardiol. 2007;49:1178–85.

69. Sato A, Hiroe M, Nozato T, Hikita H, Ito Y, Ohigashi H, Tamura M, Takahashi A, Isobe M, Aonuma K. Early validation study of 64-slice multidetector computed tomography for the assessment of myocardial viability and the prediction of left ventricular remodelling after acute myocardial infarction. Eur Heart J. 2008;29:490–8.
70. Shapiro MD, Sarwar A, Nieman K, Nasir K, Brady TJ, Cury RC. Cardiac computed tomography for prediction of myocardial viability after reperfused acute myocardial infarction. J Cardiovasc Comput Tomogr. 2010;4:267–73.
71. Goetti R, Feuchtner G, Stolzmann P, Donati OF, Wieser M, Plass A, Frauenfelder T, Leschka S, Alkadhi H. Delayed enhancement imaging of myocardial viability: low-dose high-pitch CT versus MRI. Eur Radiol. 2011;21:2091–9.
72. Mghaieth Zghal F, Boudiche S, Haboubi S, Neji H, Ben Halima M, Rekik B, Mechri M, Ouali S, Hantous S, Mourali MS. Diagnostic accuracy of strain imaging in predicting myocardial viability after an ST-elevation myocardial infarction. Medicine (Baltimore). 2020;99:e19528.
73. Lipiec P, Szymczyk E, Michalski B, Stefanczyk L, Wozniakowski B, Rotkiewicz A, Szymczyk K, Kasprzak JD. Echocardiographic quantitative analysis of resting myocardial function for the assessment of viability after myocardial infarction—comparison with magnetic resonance imaging. Kardiol Pol. 2011;69:915–22.
74. Baer FM, Voth E, LaRosee K, Schneider CA, Theissen P, Deutsch HJ, Schicha H, Erdmann E, Sechtem U. Comparison of dobutamine transesophageal echocardiography and dobutamine magnetic resonance imaging for detection of residual myocardial viability. Am J Cardiol. 1996;78:415–9.
75. Arrighi JA, Soufer R. Myocardial viability: seeking relevance and redefinition. J Nucl Cardiol. 1998;5:629–33.
76. Shibata MC. Myocardial viability. J Am Coll Cardiol. 1998;31:1215.
77. Walton S. Radionuclide techniques for myocardial viability and hibernation. Heart. 1999;81:6–7.
78. Beller GA. Noninvasive assessment of myocardial viability. N Engl J Med. 2000;343:1488–90.
79. Bax JJ, Poldermans D, Schinkel AF, Boersma E, Elhendy A, Maat A, Valkema R, Krenning EP, Roelandt JR. Perfusion and contractile reserve in chronic dysfunctional myocardium: relation to functional outcome after surgical revascularization. Circulation. 2002;106:I14–8.
80. Beller GA. The case for cardiac magnetic resonance and positron emission tomography multimodality imaging of myocardial viability. J Nucl Cardiol. 2010;17:527–8.
81. Partington SL, Kwong RY, Dorbala S. Multimodality imaging in the assessment of myocardial viability. Heart Fail Rev. 2011;16:381–95.
82. Arrighi JA, Dilsizian V. Multimodality imaging for assessment of myocardial viability: nuclear, echocardiography, MR, and CT. Curr Cardiol Rep. 2012;14:234–43.
83. Bax JJ, Wijns W, Cornel JH, Visser FC, Boersma E, Fioretti PM. Accuracy of currently available techniques for prediction of functional recovery after revascularization in patients with left ventricular dysfunction due to chronic coronary artery disease: comparison of pooled data. J Am Coll Cardiol. 1997;30:1451–60.
84. Schinkel AF, Bax JJ, Geleijnse ML, Boersma E, Elhendy A, Roelandt JR, Poldermans D. Noninvasive evaluation of ischaemic heart disease: myocardial perfusion imaging or stress echocardiography? Eur Heart J. 2003;24:789–800.
85. Schinkel AF, Bax JJ, Poldermans D, Elhendy A, Ferrari R, Rahimtoola SH. Hibernating myocardium: diagnosis and patient outcomes. Curr Probl Cardiol. 2007;32:375–410.
86. Cuocolo A, Acampa W, Nicolai E, Pace L, Petretta M, Salvatore M. Quantitative thallium-201 and technetium 99m sestamibi tomography at rest in detection of myocardial viability in patients with chronic ischemic left ventricular dysfunction. J Nucl Cardiol. 2000;7:8–15.
87. Kauffman GJ, Boyne TS, Watson DD, Smith WH, Beller GA. Comparison of rest thallium-201 imaging and rest technetium-99m sestamibi imaging for assessment of myocardial viability in patients with coronary artery disease and severe left ventricular dysfunction. J Am Coll Cardiol. 1996;27:1592–7.
88. Altehoefer C, vom Dahl J, Biedermann M, Uebis R, Beilin I, Sheehan F, Hanrath P, Buell U. Significance of defect severity in technetium-99m-MIBI SPECT at rest to assess myocardial viability: comparison with fluorine-18-FDG PET. J Nucl Med. 1994;35:569–74.
89. Altehoefer C, vom Dahl J, Buell U, Uebis R, Kleinhans E, Hanrath P. Comparison of thallium-201 single-photon emission tomography after rest injection and fluorodeoxyglucose positron emission tomography for assessment of myocardial viability in patients with chronic coronary artery disease. Eur J Nucl Med. 1994;21:37–45.
90. Lucignani G, Paolini G, Landoni C, Zuccari M, Paganelli G, Galli L, Di Credico G, Vanoli G, Rossetti C, Mariani MA, et al. Presurgical identification of hibernating myocardium by combined use of technetium-99m hexakis 2-methoxyisobutylisonitrile single photon emission tomography and fluorine-18 fluoro-2-deoxy-D-glucose positron emission tomography in patients with coronary artery disease. Eur J Nucl Med. 1992;19:874–81.
91. Tamaki N, Kawamoto M, Tadamura E, Magata Y, Yonekura Y, Nohara R, Sasayama S, Nishimura K, Ban T, Konishi J. Prediction of reversible ischemia after revascularization. Perfusion and metabolic studies with positron emission tomography. Circulation. 1995;91:1697–705.
92. vom Dahl J, Muzik O, Wolfe ER Jr, Allman C, Hutchins G, Schwaiger M. Myocardial rubidium-82

tissue kinetics assessed by dynamic positron emission tomography as a marker of myocardial cell membrane integrity and viability. Circulation. 1996;93:238–45.
93. Yoshida K, Gould KL. Quantitative relation of myocardial infarct size and myocardial viability by positron emission tomography to left ventricular ejection fraction and 3-year mortality with and without revascularization. J Am Coll Cardiol. 1993;22:984–97.
94. Allman KC, Shaw LJ, Hachamovitch R, Udelson JE. Myocardial viability testing and impact of revascularization on prognosis in patients with coronary artery disease and left ventricular dysfunction: a meta-analysis. J Am Coll Cardiol. 2002;39:1151–8.
95. deFilippi CR, Willett DL, Irani WN, Eichhorn EJ, Velasco CE, Grayburn PA. Comparison of myocardial contrast echocardiography and low-dose dobutamine stress echocardiography in predicting recovery of left ventricular function after coronary revascularization in chronic ischemic heart disease. Circulation. 1995;92:2863–8.
96. Iwakura K, Okamura A, Koyama Y, Date M, Higuchi Y, Inoue K, Kimura R, Nagai H, Imai M, Toyoshima Y, Ozawa M, Ito N, Okazaki Y, Shibuya M, Omiya S, Takagi T, Morisawa D, Fujii K. Automated assessment of myocardial viability after acute myocardial infarction by global longitudinal peak strain on low-dose dobutamine stress echocardiography. Circ J. 2010;74:2158–65.
97. Yun H, Jin H, Yang S, Huang D, Chen ZW, Zeng MS. Coronary artery angiography and myocardial viability imaging: a 3.0-T contrast-enhanced magnetic resonance coronary artery angiography with Gd-BOPTA. Int J Cardiovasc Imaging. 2014;30:99–108.
98. Gerbaud E, Faury A, Coste P, Erickson M, Corneloup O, Dos Santos P, Durrieu-Jais C, Laurent F, Montaudon M. Comparative analysis of cardiac magnetic resonance viability indexes to predict functional recovery after successful percutaneous coronary intervention in acute myocardial infarction. Am J Cardiol. 2010;105:598–604.
99. Tamaki N, Ohtani H, Yamashita K, Magata Y, Yonekura Y, Nohara R, Kambara H, Kawai C, Hirata K, Ban T, et al. Metabolic activity in the areas of new fill-in after thallium-201 reinjection: comparison with positron emission tomography using fluorine-18-deoxyglucose. J Nucl Med. 1991;32:673–8.
100. Gropler RJ, Geltman EM, Sampathkumaran K, Perez JE, Moerlein SM, Sobel BE, Bergmann SR, Siegel BA. Functional recovery after coronary revascularization for chronic coronary artery disease is dependent on maintenance of oxidative metabolism. J Am Coll Cardiol. 1992;20:569–77.
101. Dondi M, Tartagni F, Fallani F, Fanti S, Marengo M, DiTommaso I, Zheng QF, Monetti N. A comparison of rest sestamibi and rest-redistribution thallium single photon emission tomography: possible implications for myocardial viability detection in infarcted patients. Eur J Nucl Med. 1993;20:26–31.
102. Udelson JE, Coleman PS, Metherall J, Pandian NG, Gomez AR, Griffith JL, Shea NL, Oates E, Konstam MA. Predicting recovery of severe regional ventricular dysfunction. Comparison of resting scintigraphy with 201Tl and 99mTc-sestamibi. Circulation. 1994;89:2552–61.
103. Kawamoto M, Tamaki N, Yonekura Y, Tadamura E, Fujibayashi Y, Magata Y, Nohara R, Sasayama S, Ikekubo K, Kato H, et al. Combined study with I-123 fatty acid and thallium-201 to assess ischemic myocardium: comparison with thallium redistribution and glucose metabolism. Ann Nucl Med. 1994;8:47–54.
104. vom Dahl J, Altehoefer C, Sheehan FH, Buechin P, Uebis R, Messmer BJ, Buell U, Hanrath P. Recovery of regional left ventricular dysfunction after coronary revascularization. Impact of myocardial viability assessed by nuclear imaging and vessel patency at follow-up angiography. J Am Coll Cardiol. 1996;28:948–58.
105. Gerber BL, Vanoverschelde JL, Bol A, Michel C, Labar D, Wijns W, Melin JA. Myocardial blood flow, glucose uptake, and recruitment of inotropic reserve in chronic left ventricular ischemic dysfunction. Implications for the pathophysiology of chronic myocardial hibernation. Circulation. 1996;94:651–9.
106. Wolpers HG, Burchert W, van den Hoff J, Weinhardt R, Meyer GJ, Lichtlen PR. Assessment of myocardial viability by use of 11C-acetate and positron emission tomography. Threshold criteria of reversible dysfunction. Circulation. 1997;95:1417–24.
107. vom Dahl J, Altehoefer C, Sheehan FH, Buechin P, Schulz G, Schwarz ER, Koch KC, Uebis R, Messmer BJ, Buell U, Hanrath P. Effect of myocardial viability assessed by technetium-99m-sestamibi SPECT and fluorine-18-FDG PET on clinical outcome in coronary artery disease. J Nucl Med. 1997;38:742–8.
108. Cornel JH, Bax JJ, Elhendy A, Reijs AE, Fioretti PM. Dobutamine stress-redistribution-reinjection versus rest-redistribution thallium-201 SPECT in the assessment of myocardial viability. Int J Card Imaging. 1997;13:59–64.
109. Flotats A, Carrio I, Estorch M, Berna L, Catafau AM, Mari C, Ballester M. Nitrate administration to enhance the detection of myocardial viability by technetium-99m tetrofosmin single-photon emission tomography. Eur J Nucl Med. 1997;24:767–73.
110. Gerber BL, Melin JA, Bol A, Labar D, Cogneau M, Michel C, Vanoverschelde JL. Nitrogen-13-ammonia and oxygen-15-water estimates of absolute myocardial perfusion in left ventricular ischemic dysfunction. J Nucl Med. 1998;39:1655–62.
111. Fukuchi K, Katafuchi T, Fukushima K, Shimotsu Y, Toba M, Hayashida K, Takamiya M, Ishida Y. Estimation of myocardial perfusion and viability using simultaneous 99mTc-tetrofosmin—FDG collimated SPECT. J Nucl Med. 2000;41:1318–23.
112. Matsuno K, Kuwabara Y, Watanabe S, Kuroda T, Mikami Y, Fujii K, Saito T, Masuda Y. Detection of myocardial viability using rest-redistribution thal-

lium-201 imaging in a stress 99Tcm-tetrofosmin/rest thallium-201 dual-isotope protocol. Nucl Med Commun. 2001;22:165–73.
113. Acampa W, Cuocolo A, Petretta M, Bruno A, Castellani M, Finzi A, Gerundini P. Tetrofosmin imaging in the detection of myocardial viability in patients with previous myocardial infarction: comparison with sestamibi and Tl-201 scintigraphy. J Nucl Cardiol. 2002;9:33–40.
114. Maruyama A, Hasegawa S, Paul AK, Xiuli M, Yoshioka J, Maruyama K, Hori M, Nishimura T. Myocardial viability assessment with gated SPECT Tc-99m tetrofosmin % wall thickening: comparison with F-18 FDG-PET. Ann Nucl Med. 2002;16:25–32.
115. De Boer J, Slart RH, Blanksma PK, Willemsen AT, Jager PL, Paans AM, Vaalburg W, Piers DA. Comparison of 99mTc-sestamibi-18F-fluorodeoxyglucose dual isotope simultaneous acquisition and rest-stress 99mTc-sestamibi single photon emission computed tomography for the assessment of myocardial viability. Nucl Med Commun. 2003;24:251–7.
116. Yoshinaga K, Katoh C, Beanlands RS, Noriyasu K, Komuro K, Yamada S, Kuge Y, Morita K, Kitabatake A, Tamaki N. Reduced oxidative metabolic response in dysfunctional myocardium with preserved glucose metabolism but with impaired contractile reserve. J Nucl Med. 2004;45:1885–91.
117. Giorgetti A, Marzullo P, Sambuceti G, Di Quirico S, Kusch A, Landi P, Salvadori PA, Pisani P, L'Abbate A. Baseline/post-nitrate Tc-99m tetrofosmin mismatch for the assessment of myocardial viability in patients with severe left ventricular dysfunction: comparison with baseline Tc-99m tetrofosmin scintigraphy/FDG PET imaging. J Nucl Cardiol. 2004;11:142–51.
118. Orea A, Castillo L, Ochoa V, Rull JA, Gomez-Perez F, Rebollar V, Sepulveda J, Dorantes J, Asensio E, Oseguera J, Gonzalez O. Detection of myocardial viability could be improved by rest GIK (glucose-insulin-potassium solution)-Tc 99m sestamibi compared with TL-201 reinjection, in post myocardial infarction patients. Rev Invest Clin. 2004;56:321–6.
119. Slart RH, Bax JJ, Sluiter WJ, van Veldhuisen DJ, Jager PL. Added value of attenuation-corrected Tc-99m tetrofosmin SPECT for the detection of myocardial viability: comparison with FDG SPECT. J Nucl Cardiol. 2004;11:689–96.
120. Toyama T, Hoshizaki H, Seki R, Isobe N, Oshima S, Taniguchi K, Higuchi K, Seki H, Hatori T, Kurabayashi M, Endo K. Evaluation of myocardial viability following acute myocardial infarction using 201Tl SPECT after thallium-glucose-insulin infusion—comparison with 18F-FDG positron emission tomography. Ann Nucl Med. 2004;18:463–8.
121. Yamakawa Y, Takahashi N, Ishikawa T, Uchino K, Mochida Y, Ebina T, Kobayashi T, Matsushita K, Matsumoto K, Kawasaki N, Shimura M, Ohkusu Y, Sumita S, Kimura K, Inoue T, Umemura S. Clinical usefulness of ECG-gated 18F-FDG PET combined with 99mTC-MIBI gated SPECT for evaluating myocardial viability and function. Ann Nucl Med. 2004;18:375–83.
122. Matsunari I, Kanayama S, Yoneyama T, Matsudaira M, Nakajima K, Taki J, Nekolla SG, Tonami N, Hisada K. Electrocardiographic-gated dual-isotope simultaneous acquisition SPECT using 18F-FDG and 99mTc-sestamibi to assess myocardial viability and function in a single study. Eur J Nucl Med Mol Imaging. 2005;32:195–202.
123. Desideri A, Cortigiani L, Christen AI, Coscarelli S, Gregori D, Zanco P, Komorovsky R, Bax JJ. The extent of perfusion-F18-fluorodeoxyglucose positron emission tomography mismatch determines mortality in medically treated patients with chronic ischemic left ventricular dysfunction. J Am Coll Cardiol. 2005;46:1264–9.
124. Schinkel AF, Bax JJ, Biagini E, Elhendy A, van Domburg RT, Valkema R, Rizzello V, Schouten O, Simoons M, Poldermans D. Myocardial technetium-99m-tetrofosmin single-photon emission computed tomography compared with 18F-fluorodeoxyglucose imaging to assess myocardial viability. Am J Cardiol. 2005;95:1223–5.
125. Wu YW, Huang PJ, Lee CM, Ho YL, Lin LC, Wang TD, Wang SS, Chen TH, Yen RF. Assessment of myocardial viability using F-18 fluorodeoxyglucose/Tc-99m sestamibi dual-isotope simultaneous acquisition SPECT: comparison with Tl-201 stress-reinjection SPECT. J Nucl Cardiol. 2005;12:451–9.
126. Alexanderson E, Ricalde A, Romero-Ibarra JL, Meave A. Comparison of 18FDG PET with thallium SPECT in the assessment of myocardial viability. A segmental model analysis. Arch Cardiol Mex. 2006;76:9–15.
127. Roelants V, Bernard X, Walrand S, Bol A, Coppens A, Jamart J, Melin J, Vanoverschelde JL. Attenuation-corrected 99mTc-MIBI SPECT in overweight patients with chronic ischaemic dysfunction: a comparison to NH3 PET and implications for the diagnosis of myocardial viability. Nucl Med Commun. 2006;27:815–21.
128. Slart RH, Agool A, van Veldhuisen DJ, Dierckx RA, Bax JJ. Nitrate administration increases blood flow in dysfunctional but viable myocardium, leading to improved assessment of myocardial viability: a PET study. J Nucl Med. 2006;47:1307–11.
129. Gunel SE, Akgun A. Comparison of exercise-rest-reinjection Tl-201 imaging and rest sublingual isosorbide dinitrate Tc-99m MIBI imaging for the assessment of myocardial viability. Ann Nucl Med. 2009;23:451–7.
130. Raja S, Singh B, Rohit MK, Manohar K, Kashyap R, Bhattacharya A, Mittal BR. Comparison of nitrate augmented Tc-99m tetrofosmin gated SPECT imaging with FDG PET imaging for the assessment of myocardial viability in patients with severe left ventricular dysfunction. J Nucl Cardiol. 2012;19:1176–81.

131. Uebleis C, Hellweger S, Laubender RP, Becker A, Sohn HY, Lehner S, Haug A, Bartenstein P, Cumming P, Van Kriekinge SD, Slomka PJ, Hacker M. The amount of dysfunctional but viable myocardium predicts long-term survival in patients with ischemic cardiomyopathy and left ventricular dysfunction. Int J Cardiovasc Imaging. 2013;29:1645–53.
132. Dong W, Li J, Mi H, Song X, Jiao J, Li Q. Relationship between collateral circulation and myocardial viability of (18)F-FDG PET/CT subtended by chronic total occluded coronary arteries. Ann Nucl Med. 2018;32:197–205.
133. Moody JB, Hiller KM, Lee BC, Poitrasson-Riviere A, Corbett JR, Weinberg RL, Murthy VL, Ficaro EP. The utility of (82)Rb PET for myocardial viability assessment: comparison with perfusion-metabolism (82)Rb-(18)F-FDG PET. J Nucl Cardiol. 2019;26:374–86.
134. Zhang F, Wang J, Shao X, Yang M, Qian Y, Yang X, Wu Z, Li S, Xin W, Shi Y, Liu B, Yu W, He Z, Zhou W, Wang Y. Incremental value of myocardial wall motion and thickening to perfusion alone by gated SPECT myocardial perfusion imaging for viability assessment in patients with ischemic heart failure. J Nucl Cardiol. 2021;28(6):2545–56.
135. Sun XX, Li S, Fang W, Tian YQ, Shen R, Wei H, He ZX. Preserved myocardial viability in patients with chronic total occlusion of a single coronary artery. J Nucl Cardiol. 2020;28(6):2812–22.
136. Duncan BH, Ahlberg AW, Levine MG, McGill CC, Mann A, White MP, Mather JF, Waters DD, Heller GV. Comparison of electrocardiographic-gated technetium-99m sestamibi single-photon emission computed tomographic imaging and rest-redistribution thallium-201 in the prediction of myocardial viability. Am J Cardiol. 2000;85:680–4.
137. Narula J, Dawson MS, Singh BK, Amanullah A, Acio ER, Chaudhry FA, Arani RB, Iskandrian AE. Noninvasive characterization of stunned, hibernating, remodeled and nonviable myocardium in ischemic cardiomyopathy. J Am Coll Cardiol. 2000;36:1913–9.
138. Beller GA. Comparison of 201Tl scintigraphy and low-dose dobutamine echocardiography for the noninvasive assessment of myocardial viability. Circulation. 1996;94:2681–4.
139. Claeys MJ, Rademakers FE, Vrints CJ, Krug B, Bosmans JM, Conraads V, Bossaert LL, Snoeck JP, Blockx PP. Comparative study of rest technetium-99m sestamibi SPET and low-dose dobutamine stress echocardiography for the early assessment of myocardial viability after acute myocardial infarction: importance of the severity of the infarct-related stenosis. Eur J Nucl Med. 1996;23:748–55.
140. Perrone-Filardi P, Pace L, Prastaro M, Squame F, Betocchi S, Soricelli A, Piscione F, Indolfi C, Crisci T, Salvatore M, Chiariello M. Assessment of myocardial viability in patients with chronic coronary artery disease. Rest-4-hour-24-hour 201Tl tomography versus dobutamine echocardiography. Circulation. 1996;94:2712–9.
141. Bax JJ, Valkema R, Visser FC, van Lingen A, Cornel JH, Poldermans D, Rambaldi R, Krenning EP, Fioretti PM. FDG SPECT in the assessment of myocardial viability. Comparison with dobutamine echo. Eur Heart J. 1997;18 Suppl D:D124–9.
142. Nagueh SF. Dobutamine echocardiography versus nuclear cardiac imaging for evaluation of myocardial viability. Curr Opin Cardiol. 1997;12:547–52.
143. Baumgartner H, Porenta G, Lau YK, Wutte M, Klaar U, Mehrabi M, Siegel RJ, Czernin J, Laufer G, Sochor H, Schelbert H, Fishbein MC, Maurer G. Assessment of myocardial viability by dobutamine echocardiography, positron emission tomography and thallium-201 SPECT: correlation with histopathology in explanted hearts. J Am Coll Cardiol. 1998;32:1701–8.
144. Elsasser A, Muller KD, Vogt A, Strasser R, Gagel C, Schlepper M, Klovekorn WP. Assessment of myocardial viability: dobutamine echocardiography and thallium-201 single-photon emission computed tomographic imaging predict the postoperative improvement of left ventricular function after bypass surgery. Am Heart J. 1998;135:463–75.
145. Castini D, Bestetti A, Garbin M, Di Leo C, Bigi R, Sponzilli C, Concardi G, Gioventu M, Tarolo GL, Lombardi F, Fiorentini C. Myocardial viability assessment after acute myocardial infarction: low-dose dobutamine echocardiography versus rest-redistribution thallium-201 SPECT. Cardiologia. 1999;44:817–23.
146. Sicari R, Varga A, Picano E, Borges AC, Gimelli A, Marzullo P. Comparison of combination of dipyridamole and dobutamine during echocardiography with thallium scintigraphy with thallium scintigraphy to improve viability detection. Am J Cardiol. 1999;83:6–10.
147. Leoncini M, Marcucci G, Sciagra R, Mondanelli D, Traini AM, Magni M, Frascarelli F, Mennuti A, Dabizzi RP. Comparison of baseline and low-dose dobutamine technetium-99m sestamibi scintigraphy with low-dose dobutamine echocardiography for predicting functional recovery after revascularization. Am J Cardiol. 2000;86:153–7.
148. Picano E, Ostojic M, Varga A, Sicari R, Djordjevic-Dikic A, Nedeljkovic I, Torres M. Combined low dose dipyridamole-dobutamine stress echocardiography to identify myocardial viability. J Am Coll Cardiol. 1996;27:1422–8.
149. He ZX, Darcourt J, Guignier A, Ferrari E, Bussiere F, Baudouy M, Morand P. Nitrates improve detection of ischemic but viable myocardium by thallium-201 reinjection SPECT. J Nucl Med. 1993;34:1472–7.
150. Bisi G, Sciagra R, Santoro GM, Fazzini PF. Rest technetium-99m sestamibi tomography in combination with short-term administration of nitrates: feasibility and reliability for prediction of postrevascularization outcome of asynergic territories. J Am Coll Cardiol. 1994;24:1282–9.

151. Wahba FF, Lamb HJ, Bax JJ, Dibbets-Schneider P, Bavelaar-Croon CD, Zwinderman AH, Pauwels EK, Van Der Wall EE. Assessment of regional myocardial wall motion and thickening by gated 99Tcm-tetrofosmin SPECT: a comparison with magnetic resonance imaging. Nucl Med Commun. 2001;22:663–71.
152. Gardner BI, Bingham SE, Allen MR, Blatter DD, Anderson JL. Cardiac magnetic resonance versus transthoracic echocardiography for the assessment of cardiac volumes and regional function after myocardial infarction: an intrasubject comparison using simultaneous intrasubject recordings. Cardiovasc Ultrasound. 2009;7:38.
153. Romero J, Xue X, Gonzalez W, Garcia MJ. CMR imaging assessing viability in patients with chronic ventricular dysfunction due to coronary artery disease: a meta-analysis of prospective trials. JACC Cardiovasc Imaging. 2012;5:494–508.
154. Orlandini A, Castellana N, Pascual A, Botto F, Cecilia Bahit M, Chacon C, Luz Diaz M, Diaz R. Myocardial viability for decision-making concerning revascularization in patients with left ventricular dysfunction and coronary artery disease: a meta-analysis of non-randomized and randomized studies. Int J Cardiol. 2015;182:494–9.
155. Tsai JP, Yun CH, Wu TH, Yen CH, Hou CJ, Kuo JY, Hung CL. A meta-analysis comparing SPECT with PET for the assessment of myocardial viability in patients with coronary artery disease. Nucl Med Commun. 2014;35:947–54.
156. Inaba Y, Chen JA, Bergmann SR. Quantity of viable myocardium required to improve survival with revascularization in patients with ischemic cardiomyopathy: a meta-analysis. J Nucl Cardiol. 2010;17:646–54.
157. Bourque JM, Hasselblad V, Velazquez EJ, Borges-Neto S, O'Connor CM. Revascularization in patients with coronary artery disease, left ventricular dysfunction, and viability: a meta-analysis. 2003;146:621–Am Heart J, 627.
158. Beanlands RS, Nichol G, Huszti E, Humen D, Racine N, Freeman M, Gulenchyn KY, Garrard L, deKemp R, Guo A, Ruddy TD, Benard F, Lamy A, Iwanochko RM, PARR-2 Investigators. F-18-fluorodeoxyglucose positron emission tomography imaging-assisted management of patients with severe left ventricular dysfunction and suspected coronary disease: a randomized, controlled trial (PARR-2). J Am Coll Cardiol. 2007;50:2002–12.
159. Abraham A, Nichol G, Williams KA, Guo A, deKemp RA, Garrard L, Davies RA, Duchesne L, Haddad H, Chow B, DaSilva J, Beanlands RS, PARR-2 Investigators. 18F-FDG PET imaging of myocardial viability in an experienced center with access to 18F-FDG and integration with clinical management teams: the Ottawa-FIVE substudy of the PARR 2 trial. J Nucl Med. 2010;51:567–74.
160. Bonow RO, Maurer G, Lee KL, Holly TA, Binkley PF, Desvigne-Nickens P, Drozdz J, Farsky PS, Feldman AM, Doenst T, Michler RE, Berman DS, Nicolau JC, Pellikka PA, Wrobel K, Alotti N, Asch FM, Favaloro LE, She L, Velazquez EJ, Jones RH, Panza JA, Investigators ST. Myocardial viability and survival in ischemic left ventricular dysfunction. N Engl J Med. 2011;364:1617–25.
161. Cleland JG, Pennell DJ, Ray SG, Coats AJ, Macfarlane PW, Murray GD, Mule JD, Vered Z, Lahiri A, Carvedilol hibernating reversible ischaemia trial: marker of success investigators. Myocardial viability as a determinant of the ejection fraction response to carvedilol in patients with heart failure (CHRISTMAS trial): randomised controlled trial. Lancet. 2003;362:14–21.
162. Udelson JE, Pearte CA, Kimmelstiel CD, Kruk M, Kufera JA, Forman SA, Teresinska A, Bychowiec B, Marin-Neto JA, Hochtl T, Cohen EA, Caramori P, Busz-Papiez B, Adlbrecht C, Sadowski ZP, Ruzyllo W, Kinan DJ, Lamas GA, Hochman JS. The Occluded Artery Trial (OAT) Viability Ancillary Study (OAT-NUC): influence of infarct zone viability on left ventricular remodeling after percutaneous coronary intervention versus optimal medical therapy alone. Am Heart J. 2011;161:611–21.
163. Cleland JG, Calvert M, Freemantle N, Arrow Y, Ball SG, Bonser RS, Chattopadhyay S, Norell MS, Pennell DJ, Senior R. The Heart Failure Revascularisation Trial (HEART). Eur J Heart Fail. 2011;13:227–33.
164. D'Egidio G, Nichol G, Williams KA, Guo A, Garrard L, deKemp R, Ruddy TD, DaSilva J, Humen D, Gulenchyn KY, Freeman M, Racine N, Benard F, Hendry P, Beanlands RS, PARR-2 Investigators. Increasing benefit from revascularization is associated with increasing amounts of myocardial hibernation: a substudy of the PARR-2 trial. JACC Cardiovasc Imaging. 2009;2:1060–8.
165. Di Carli M, Sherman T, Khanna S, Davidson M, Rokhsar S, Hawkins R, Phelps M, Schelbert H, Maddahi J. Myocardial viability in asynergic regions subtended by occluded coronary arteries: relation to the status of collateral flow in patients with chronic coronary artery disease. J Am Coll Cardiol. 1994;23:860–8.
166. Di Carli MF, Asgarzadie F, Schelbert HR, Brunken RC, Rokhsar S, Maddahi J. Relation of myocardial perfusion at rest and during pharmacologic stress to the PET patterns of tissue viability in patients with severe left ventricular dysfunction. J Nucl Cardiol. 1998;5:558–66.
167. Lee HH, Davila-Roman VG, Ludbrook PA, Courtois M, Walsh JF, Delano DA, Rubin PJ, Gropler RJ. Dependency of contractile reserve on myocardial blood flow: implications for the assessment of myocardial viability with dobutamine stress echocardiography. Circulation. 1997;96:2884–91.
168. Bonow RO, Castelvecchio S, Panza JA, Berman DS, Velazquez EJ, Michler RE, She L, Holly TA, Desvigne-Nickens P, Kosevic D, Rajda M, Chrzanowski L, Deja M, Lee KL, White H, Oh

JK, Doenst T, Hill JA, Rouleau JL, Menicanti L, Investigators ST. Severity of remodeling, myocardial viability, and survival in ischemic LV dysfunction after surgical revascularization. JACC Cardiovasc Imaging. 2015;8:1121–9.
169. Carson P, Wertheimer J, Miller A, O'Connor CM, Pina IL, Selzman C, Sueta C, She L, Greene D, Lee KL, Jones RH, Velazquez EJ, Investigators S. The STICH trial (Surgical Treatment for Ischemic Heart Failure): mode-of-death results. JACC Heart Fail. 2013;1:400–8.
170. Bonow RO, Holly TA. Myocardial viability testing: still viable after stich? J Nucl Cardiol. 2011;18:991–4.
171. Perrone-Filardi P, Pinto FJ. Looking for myocardial viability after a STICH trial: not enough to close the door. J Nucl Med. 2012;53:349–52.
172. Shah BN, Khattar RS, Senior R. The hibernating myocardium: current concepts, diagnostic dilemmas, and clinical challenges in the post-STICH era. Eur Heart J. 2013;34:1323–36.
173. Panza JA, Ellis AM, Al-Khalidi HR, Holly TA, Berman DS, Oh JK, Pohost GM, Sopko G, Chrzanowski L, Mark DB, Kukulski T, Favaloro LE, Maurer G, Farsky PS, Tan RS, Asch FM, Velazquez EJ, Rouleau JL, Lee KL, Bonow RO. Myocardial viability and long-term outcomes in ischemic cardiomyopathy. N Engl J Med. 2019;381:739–48.
174. Petrie MC, Jhund PS, She L, Adlbrecht C, Doenst T, Panza JA, Hill JA, Lee KL, Rouleau JL, Prior DL, Ali IS, Maddury J, Golba KS, White HD, Carson P, Chrzanowski L, Romanov A, Miller AB, Velazquez EJ, STICH Trial Investigators. Ten-year outcomes after coronary artery bypass grafting according to age in patients with heart failure and left ventricular systolic dysfunction: an analysis of the extended follow-up of the STICH trial (Surgical Treatment for Ischemic Heart Failure). Circulation. 2016;134:1314–24.
175. Wu WY, Biery DW, Singh A, Divakaran S, Berman AN, Ayuba G, DeFilippis EM, Nasir K, Januzzi JL, Di Carli MF, Bhatt DL, Blankstein R. Recovery of left ventricular systolic function and clinical outcomes in young adults with myocardial infarction. J Am Coll Cardiol. 2020;75:2804–15.
176. Sicari R, Nihoyannopoulos P, Evangelista A, Kasprzak J, Lancellotti P, Poldermans D, Voigt JU, Zamorano JL, European Association of Echocardiography. Stress echocardiography expert consensus statement—executive summary: European Association of Echocardiography (EAE) (a registered branch of the ESC). Eur Heart J. 2009;30:278–89.
177. Lepper W, Belcik T, Wei K, Lindner JR, Sklenar J, Kaul S. Myocardial contrast echocardiography. Circulation. 2004;109:3132–5.
178. Ito H, Iwakura K, Oh H, Masuyama T, Hori M, Higashino Y, Fujii K, Minamino T. Temporal changes in myocardial perfusion patterns in patients with reperfused anterior wall myocardial infarction. Their relation to myocardial viability. Circulation. 1995;91:656–62.
179. Ragosta M, Camarano G, Kaul S, Powers ER, Sarembock IJ, Gimple LW. Microvascular integrity indicates myocellular viability in patients with recent myocardial infarction. New insights using myocardial contrast echocardiography. Circulation. 1994;89:2562–9.
180. Bansal M, Jeffriess L, Leano R, Mundy J, Marwick TH. Assessment of myocardial viability at dobutamine echocardiography by deformation analysis using tissue velocity and speckle-tracking. JACC Cardiovasc Imaging. 2010;3:121–31.
181. Ran H, Zhang PY, Zhang YX, Zhang JX, Wu WF, Dong J, Ma XW. Assessment of left ventricular myocardial viability by 3-dimensional speckle-tracking echocardiography in patients with myocardial infarction. J Ultrasound Med. 2016;35:1631–8.
182. Kiat H, Berman DS. Clinical radionuclide imaging of myocardial viability. Curr Opin Radiol. 1989;1:435–9.
183. Dilsizian V, Rocco TP, Freedman NM, Leon MB, Bonow RO. Enhanced detection of ischemic but viable myocardium by the reinjection of thallium after stress-redistribution imaging. N Engl J Med. 1990;323:141–6.
184. Inglese E, Brambilla M, Dondi M, Pieri P, Bisi G, Sara R, Cannizzaro G, Cappagli M, Giordano A, Moscatelli G, et al. Assessment of myocardial viability after thallium-201 reinjection or rest-redistribution imaging: a multicenter study. The Italian Group of Nuclear Cardiology. J Nucl Med. 1995;36:555–63.
185. Ohtani H, Tamaki N, Yonekura Y, Mohiuddin IH, Hirata K, Ban T, Konishi J. Value of thallium-201 reinjection after delayed SPECT imaging for predicting reversible ischemia after coronary artery bypass grafting. Am J Cardiol. 1990;66:394–9.
186. Gibson RS, Watson DD, Taylor GJ, Crosby IK, Wellons HL, Holt ND, Beller GA. Prospective assessment of regional myocardial perfusion before and after coronary revascularization surgery by quantitative thallium-201 scintigraphy. J Am Coll Cardiol. 1983;1:804–15.
187. Pohost GM, Zir LM, Moore RH, McKusick KA, Guiney TE, Beller GA. Differentiation of transiently ischemic from infarcted myocardium by serial imaging after a single dose of thallium-201. Circulation. 1977;55:294–302.
188. Rozanski A, Berman DS, Gray R, Levy R, Raymond M, Maddahi J, Pantaleo N, Waxman AD, Swan HJ, Matloff J. Use of thallium-201 redistribution scintigraphy in the preoperative differentiation of reversible and nonreversible myocardial asynergy. Circulation. 1981;64:936–44.
189. Einstein AJ, Pascual TN, Mercuri M, Karthikeyan G, Vitola JV, Mahmarian JJ, Better N, Bouyoucef SE, Hee-Seung Bom H, Lele V, Magboo VP, Alexanderson E, Allam AH, Al-Mallah MH, Flotats A, Jerome S, Kaufmann PA, Luxenburg O, Shaw

LJ, Underwood SR, Rehani MM, Kashyap R, Paez D, Dondi M, INCAPS Investigators Group. Current worldwide nuclear cardiology practices and radiation exposure: results from the 65 country IAEA Nuclear Cardiology Protocols Cross-Sectional Study (INCAPS). Eur Heart J. 2015;36:1689–96.
190. Marzullo P, Sambuceti G, Parodi O. The role of sestamibi scintigraphy in the radioisotopic assessment of myocardial viability. J Nucl Med. 1992;33:1925–30.
191. Udelson JE. Can technetium 99m-labeled sestamibi track myocardial viability? J Nucl Cardiol. 1994;1:571–5.
192. Maurea S, Cuocolo A, Soricelli A, Castelli L, Squame F, Imbriaco M, De Luca N, Trimarco B, Salvatore M. Myocardial viability index in chronic coronary artery disease: technetium-99m-methoxy isobutyl isonitrile redistribution. J Nucl Med. 1995;36:1953–60.
193. Chua T, Kiat H, Germano G, Maurer G, van Train K, Friedman J, Berman D. Gated technetium-99m sestamibi for simultaneous assessment of stress myocardial perfusion, postexercise regional ventricular function and myocardial viability. Correlation with echocardiography and rest thallium-201 scintigraphy. J Am Coll Cardiol. 1994;23:1107–14.
194. Dilsizian V, Arrighi JA, Diodati JG, Quyyumi AA, Alavi K, Bacharach SL, Marin-Neto JA, Katsiyiannis PT, Bonow RO. Myocardial viability in patients with chronic coronary artery disease. Comparison of 99mTc-sestamibi with thallium reinjection and [18F]fluorodeoxyglucose. Circulation. 1994;89:578–87.
195. Everaert H, Vanhove C, Franken PR. Assessment of perfusion, function, and myocardial metabolism after infarction with a combination of low-dose dobutamine tetrofosmin gated SPECT perfusion scintigraphy and BMIPP SPECT imaging. J Nucl Cardiol. 2000;7:29–36.
196. Leoncini M, Marcucci G, Sciagra R, Frascarelli F, Traini AM, Mondanelli D, Magni M, Bini L, Bellandi F, Mennuti A, Dabizzi RP. Nitrate-enhanced gated technetium 99m sestamibi SPECT for evaluating regional wall motion at baseline and during low-dose dobutamine infusion in patients with chronic coronary artery disease and left ventricular dysfunction: comparison with two-dimensional echocardiography. J Nucl Cardiol. 2000;7:426–31.
197. Yamagishi H, Akioka K, Hirata K, Sakanoue Y, Toda I, Yoshiyama M, Teragaki M, Takeuchi K, Yoshikawa J, Ochi H. Dobutamine stress electrocardiography-gated Tc-99m tetrofosmin SPECT for detection of viable but dysfunctional myocardium. J Nucl Cardiol. 2001;8:58–67.
198. Knapp FF Jr, Franken P, Kropp J. Cardiac SPECT with iodine-123-labeled fatty acids: evaluation of myocardial viability with BMIPP. J Nucl Med. 1995;36:1022–30.
199. Dobbeleir AA, Hambye AS, Franken PR. Influence of methodology on the presence and extent of mismatching between 99mTc-MIBI and 123I-BMIPP in myocardial viability studies. J Nucl Med. 1999;40:707–14.
200. Katsunuma E, Kurokawa S, Takahashi M, Fukuda N, Kurosawa T, Izumi T. Usefulness of BMIPP SPECT to evaluate myocardial viability, contractile reserve and coronary stenotic progression after reperfusion in acute myocardial infarction. Jpn Heart J. 2001;42:435–49.
201. Mielniczuk LM, Toth GG, Xie JX, De Bruyne B, Shaw LJ, Beanlands RS. Can functional testing for ischemia and viability guide revascularization? JACC Cardiovasc Imaging. 2017;10:354–64.
202. Burt RW, Perkins OW, Oppenheim BE, Schauwecker DS, Stein L, Wellman HN, Witt RM. Direct comparison of fluorine-18-FDG SPECT, fluorine-18-FDG PET and rest thallium-201 SPECT for detection of myocardial viability. J Nucl Med. 1995;36:176–9.
203. Chen EQ, MacIntyre WJ, Go RT, Brunken RC, Saha GB, Wong CY, Neumann DR, Cook SA, Khandekar SP. Myocardial viability studies using fluorine-18-FDG SPECT: a comparison with fluorine-18-FDG PET. J Nucl Med. 1997;38:582–6.
204. Landoni C, Lucignani G, Paolini G, Zuccari M, Galli L, Di Credico G, Rossetti C, Pelenghi S, Gilardi MC, Fazio F, Grossi A. Assessment of CABG-related risk in patients with CAD and LVD. Contribution of PET with [18F]FDG to the assessment of myocardial viability. J Cardiovasc Surg (Torino). 1999;40:363–72.
205. Lauerma K, Niemi P, Hanninen H, Janatuinen T, Voipio-Pulkki LM, Knuuti J, Toivonen L, Makela T, Makijarvi MA, Aronen HJ. Multimodality MR imaging assessment of myocardial viability: combination of first-pass and late contrast enhancement to wall motion dynamics and comparison with FDG PET-initial experience. Radiology. 2000;217:729–36.
206. Thorley PJ, Beacock DJ, Trickett CA, Sivananthan UM. 18FDG SPECT to assess myocardial viability: initial experience at a hospital remote from a cyclotron. Nucl Med Commun. 2000;21:715–8.
207. Kuhl HP, van de Weert AP, Beek AM, Visser FC, van Rossum AC. Myocardial viability by contrast enhanced MRI in a patient with left bundle branch block showing a severe defect on FDG-PET. Heart. 2002;87:319.
208. Beanlands R, Nichol G, Ruddy TD, deKemp RA, Hendry P, Humen D, Racine N, Ross H, Benard F, Coates G, Iwanochko RM, Fallen E, Wells G, PARR-2 Investigators. Evaluation of outcome and cost-effectiveness using an FDG PET-guided approach to management of patients with coronary disease and severe left ventricular dysfunction (PARR-2): rationale, design, and methods. Control Clin Trials. 2003;24:776–94.
209. Schinkel AF, Bax JJ, Valkema R, Elhendy A, van Domburg RT, Vourvouri EC, Bountioukos MA, Krenning EP, Roelandt JR, Poldermans D. Effect of diabetes mellitus on myocardial 18F-FDG SPECT using acipimox for the assessment of myocardial viability. J Nucl Med. 2003;44:877–83.

210. Maddahi J. Factors influencing predictive value of FDG imaging for evaluating myocardial viability. J Nucl Cardiol. 2004;11:524–6.
211. Karamitsos TD, Francis JM, Myerson S, Selvanayagam JB, Neubauer S. The role of cardiovascular magnetic resonance imaging in heart failure. J Am Coll Cardiol. 2009;54:1407–24.
212. Charoenpanichkit C, Hundley WG. The 20 year evolution of dobutamine stress cardiovascular magnetic resonance. J Cardiovasc Magn Reson. 2010;12:59.
213. Ichikawa Y, Sakuma H, Suzawa N, Kitagawa K, Makino K, Hirano T, Takeda K. Late gadolinium-enhanced magnetic resonance imaging in acute and chronic myocardial infarction. Improved prediction of regional myocardial contraction in the chronic state by measuring thickness of nonenhanced myocardium. J Am Coll Cardiol. 2005;45:901–9.
214. Bondarenko O, Beek AM, Hofman MB, Kuhl HP, Twisk JW, van Dockum WG, Visser CA, van Rossum AC. Standardizing the definition of hyperenhancement in the quantitative assessment of infarct size and myocardial viability using delayed contrast-enhanced CMR. J Cardiovasc Magn Reson. 2005;7:481–5.
215. Arai AE. The cardiac magnetic resonance (CMR) approach to assessing myocardial viability. J Nucl Cardiol. 2011;18:1095–102.
216. Ryf S, Rutz AK, Boesiger P, Schwitter J. Is post-systolic shortening a reliable indicator of myocardial viability? An MR tagging and late-enhancement study. J Cardiovasc Magn Reson. 2006;8:445–51.
217. Cupps BP, Bree DR, Wollmuth JR, Howells AC, Voeller RK, Rogers JG, Pasque MK. Myocardial viability mapping by magnetic resonance-based multiparametric systolic strain analysis. Ann Thorac Surg. 2008;86:1546–53.
218. Garot P, Pascal O, Simon M, Monin JL, Teiger E, Garot J, Gueret P, Dubois-Rande JL. Impact of microvascular integrity and local viability on left ventricular remodelling after reperfused acute myocardial infarction. Heart. 2003;89:393–7.
219. Sasaki T, Hansford R, Zviman MM, Kolandaivelu A, Bluemke DA, Berger RD, Calkins H, Halperin HR, Nazarian S. Quantitative assessment of artifacts on cardiac magnetic resonance imaging of patients with pacemakers and implantable cardioverter-defibrillators. Circ Cardiovasc Imaging. 2011;4:662–70.

10 Hybrid Cardiac Imaging in Clinical Practice: From Diagnosis to Prognosis and Management

Cigdem Akincioglu and Saurabh Malhotra

Cardiovascular diseases remain the leading cause of morbidity and mortality worldwide. While coronary artery disease (CAD) continues to pose the greatest healthcare burden among cardiovascular diseases, infiltrative cardiomyopathies, such as sarcoidosis and amyloidosis, are being recognized with greater frequency due to the increasing awareness and robust imaging tools for accurate diagnosis. Finally, among those with heart failure (HF), implantable cardiac devices improve survival from HF and arrhythmias, as circulatory support devices provide a bridge to transplant. These implanted artificial devices, along with prosthetic valves are at a high-risk of infections which can be life-threatening. Advances in cardiovascular imaging have allowed for the availability of complimentary imaging modalities to be applied in a hybrid fashion for accurate diagnosis, prognosis, and management of patients with various cardiovascular conditions.

C. Akincioglu
Division of Nuclear Medicine, Department of Medical Imaging, University of Western Ontario, London, ON, Canada
e-mail: Cigdem.Akincioglu@lhsc.on.ca

S. Malhotra (✉)
Division of Cardiology, Cook County Health, Chicago, IL, USA

Division of Cardiology, Rush Medical College, Chicago, IL, USA
e-mail: saurabh.malhotra@cookcountyhhs.org

10.1 Hybrid Imaging for Coronary Artery Disease

Advances in cardiovascular imaging have allowed for the determination of myocardial ischemia and myocardial blood flow via perfusion imaging, and the determination of coronary stenosis with high spatial resolution using cardiac computed tomography angiography (CCTA). Individually each of these anatomic [1] and physiologic alterations [2, 3] from CAD have an established prognostic value, based on decades of observational and randomized trial data. Technological advances in camera technology have allowed for the fusion of these techniques via hybrid SPECT/CT and PET/CT systems. While initial systems with low resolution hybrid CT technology were only used for attenuation correction, more recent cameras with up to 64-slice CT technology allow for additional diagnostic cardiac imaging. Hybrid SPECT/CT and PET/CT technology allow for functional and anatomical imaging to complement each other and have paved the way for improved diagnostics for CAD with incremental prognostic guidance.

A meta-analysis of 20 studies compared stress-induced ischemia on SPECT or PET myocardial perfusion imaging (MPI) to the presence of coronary artery calcium score (CACS) [4]. MPI and CACS data from a total of 2123 patients were evaluated in this meta-analysis. Interestingly, in this analysis ischemia on MPI increased with

F. Nudi et al. (eds.), *Hybrid Cardiac Imaging for Clinical Decision-Making*,
https://doi.org/10.1007/978-3-030-99391-7_10

increasing CACS burden, which was also present in 6.6% of patients with CACS of 0 and increased to 8.5%, 10.5%, and 23.6%, among those with CACS between 1–100, 101–399, and >400, respectively. Although the prevalence of ischemia on MPI increased with increasing burden of CACS, there was a wide range of the severity of ischemia across CACS categories, with prognostically significant ischemia (>10% ischemic myocardium) being present in all CACS categories. While the image acquisition was not always performed on a hybrid system, this analysis suggests the ability of hybrid functional and anatomic data to diagnose the presence of ischemia and even possibly prognosticate across a distribution of CACS. Similarly, Chang et al. studied the complimentary role of perfusion defects on SPECT myocardial perfusion MPI and CACS, in a hybrid manner by acquiring MPI and CACS data from two different examinations [5]. They retrospectively reviewed clinical, MPI and CACS data on 1126 patients without prior CAD who underwent both electron beam computed tomography (EBCT) and SPECT MPI on two separate occasions, within an average of 2 months of each other. Analysis of the SPECT and CACS data in this study showed that the prevalence of an abnormal SPECT increased with increasing CACS. Among those with a CACS < 100 prevalence of an abnormal SPECT was <2%, and increased to 9.8% and 31% among those with CACS between 101–400 and >400, respectively ($p < 0.001$) (Fig. 10.1). Even when an abnormal SPECT was present, prognostically significant ischemia (>10% ischemic myocardium) was not noted in patients with a CACS < 100, while it was present in 1.7% and 8.9% of patients with CACS between 101–400 and >400, respectively ($p < 0.001$). The authors also studied the occurrence of all-cause mortality or myocardial infarction in relation to MPI defect and CACS severity. With the increasing CACS burden, there was an increase in the annualized event rate from <1% among those with CACS <100, to 1.25% and 2.05% among those with CACS between 101–400 and >400, respectively. However, the presence of an abnormal SPECT MPI among those with CACS >100 predicted a greater event rate of

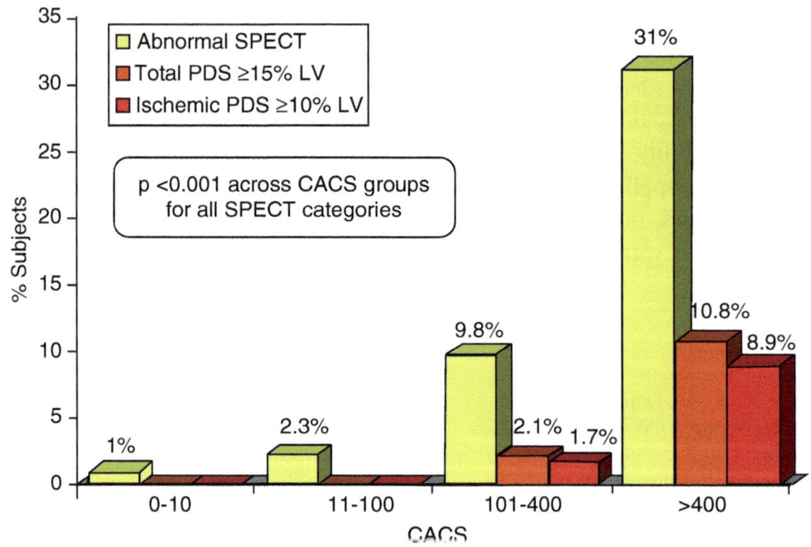

Fig. 10.1 Distribution of Abnormality on SPECT Myocardial Perfusion Imaging Across Increasing Burden of Coronary Artery Calcium Score ($n = 1126$). *PDS* perfusion defect score, *CACS* coronary artery calcium score, *LV* left ventricle. (Reproduced with permission from, Chang et al., The Coronary Artery Calcium Score and Stress Myocardial Perfusion Imaging Provide Independent and Complementary Prediction of Cardiac. Risk J Am Coll Cardiol 2009;54:1872–82)

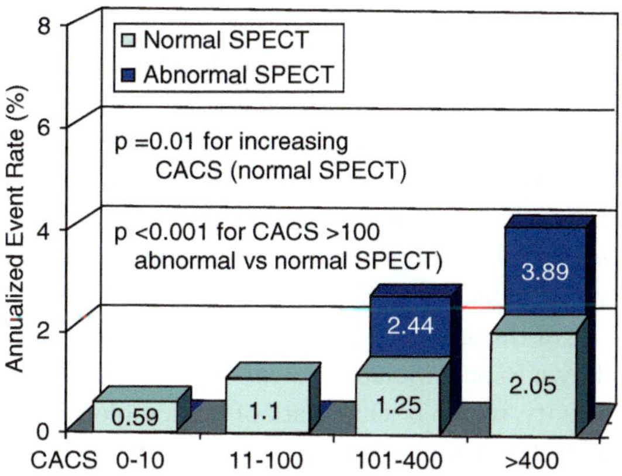

Fig. 10.2 Annualized Rates of All-Cause Mortality and Myocardial Infarction Stratified by Coronary Artery Calcium Burden and Abnormality on SPECT Myocardial Perfusion Imaging ($n = 1126$). *CACS* coronary artery calcium score. (Reproduced with permission from, Chang et al., The Coronary Artery Calcium Score and Stress Myocardial Perfusion Imaging Provide Independent and Complementary Prediction of Cardiac. Risk J Am Coll Cardiol 2009;54:1872–82)

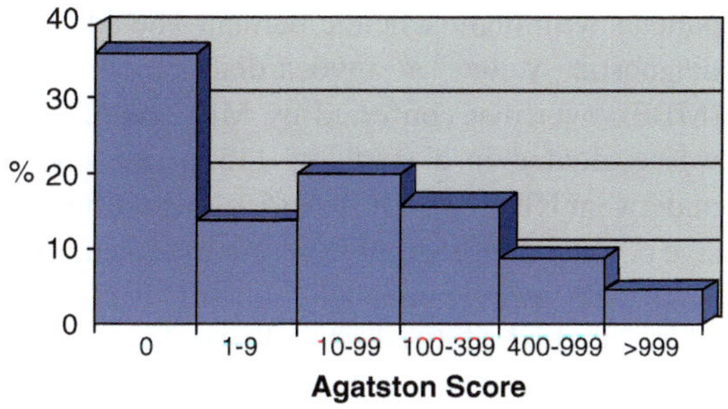

Fig. 10.3 Prevalence of Coronary Artery Calcium Burden Among Patients with Normal PET Myocardial Perfusion Imaging ($n = 760$). (Reproduced with permission from, Bybee et al., Diagnostic and clinical benefit of combined coronary calcium and perfusion assessment in patients undergoing PET/CT myocardial perfusion stress imaging. J Nucl Cardiol 2010;17:188–96)

2.44% and 3.89% among those with CACS between 101–400 and those with CACS > 400, respectively (Fig. 10.2). This study highlights that abnormal myocardial perfusion and CACS are not only complimentary in their ability to diagnose disease presence and severity, but also in their ability to predict clinically significant outcomes. While two separate studies were performed to determine myocardial perfusion and CACS, implementation of hybrid SPECT/CT in practice will allow for simultaneous assessment of perfusion and CACS data and provide incremental diagnostic and prognostic values, above that provided by each of them individually.

The value of simultaneous assessment of functional and anatomic components of CAD utilizing hybrid PET/CT was reported by Bybee and colleagues [6]. The authors studied the complimentary diagnostic and therapeutic value of coronary artery calcium score (CACS) among patients without known CAD [6]. In this retrospective observational study, hybrid imaging data from 760 consecutive patients with a normal Rubidium (Rb)-82 PET/CT perfusion study was evaluated for the presence of CAD defined by CACS. Despite normal relative perfusion on Rb-82 PET/CT, 64% of the patients were noted to have CACS thus identifying CAD in a substantial proportion of patients which would have been otherwise missed if only perfusion data was relied upon (Fig. 10.3). Additionally, among those with CACS, there was a greater likelihood of optimization of medical therapy when compared to those without CACS (53% vs. 34%, $p < 0.001$), with a sequential increase in medical therapy optimization with increasing CAC burden. A recent study employing hybrid PET/CT further evaluated the value of hybrid imaging in the determination of risk for revascularization [7]. Of the 5528 patients who underwent Rb-82 PET/CT, CAC was present in 2510 (45.4%) patients. Those with CAC were significantly more likely to have severe CAD, more likely to undergo invasive coronary angiography, and more likely to receive revascularization when compared to those without CAC. Even among those with a prognostically significant ischemic burden of >10%, those without CAC had a lower risk of revascularization (adjusted OR = 0.14; 95% CI, 0.06–0.31, $p < 0.0001$), when compared to those with any CAC burden. This study highlights that CAC assessment from low dose attenuation-correction CT performed during PET MPI aids in the identification of severe CAD and those who are more likely to undergo revascularization. This prognostic value of CAC obtained during hybrid imaging is preserved even among patients with high ischemic burden. The additive diagnostic value of myocardial blood flow (MBF), over that conferred by MPI and CACS, was evaluated in a study of 113 patients who underwent RB-82 PET/CT MPI, along with invasive coronary angiography [8]. As expected, vessels with angiographically obstructive CAD ($n = 71$) had higher ischemic total perfusion defect (ITPD; 4.6 ± 6.2 vs. 0.6 ± 1.3), lower hyperemic MBF (1.01 ± 0.5 vs. 1.75 ± 0.6 mL/min/g), and coronary flow reserve (CFR; 1.56 ± 0.6 vs. 2.38 ± 0.7; all $p < 0.001$) than those without. However, prediction of per-vessel CAD was superior when MBF and CFR were incrementally added to models predicting the accuracy for anatomical CAD: area under the curve for (a) model including CAC/ITPD/hyperemic MBF = 0.87, (b) CAC/ITPD/CFR = 0.88, and (c) for the model including CAC/ITPD = 0.79; all $p < 0.001$. Thus, MBF and CFR, which are now routinely assessed on hybrid PET/CT perfusion imaging, provide incremental diagnostic value to that conferred by relative perfusion data and CACS. This underscores the multitude of advantages offered by advancements in hybrid imaging, all of which are now available in routine clinical practice.

10.2 Hybrid Imaging of Vulnerable Atherosclerotic Lesions

In routine clinical practice, the major focus is often on anatomic or physiologic assessment of atherosclerosis—such as in CAD. However, it is well known that high-risk plaque features predispose to plaque rupture that is responsible for acute cardiovascular events—such as myocardial infarction and cerebrovascular accidents (CVA). Though patients perceived to be at high clinical risk are recommended to be treated aggressively with medical therapy, imaging of vulnerable atherosclerotic lesions can further facilitate early aggressive medical therapy, intensification of medical therapy and may also allow for prognostication from cardiovascular outcomes. In this regard, a modality with the high spatial and temporal resolution is required for anatomical localization of these small, focal lesions, but also requires an ability to determine the plaque biology and disease process. Hybrid imaging with the utilization of computed tomography (CT) or magnetic resonance (MR) in conjunction with advanced radiotracers is at the forefront of imaging of vulnerable plaques.

18F-fluorodeoxyglucose (FDG) has been shown to accumulate in areas with inflammatory activity, which is a hallmark of vulnerable atherosclerotic plaques. Among patients with vasculitis, there is evidence of FDG uptake in large arteries and also in the arteries of patients with malignancies. Such vascular uptake of FDG has been shown to be related to cardiovascular risk factors, such as age, hypercholesterolemia, and hypertension. These seminal findings have fueled the investigations of the use of FDG PET for the identification of vulnerable plaques. In an early study of 50 patients undergoing FDG PET/CT following a cerebrovascular accident (CVA), there was a significantly greater FDG uptake in ipsilateral carotid arteries when compared to the contralateral side among those patients imaged early after the CVA [9]. Recurrent strokes have also been shown to be associated with carotid plaque inflammation which was evaluated in 109 patients with carotid stenosis and recent CVA in the Biomarkers/Imaging Vulnerable Atherosclerosis in Symptomatic Carotid disease (BIOVASC) study. Plaque FDG maximum standardized uptake value (SUV_{max}) was greater among patients with recurrent strokes, and the risk of recurrent strokes increased across increasing quartiles of SUV_{max}, which predicted the occurrence of recurrent stroke with modest accuracy (area under the curve; AUC = 0.70). In addition to the ability to image vulnerable plaques, assessment of arterial inflammation with hybrid FDG PET/CT allows to quantify the effect of medical therapy on plaque inflammatory activity. Among 67 patients with risk factors for or established atherosclerosis, FDG PET/CT was performed at baseline and after randomization to either 10 mg or 80 mg of atorvastatin [10]. When compared to baseline, those on 80 mg of atorvastatin showed a significant reduction in arterial

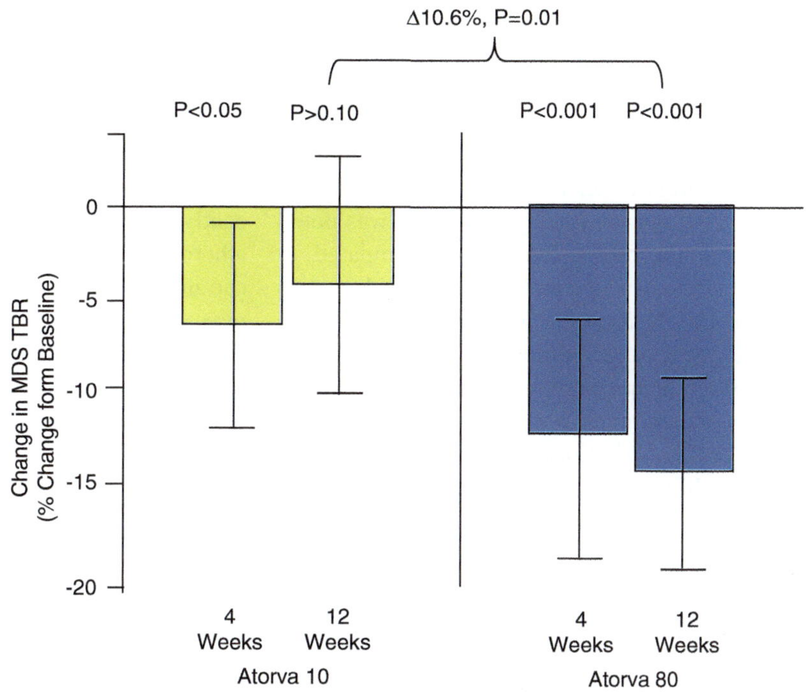

Fig. 10.4 Change in Arterial Inflammation on ^{18}F-FDG PET/CT Among Patients Receiving Atorvastatin. *MDS TBR* most diseased segment target-to-background ratio, *Atorva* atorvastatin. (Reproduced with permission from, Tawakol et al., Intensification of Statin Therapy Results in a Rapid Reduction in Atherosclerotic Inflammation: Results of a Multicenter Fluorodeoxyglucose-Positron Emission Tomography/Computed Tomography Feasibility Study. J Am Coll Cardiol. 2013;62(10): 909–17)

inflammation at 12 weeks, as measured by target-to-background ratio (TBR) (average of 14% reduction) (Fig. 10.4). This degree of reduction in inflammation was not noted among those on 10 mg of atorvastatin. Among patients with known atherosclerosis, but no clinical events (subclinical disease), arterial inflammation was studied in the carotid, aortic and iliofemoral vessels with hybrid FDG PET/MRI [11]. Among 755 individuals imaged (age range 40–54 years), arterial inflammation was present in 48.2% individuals (24.4% femorals, 19.3% aorta, 15.8% carotids, and 9.3% iliacs) and plaques in 90.1% (73.9% femorals, 55.8% iliacs, and 53.1% carotids). In these patients with subclinical disease, FDG uptake in arteries and plaques increased significantly with cardiovascular risk factors ($p < 0.01$). Arterial inflammation is highly prevalent in middle-aged individuals with known subclinical atherosclerosis. Thus, hybrid imaging with FDG PET allows for multiterritorial assessment of atherosclerosis-related subclinical arterial inflammation, identification of vulnerable plaques, and has the ability to guide medical management.

Despite the ability of hybrid FDG PET imaging for diagnosis of atherosclerosis and for assessment of its vulnerability, several disadvantages of FDG PET have been noted. A significant proportion of FDG-avid plaques may not have any calcifications on CT. Similarly, calcified atherosclerotic lesions and conversely, calcified lesions detected on CT do not avidly accumulate FDG. Concomitant FDG uptake and calcification on CT were observed in anywhere between 2 and 14% of plaques [12–14]. While this could be due to different stages of atherosclerosis, with transient arterial/plaque inflammation, it does highlight a limitation of FDG PET/CT to detect vulnerable plaques. Additionally, background FDG activity in the myocardium also obscures activity in the plaque. In this regard, ^{18}F-sodium fluoride (NaF) PET/CT may provide superior diagnostic accuracy. As opposed to FDG, NaF has negligible background activity, and is a marker of active mineralization and thus can detect active arterial osteogenic activity. In a study of 119 patients, there was a good correlation between NaF uptake and CACS ($r = 0.652$, $p < 0.001$), with an intra-class correlation coefficient of 0.99, highlighting excellent repeatability of NaF uptake measurement [12]. Additionally, NaF signal was greatest in patients with CAD risk factors, and prior cardiovascular events. In a study of 26 patients with recent transient ischemic attacks (18 awaiting endarterectomy), NaF uptake on culprit plaques was noted to be significantly greater when compared to uptake in plaques in contralateral carotid arteries ($p = 0.001$). NaF uptake is correlated with high-risk plaque features (remodeling index [$r = 0.53$, $P = 0.003$], plaque burden [$r = 0.51$, $P = 0.004$]), and predicted cardiovascular risk [$r = 0.65$, $P = 0.002$]). Additionally, NaF activity selectively highlights microcalcifications in the histopathology of excised plaques. This relationship of NaF uptake with high-risk plaques was further evaluated in a study of 32 patients who underwent NaF PET/CT and intravascular ultrasound (IVUS) [13]. NaF and IVUS of a total of 69 plaques were correlated. NaF uptake was significantly greater in fibrocalcific lesions, thin-cap atheroma with spotty calcifications, and thick-cap mixed atheroma, when compared to fibrotic plaques (Fig. 10.5). NaF uptake ratio was consistently higher in atherosclerotic lesions with severe calcification, and lesions with NaF uptake correlated with high-risk anatomical features on IVUS, such as severe plaque burden, positive remodeling, and a higher percentage of necrotic

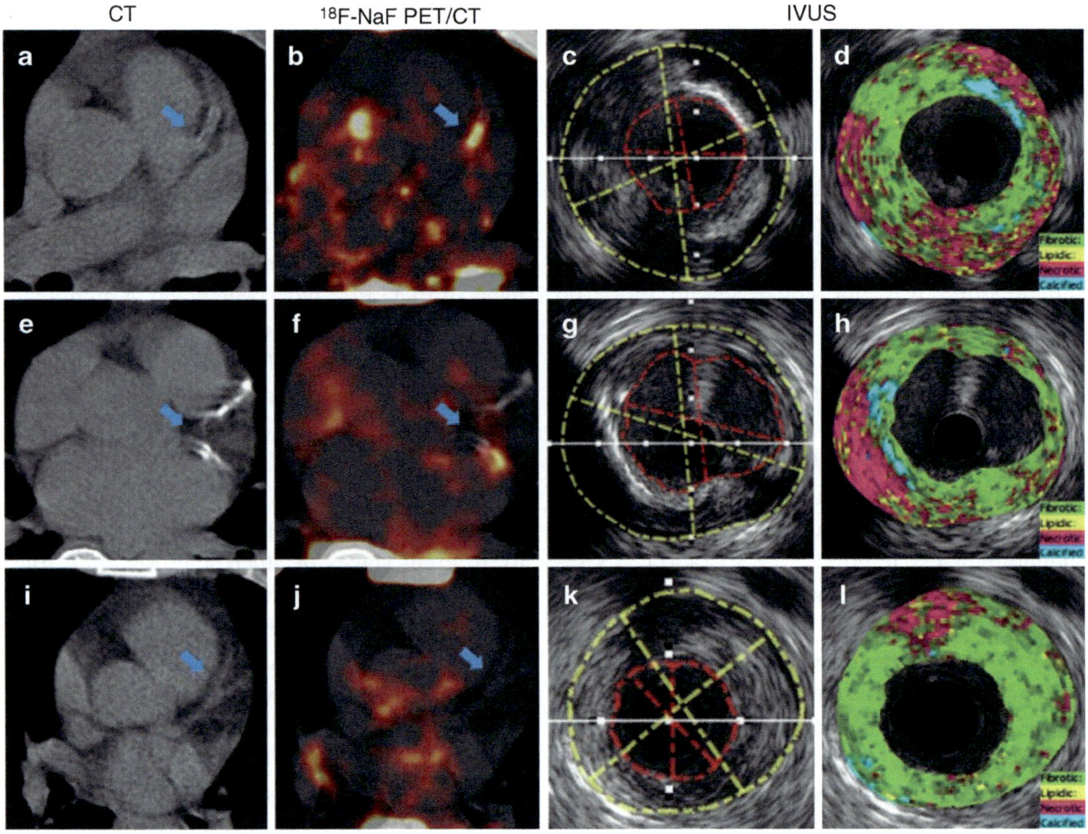

Fig. 10.5 Correlation between Plaque Characteristics on ^{18}F-NaF PET/CT and Intravascular Ultrasound. Representative images of PET/CT and IVUS from three patients with unstable angina. Increased 18F-NaF focal uptake was seen at atheromatous lesions with spotty calcification (**a**–**d**) in segments of the LAD, and thin-cap fibrocalcified lesions with a large necrotic core (**e**–**h**) in segments of the LCX. But, there was no uptake in fibrotic lesions (**i**–**l**) in segments of the LAD. (Reproduced from, Li et al., Sodium-fluoride PET-CT for the noninvasive evaluation of coronary plaques in symptomatic patients with coronary artery disease: a cross-correlation study with intravascular ultrasound. Eur J Nucl Med Mol Imaging. 2018;45(12):2181–2189)

tissue. Thus, in patients with known atherosclerosis, NaF PET/CT may assist in risk stratification and selection of patients for more intensive therapy.

10.3 Hybrid Imaging of Cardiac Infections

Cardiac infections can present with varied clinical features. The presence of multiple potential causative microorganisms, comorbidities such as known heart disease, cardiac devices, prosthetic valves, and nonspecific nature of initial symptoms all present a challenge. Early diagnosis is crucial for a favorable outcome, and cardiac imaging plays an essential role in diagnosis and management.

Duke criteria was developed based on clinical, echocardiographic, and biological findings in addition to blood cultures and serologies in the diagnosis of infective endocarditis (IE), and showed an overall sensitivity of 80% [14]. Echocardiography is part of Duke criteria and utilized as first-line in the diagnosis of IE (as per the guidelines, class I indication, level of evidence B) [15]. Sensitivity of TEE for identification of vegetations is superior to TTE (85–90% versus 75%); however, a negative echocardiography does not rule out IE and in addition, noninfected vegetations such as strands or thrombi on valvular prosthesis or leads can case false diagnosis in IE up to 15% of cases [16]. In this regard, the diagnostic accuracy of Duke criteria was lower for early diagnosis in clinical practice, particularly in the assessment of prosthetic valve endocarditis (PVE), pacemaker (PM) or defibrillator lead IE, where echocardiography was normal or inconclusive in up to 30% of cases. Radionuclide imaging of CIED infection, as well as associated IE, has been mainly been diagnosed by utilizing FDG PET/CT, or with Tc-99m HMPAO labeled white blood cell (WBC) SPECT/CT when PET/CT is not available. The 2015 European Society of Cardiology Guidelines incorporated these two hybrid imaging methods as a part of diagnostic algorithm for PVE with class 2b recommendation, evidence level C [15]. Since then, more studies are published on diagnostic value of FDG in cardiovascular implantable electronic device (CIED)-related infections.

There is a concern for disproportionate increase of CIED infections compared to the growth of newly implanted devices [17]. Since early detection is crucial for a favorable outcome, the use of hybrid imaging has been increasing with the growing evidence of its potential in particularly challenging scenarios as an adjunctive diagnostic test. CIED infections can include superficial or deep generator pocket infection, lead infection, CIED-IE where a lead and/or cardiac valve or both are involved [18]. It is crucial to differentiate between superficial skin infection and deep pocket infections as the treatment can vary from long-term antibiotics to device removal. FDG is actively incorporated by leukocytes, macrophages, and CD4 T-lymphocytes at the site of infection via glucose transporters GLUT-1 and GLUT-3, which are insulin sensitive and present in the myocardium [19, 20]. A meta-analysis of 14 studies involving 495 patients showed a pooled sensitivity of 83% and pooled specificity of 89% for FDG PET/CT in identification of the CIED infection [21]. This study also demonstrated that PET/CT had higher diagnostic accuracy in generator pocket infection than lead infection or CIED-IE. The preparatory protocols, motion correction methods were shown to significantly improve image quality and possibly diagnostic accuracy for lead infection. Sarrazin et al. evaluated the usefulness of FDG PET-CT for identification of CIED infection [22]. They compared three groups: 42 patients with suspected CIED infection, 12 patients with recent device implantation (4–8 weeks postoperatively) and no clinical signs of infection, and 12 patients with devices implanted more than 6 months and also have no signs of device infection. Using a qualitative score, FDG PET/CT had a sensitivity and specificity of 89% and 86%, respectively for the diagnosis of CIED infection. FDG PET/CT was also able to identify superficial infection versus deep generator or lead infection. Using a semiquantitative ratio (maximal uptake/normal lung parenchyma) threshold of 1.5 was useful in differentiating between CIED infection and post-operative changes. Although other studies confirmed the high accuracy of FDG PET/CT in diagnosis of skin and pocket CIED infections, additional information gained was that it had lower sensitivity (86.7% versus 30.8%) and specificity (100% versus 62.5%) for lead and cardiac involvement [23]. This study also showed that many patients with a false-negative test were already on antibiotics and that not every patient was prepared properly for normal myocardial suppression. It is recommended that all patients would have low carbohydrate-high fat diet preparation, with 12 h fast prior to FDG PET/CT study to suppress normal myocardium and improve the diagnostic accuracy [24]. Injection of 50 IU/kg iv heparin is also shown to improve image quality [25]. A review of the non-attenuation corrected images is recommended to mitigate metal artifacts from the leads and associated falsely increased FDG uptake values [26]. Saby et al. demonstrated that FDG PET/CT increased the sensitivity of PVE-IE diagnosis from 70% to 97%, when added to Duke criteria, and showed that abnormal FDG uptake could be seen prior to valvular damage on echocardiography [27]. An example of hybrid FDG PET/CT for diagnosis of infection in a left ventricular assist device is shown in Fig. 10.6.

Radiolabelled WBC scintigraphy is a valuable option, particularly with the availability of hybrid SPECT/CT imaging. Tc-99m HMPAO WBC scan can differentiate between inflammatory changes and active infection. Although there are fewer studies using Tc-99m HMPAO WBC scan for CIED infection, the results are encouraging. Erba et al. investigated the performance of Tc-99m HMPAO WBC scan with SPECT/CT in 63 patients with suspected infections associated with CIEDs [28]. Tc-99m HMPAO WBC scan showed a 94% sensitivity in both detection and localization of CIED-associated infections. Acquisition of whole body and SPECT/CT images helped not only confirmation of CIED-associated infection but also definition of the extent of device involvement and detection of associated complications. Tc-99m HMPAO WBC scan reliably excluded device-associated infection during a febrile episode and sepsis with a negative predictive value of 95%. SPECT/CT had a definite added diagnostic value over both planar and stand-alone SPECT [26–28]. In a study comparing the ability of FDG PET/CT and Tc-99m HMPAO WBC SPECT/CT to diagnose PVE in patients with inconclusive echocardiography findings, PET had higher sensitivity (93% versus 64%) but WBC scan had a higher specificity (100% versus 71%) [29]. It is suggested that WBC scan could be used in cases of equivocal PET or within an early time frame (2–8 weeks) after surgery.

Knowledge of the pitfalls of hybrid imaging for cardiac infections is important. In case of PET/CT, false-positive results can be due to post-surgical inflammation, active thrombi, tumors or metastases, and foreign body reactions such as vascular grafts as well as BioGlue surgical adhesive [30]. One common challenge for both FDG PET-CT and Tc-99m HMPAO WBC scan is the long-term use of antibiotics prior to the performance of these tests which produces falsely negative results. Although Tc99m HMPAO WBC scan with SPECT/CT systems are more available than FDG PET/CT, it should be kept in mind that the Tc99m HMPAO WBC scan involves time-consuming manipulation, separation, and labeling of leukocytes. In addition, the imaging protocol is over 24 h with the initial 3–4 h images for assessment of the blood pool and 20–24 h images for detection of specific WBC accumulation at the suspected infection sites. FDG PET/CT study can be completed as early as 90 min post radiotracer injection and there are studies suggesting delayed imaging up to 180 min with further improved sensitivity [31]. The choice of hybrid modality is dependent on the local expertise and availability of these modalities.

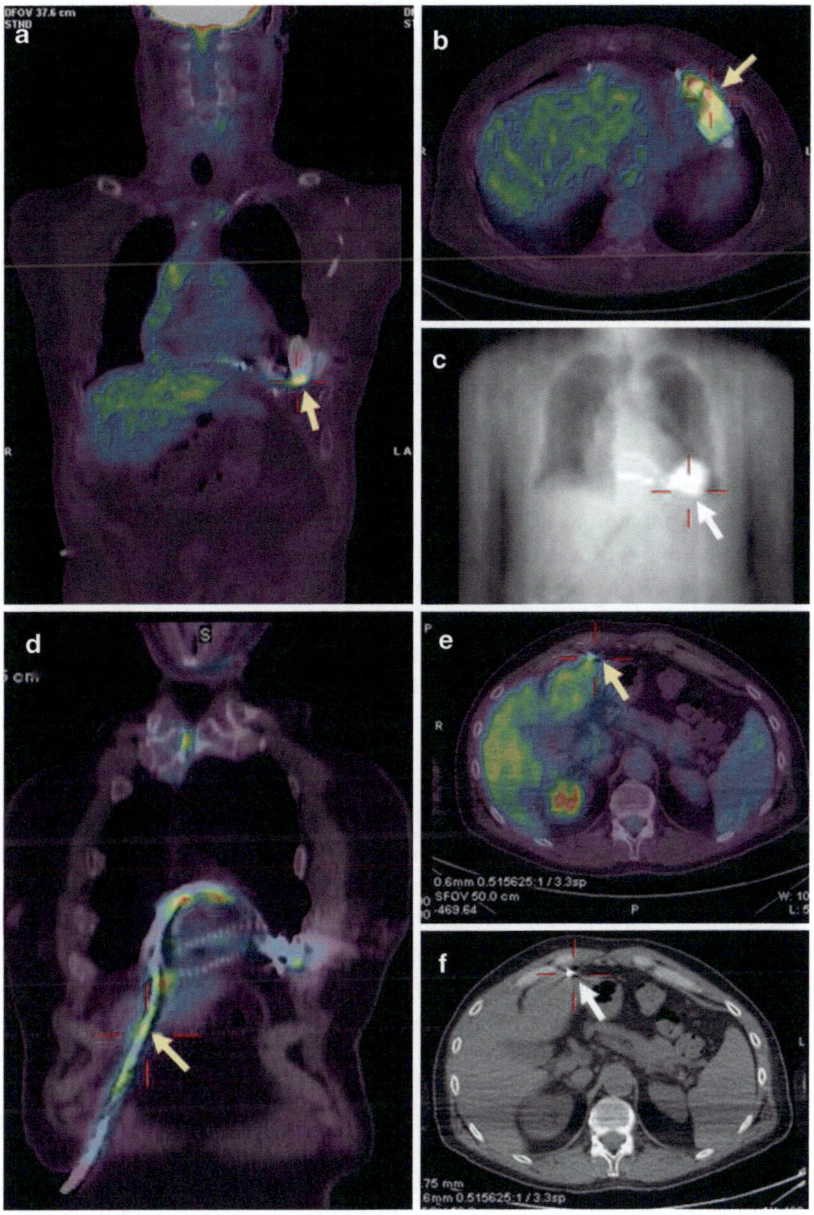

Fig. 10.6 ^{18}F-FDG PET/CT for Diagnosis of Left Ventricular Assist Device Infection. A 55-year-old male patient with heart failure and left ventricular assist device was admitted with sepsis. FDG PET/CT images depict deep pocket infection (**a**, **b**; yellow arrows), with co-registration with the CT image (**c**), and external line infection (**d**, **e**; yellow arrows), with anatomical co-registration on CT (**f**)

10.4 Hybrid Imaging for Infiltrative Cardiomyopathies

10.4.1 Cardiac Sarcoidosis

Sarcoidosis is a granulomatous disease of unknown etiology. The hypothesis of its development is to be an exaggerated immunological response with granuloma formation in various organs to an unidentified antigenic trigger [32]. Clinical manifestations of cardiac sarcoidosis (CS) depend on the location, extent, and activity of the disease. Main signs include conduction abnormalities, ventricular arrhythmias, and heart failure. It is important to determine cardiac involvement as the presence of cardiac disease is associated with significant morbidity and mortality. The only absolute test for cardiac involvement in sarcoidosis is histological examination of tissue for the presence of granulomatous inflammation and exclusion of other known causes of granuloma. However, due to the patchy involvement of the disease, the diagnostic yield of biopsy is low [33]. Over the past few decades, the nuclear imaging modality of choice for CS has evolved from planar scintigraphy and SPECT with ^{67}Gallium (^{67}Ga), to ^{18}FDG PET/CT combined with perfusion imaging to detect inflammation and fibro-granulomatous replacement of the myocardium [34, 35].

^{67}Ga-citrate is specific for inflammation but has relatively low sensitivity and poor spatial resolution compared to FDG PET/CT, especially for detecting extra-pulmonary sarcoidosis involvement. With the development of hybrid SPECT/CT systems, ^{67}Ga imaging is still considered a valuable diagnostic tool for pulmonary and extra-pulmonary sarcoidosis in centers without access to PET. In a study of 37 patients, 13 with and 24 without a diagnosis of CS, the sensitivity of ^{67}Ga without CT fusion was 77%, the specificity 54%, and the accuracy 62%. Utilization of hybrid imaging data SPECT/CT improved the specificity to 79%, and the accuracy to 76% [36]. Another study reported the value of hybrid ^{67}Ga–Tc-99m sestamibi SPECT in 14 patients with known CS, by superimposing a Ga-SPECT image on the myocardial outline traced with Tc-99m SPECT [37]. Abnormal ^{67}Ga uptake in the myocardium was observed in 9 of the 14 subjects. In seven of these nine subjects, the location of the abnormal myocardial ^{67}Ga uptake was identical to the resting perfusion defect on Tc-99m MPI, which resolved in all cases after institution of steroid therapy. Among the five subjects with no ^{67}Ga uptake, only two patients had resting perfusion defect on perfusion imaging and both had been receiving steroid therapy. These results suggest that hybrid dual ^{67}Ga-Tc-99m SPECT may improve the ability of ^{67}Ga for diagnosis of CS, which can be particularly useful among those without access to a hybrid SPECT/CT system.

FDG PET has emerged as a superior technique, as it provides improved sensitivity and spatial resolution over ^{67}Ga imaging in the assessment of both systemic sarcoidosis and its myocardial involvement [38, 39]. Overall, the sensitivity of FDG PET for systemic sarcoidosis is 80%–100% [40]. In addition, recent studies have demonstrated the importance of identifying perfusion defects in patients with cardiac sarcoidosis, as this group of patients is at the highest risk for death or ventricular arrhythmia [41, 42]. The presence of FDG alone is not specific to CS. Hibernating myocardium, myocarditis, and rheumatologic conditions with cardiac involvement also may be associated with FDG uptake [43]. Also, absence of FDG uptake does not rule out the presence of previous CS, especially if a perfusion defect is present, this could be a sign of CS without active inflammation (or a scar from another etiology). Thus, FDG PET/CT in conjunction with MPI is currently the recommended method for the evaluation of cardiac sarcoidosis in clinical practice [25].

Hybrid PET/CT has allowed for the identification of three basic patterns of FDG uptake that are typically described in patients with CS: diffuse, focal, and focal on diffuse. CS is most typically associated with focal FDG uptake either in isolation or on a background of mild diffuse uptake with or without resting perfusion defects and wall motion abnormalities [44] (Fig. 10.7). Among patients who have focal FDG uptake without a perfusion defect, co-registration with CT allows for localization of such focal uptake, which when noted along the lateral wall without a perfusion defect is often a nonspecific finding. On the other hand, the presence of multiple noncontiguous focal areas of uptake (i.e., simultaneously involving the basal anteroseptal, the basal inferior, and the basal lateral segments), is more likely to be pathologic [25]. In addition to evaluating for abnormal FDG uptake in the LV, PET/CT also allows for the identification of and localization of FDG uptake in the right ventricle, which could be associated with a worse prognosis [45]. One study reported that the presence of focal uptake within the right ventricle is associated with an extremely high event rate [42]. Some studies used quantitative metrics of SUV_{max} as well as the volume of myocardial pixels with SUV above a certain threshold, and changes in

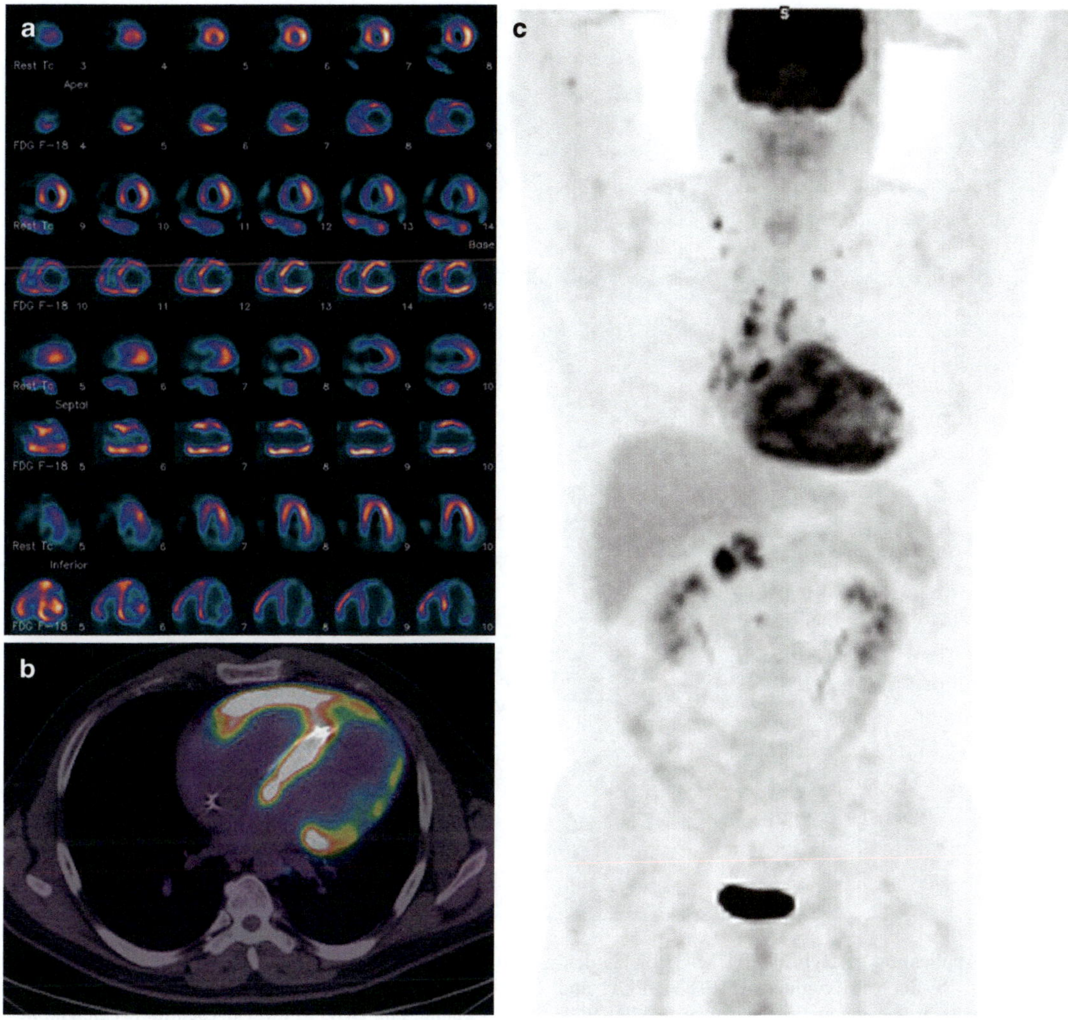

Fig. 10.7 Hybrid ^{18}F-FDG PET/CT of a Patient with Sarcoidosis. A 44-year-old male patient was admitted with complete heart block and left ventricular ejection fraction of 30%. Hybrid imaging with Tc-99m SPECT/CT and ^{18}F-FDG PET/CT shows (**a**) areas of reduced perfusion matched with areas of increased FDG uptake, with (**b**) evidence of right ventricular uptake on ^{18}F-FDG PET/CT, along with (**c**) multiple foci of extra-cardiac ^{18}F-FDG uptake. The patient was diagnosed with active cardiac and extra-cardiac sarcoid

extent and severity of myocardial perfusion [46]. Serial assessment of quantitative metrics may allow for assessment of disease response to therapy and prognosis. In a small study of 15 patients with histopathological diagnosis of CS, SUV_{max} decreased significantly among steroid responders, with an increase in SUV_{max} among nonresponders. Heterogeneous FDG uptake on baseline PET/CT, increase in intensity and the area of myocardial inflammation on follow-up PET/CT were all associated with poor prognosis despite steroid therapy. The duration and intensity of therapy for CS are guided by clinical response based on disease activity on FDG PET/CT, and though the optimal timing to repeat FDG PET/CT is not known, it is generally recommended to repeat imaging approximately 4–6 months after initiation of therapy [47]. In addition to the dedicated cardiac images, one can perform whole body PET/CT and assess for extra-cardiac uptake for diagnosis, prognosis, and identification of possible biopsy sites. Furthermore, presence of

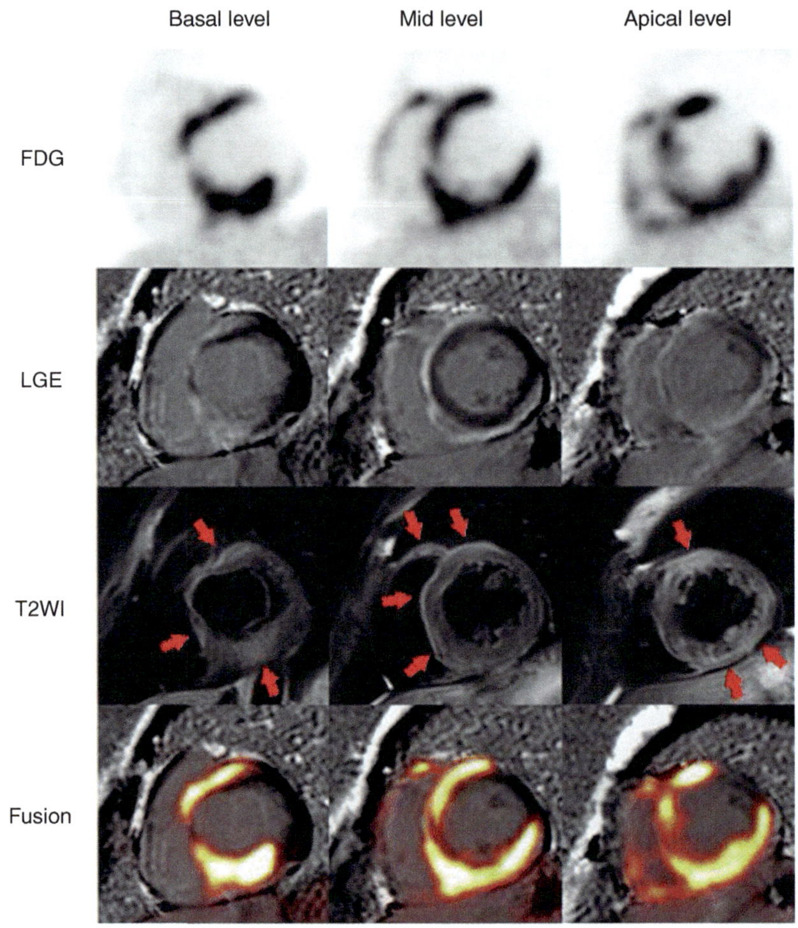

Fig. 10.8 Application of Hybrid PET/MRI for Cardiac Sarcoidosis. ^{18}F-fluorodeoxyglucose (FDG) PET and multisequence cardiac magnetic resonance (CMR) with representative images corresponding to the base, mid, and apical left ventricle. FDG uptake was observed on anterior, septal, inferior, and lateral walls in the left ventricle and in the right ventricle. Late gadolinium enhancement (LGE) was also detected on anterior, septal, inferior, and lateral walls in the left ventricle and in the right ventricle. T2-weighted images (T2WI) showed high-intensity signal (arrows) concordant with the FDG uptake and LGE regions. Fusion images clearly showed the overlap of FDG uptake and LGE in most myocardial regions, but it should be noted that there was a subtle discrepancy between these images (With permission from Wada et al. Simultaneous cardiac imaging to detect inflammation and scar tissue with (18)F-fluorodeoxyglucose PET/MRI in cardiac sarcoidosis. J Nucl Cardiol. 2016;23(5): 1180–1182)

any extra CS may be helpful when deciding on the role of systemic immunosuppressive therapy.

Similar to PET/CT with hybrid metabolic and perfusion imaging, novel hybrid imaging systems combining PET and MRI (PET/MRI) provide highly complementary information on tissue characterization and metabolic information in one single session [48, 49]. The findings of fibrosis by late gadolinium enhancement on cardiac magnetic resonance (CMR) and increased glucose uptake due to increased macrophage infiltration/inflammation are complementary as they identify different pathologies (Fig. 10.8). There is no specific pattern of LGE that is pathognomonic for CS; therefore, images must be interpreted in the context of the patient's history. Mid-wall or subepicardial enhancement in the basal ventricular wall, the lateral wall, and the septum is considered the most common pattern in cardiac sarcoidosis, but subendocardial or transmural enhancement in other myocardial locations have also been described [50]. The absence of LGE is associated with a high negative predictive value for excluding disease as well as with an excellent prognosis. CMR also can be useful in the assessment of LV remodeling, LV and RV function, pulmonary arterial hypertension, and follow-up for end-stage CS (before and after transplantation). Although some studies have shown CMR to be more sensitive for initial diagnosis whereas FDG PET/CT likely has greater utility for serial imaging of inflammation and response to anti-inflammatory therapy. In addition, the presence of pacemakers or defibrillators is not rare in this population and limits the use of CMR, particularly in for follow-up assessments.

10.4.2 Cardiac Amyloidosis

Cardiac amyloidosis (CA) is a disease resulting from deposition of insoluble amyloid fibrils in myocardial interstitium. This can occur from deposition of amyloid light chains (light-chain amyloidosis, AL) or from deposition of amyloid fibrils resulting from abnormal transthyretin protein (TTR). Radionuclide imaging is paving the way for accurate diagnosis of these infiltrative cardiomyopathies. Bone avid tracers, specifically Tc-99m pyrophosphate (PYP), have high diagnostic accuracy for TTR-CA, in the absence of paraproteinemia which is noted among those with AL-CA [51]. While the specifics of imaging protocol are beyond the purview of this chapter, semiquantitative and quantitative assessments of myocardial PYP uptake on planar imaging have shown to have high specificity for TTR-CA. Recent data suggests, limitations of the planar technique with a growing evidence favoring the use of routine SPECT imaging for all cases [52]. Though diagnostic certainty is improved with PYP SPECT, at times it is difficult to differentiate blood pool activity from myocardial uptake. This could be particularly problematic among patients with early disease, in whom PYP uptake may only be focal and thus could be missed on SPECT-only imaging. The use of SPECT/CT in this regard has the potential of enhancing diagnostic certainty, in cases of focal uptake and also may allow for superior differentiation of blood pool activity from myocardial uptake. While no studies have systematically evaluated the superiority of hybrid PYP SPECT/CT, Fig. 10.9 shows clinical examples that highlight the possible advantage of SPECT/CT for diagnosis of TTR-CA.

While PYP scintigraphy has a high diagnostic accuracy for TTR-CA, it is not diagnostic of AL-CA. In this regard, novel PET tracers have shown promise in diagnosis of both AL-CA and TTR-CA, and also for the understanding of the disease process. Emerging data shows promise for targeted amyloid-binding radiotracers, ^{18}F-florbetapir, -flutemetamol, -florbetaben, and ^{11}C-Pittsburgh Compound-B (^{11}C-PIB), that can be employed with hybrid PET/CT [53]. The possible binding of these tracers to the beta-pleated motif of amyloid fibrils has been proposed to explain their ability to detect all amyloid deposits, independent of the precursor protein, and thus these PET radiotracers are the only clinically applicable tracers for imaging of AL-CA. Hybrid PET/CT imaging of CA provides quantitative data that is not only valuable for diagnosis of early CA but may also help in assessment of myocardial amyloid burden. In a seminal study of nine subjects with CA (biopsy-proven or cardiac morphology on echocardiogram) and four controls, left and right ventricular myocardial uptake of ^{18}F-florbetapir was noted in all patients with amyloidosis and in none of the controls [54]. Additionally, the retention index was significantly greater among those with amyloidosis, with a clear distinction from those without amyloidosis (Fig. 10.10). Furthermore, in another prospective study of 32 patients with AL-CA, a base to apex gradient of total florbetapir binding was noted on ^{18}F-Florbetapir PET/CT, which correlated with a base to apex gradient in extracellular mass assessed on CMR [55]. Only, 15% of the total amyloid load was noted to be present in the apical segments, which likely explains the finding of relative apical sparing of longitudinal strain on echocardiography that is observed in CA. Another prospective ^{18}F-Florbetapir PET/CT study evaluated the

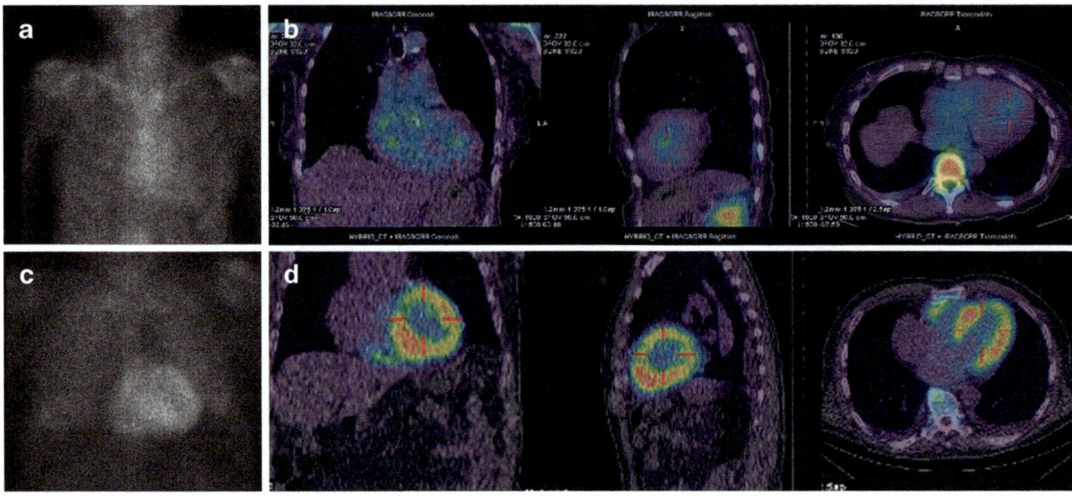

Fig. 10.9 Discrimination of Blood pool from Myocardial Pyrophosphate Uptake by Hybrid Pyrophosphate SPECT/CT. Representative images from two patients with heart failure. Patient 1 has a visual score of 1 (panel **a**) on anterior planar view, which is confirmed as blood pool activity (panel **b**) on SPECT/CT. Patient 2 has a visual score of 3 (panel **c**), with confirmation of myocardial uptake (both left and right ventricle) on SPECT/CT images (panel **d**)

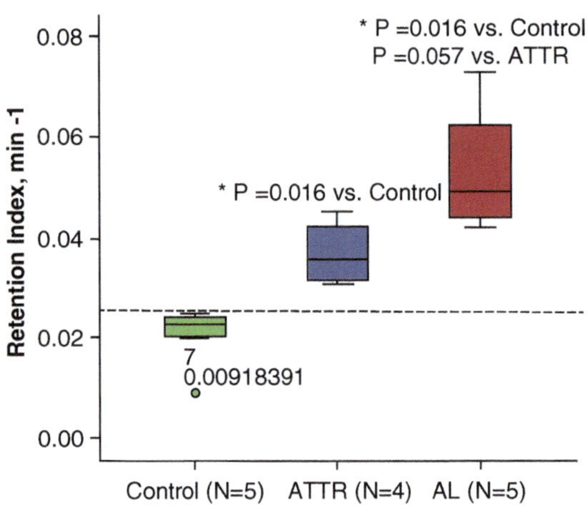

Fig. 10.10 Myocardial 18F-Florbetapir Retention Among Controls and Patients with Amyloidosis. *ATTR* transthyretin amyloidosis, *AL* light-chain amyloidosis. (Reproduced with permission from, Dorbala et al., Imaging Cardiac Amyloidosis: A Pilot Study Using ^{18}F-florbetapir Positron Emission Tomography. Eur J Nucl Med Mol Imaging (2014) 41:1652–1662)

imaging data from 40 subjects with biopsy-proven AL (active AL = 30; remission for >1 year =10) [56]. In these patients, hybrid PET/CT was performed from the skull base to below the kidney, with tracer uptake being measured in several organs—the parotid gland, tongue, thyroid, lung, gastric wall, pancreas, spleen, kidney, muscle, abdominal fat, lower thoracic spine, vertebral body, and humeral head. Compared with the international consensus definition of organ involvement, hybrid florbetapir PET/CT identified amyloid deposits in substantially higher percentages of subjects for several organ systems, including parotid gland (50% vs. 3%), tongue (53% vs. 10%), and lung (35% vs. 10%). Quantitative analysis of hybrid PET/CT revealed more frequent organ involvement than did visual analysis in the tongue, thyroid, lung, pancreas, kidney, muscle, and humeral head, with extensive organ amyloid deposits observed in active AL patients and among those in remission. This study showcases the ability of hybrid florbetapir PET/CT to identify widespread organ amyloid deposition among patients with AL. Hybrid PET/CT identified amyloid deposits in organs associated with no clinical symptoms, suggesting its ability to recognize the disease early which may guide timely therapeutic intervention.

References

1. Cheruvu C, Precious B, Naoum C, Blanke P, Ahmadi A, Soon J, et al. Long term prognostic utility of coronary CT angiography in patients with no modifiable coronary artery disease risk factors: results from the 5 year follow-up of the CONFIRM International Multicenter Registry. J Cardiovasc Comput Tomogr. 2016;10(1):22–7.
2. Majmudar MD, Murthy VL, Shah RV, Kolli S, Mousavi N, Foster CR, et al. Quantification of coronary flow reserve in patients with ischaemic and non-ischaemic cardiomyopathy and its association with clinical outcomes. Eur Heart J Cardiovasc Imaging. 2015;16(8):900–9.
3. Al Badarin FJ, Malhotra S. Diagnosis and prognosis of coronary artery disease with SPECT and PET. Curr Cardiol Rep. 2019;21(7):57.
4. Bavishi C, Argulian E, Chatterjee S, Rozanski A. CACS and the frequency of stress-induced myocardial ischemia during MPI: a meta-analysis. JACC Cardiovasc Imaging. 2016;9(5):580–9.
5. Chang SM, Nabi F, Xu J, Peterson LE, Achari A, Pratt CM, et al. The coronary artery calcium score and stress myocardial perfusion imaging provide independent and complementary prediction of cardiac risk. J Am Coll Cardiol. 2009;54(20):1872–82.
6. Bybee KA, Lee J, Markiewicz R, Longmore R, McGhie AI, O'Keefe JH, et al. Diagnostic and clinical benefit of combined coronary calcium and perfusion assessment in patients undergoing PET/CT myocardial perfusion stress imaging. J Nucl Cardiol. 2010;17(2):188–96.
7. Le VT, Knight S, Min DB, McCubrey RO, Horne BD, Jensen KR, et al. Absence of coronary artery calcium during positron emission tomography stress testing in patients without known coronary artery disease identifies individuals with very low risk of cardiac events. Circ Cardiovasc Imaging. 2020;13(1):e009907.
8. Zampella E, Acampa W, Assante R, Nappi C, Gaudieri V, Mainolfi CG, et al. Combined evaluation of regional coronary artery calcium and myocardial perfusion by (82)Rb PET/CT in the identification of obstructive coronary artery disease. Eur J Nucl Med Mol Imaging. 2018;45(4):521–9.
9. Kwee RM, Truijman MT, Mess WH, Teule GJ, ter Berg JW, Franke CL, et al. Potential of integrated [18F] fluorodeoxyglucose positron-emission tomography/CT in identifying vulnerable carotid plaques. AJNR Am J Neuroradiol. 2011;32(5):950–4.
10. Tawakol A, Fayad ZA, Mogg R, Alon A, Klimas MT, Dansky H, et al. Intensification of statin therapy results in a rapid reduction in atherosclerotic inflammation: results of a multicenter fluorodeoxyglucose-positron emission tomography/computed tomography feasibility study. J Am Coll Cardiol. 2013;62(10):909–17.
11. Fernandez-Friera L, Fuster V, Lopez-Melgar B, Oliva B, Sanchez-Gonzalez J, Macias A, et al. Vascular inflammation in subclinical atherosclerosis detected by hybrid PET/MRI. J Am Coll Cardiol. 2019;73(12):1371–82.
12. Dweck MR, Chow MW, Joshi NV, Williams MC, Jones C, Fletcher AM, et al. Coronary arterial 18F-sodium fluoride uptake: a novel marker of plaque biology. J Am Coll Cardiol. 2012;59(17):1539–48.
13. Li L, Li X, Jia Y, Fan J, Wang H, Fan C, et al. Sodium-fluoride PET-CT for the non-invasive evaluation of coronary plaques in symptomatic patients with coronary artery disease: a cross-correlation study with intravascular ultrasound. Eur J Nucl Med Mol Imaging. 2018;45(12):2181–9.
14. Li JS, Sexton DJ, Mick N, Nettles R, Fowler VG Jr, Ryan T, et al. Proposed modifications to the Duke criteria for the diagnosis of infective endocarditis. Clin Infect Dis. 2000;30(4):633–8.
15. Habib G, Lancellotti P, Antunes MJ, Bongiorni MG, Casalta JP, Del Zotti F, et al. 2015 ESC guidelines for the management of infective endocarditis: the task force for the Management of Infective Endocarditis of the European Society of Cardiology (ESC). Endorsed by: European Association for Cardio-Thoracic Surgery (EACTS), the European Association of Nuclear Medicine (EANM). Eur Heart J. 2015;36(44):3075–128.
16. Habib G, Derumeaux G, Avierinos JF, Casalta JP, Jamal F, Volot F, et al. Value and limitations of the Duke criteria for the diagnosis of infective endocarditis. J Am Coll Cardiol. 1999;33(7):2023–9.
17. Voigt A, Shalaby A, Saba S. Continued rise in rates of cardiovascular implantable electronic device infections in the United States: temporal trends and causative insights. Pacing Clin Electrophysiol. 2010;33(4):414–9.
18. Sohail MR, Uslan DZ, Khan AH, Friedman PA, Hayes DL, Wilson WR, et al. Management and outcome of permanent pacemaker and implantable cardioverter-defibrillator infections. J Am Coll Cardiol. 2007;49(18):1851–9.
19. Kubota R, Yamada S, Kubota K, Ishiwata K, Tamahashi N, Ido T. Intratumoral distribution of fluorine-18-fluorodeoxyglucose in vivo: high accumulation in macrophages and granulation tissues studied by microautoradiography. J Nucl Med. 1992;33(11):1972–80.
20. Mochizuki T, Tsukamoto E, Kuge Y, Kanegae K, Zhao S, Hikosaka K, et al. FDG uptake and glucose transporter subtype expressions in experimental tumor and inflammation models. J Nucl Med. 2001;42(10):1551–5.
21. Mahmood M, Kendi AT, Farid S, Ajmal S, Johnson GB, Baddour LM, et al. Role of (18)F-FDG PET/CT in the diagnosis of cardiovascular implantable electronic device infections: a meta-analysis. J Nucl Cardiol. 2019;26(3):958–70.
22. Sarrazin JF, Philippon F, Tessier M, Guimond J, Molin F, Champagne J, et al. Usefulness of fluorine-18 positron emission tomography/computed tomography for identification of cardiovascular implantable electronic device infections. J Am Coll Cardiol. 2012;59(18):1616–25.

23. Cautela J, Alessandrini S, Cammilleri S, Giorgi R, Richet H, Casalta JP, et al. Diagnostic yield of FDG positron-emission tomography/computed tomography in patients with CEID infection: a pilot study. Europace. 2013;15(2):252–7.
24. Dilsizian V, Bacharach SL, Beanlands RS, Bergmann SR, Delbeke D, Dorbala S, et al. ASNC imaging guidelines/SNMMI procedure standard for positron emission tomography (PET) nuclear cardiology procedures. J Nucl Cardiol. 2016;23(5):1187–226.
25. Chareonthaitawee P, Beanlands RS, Chen W, Dorbala S, Miller EJ, Murthy VL, et al. Joint SNMMI-ASNC expert consensus document on the role of (18)F-FDG PET/CT in cardiac sarcoid detection and therapy monitoring. J Nucl Med. 2017;58(8):1341–53.
26. DiFilippo FP, Brunken RC. Do implanted pacemaker leads and ICD leads cause metal-related artifact in cardiac PET/CT? J Nucl Med. 2005;46(3):436–43.
27. Saby L, Laas O, Habib G, Cammilleri S, Mancini J, Tessonnier L, et al. Positron emission tomography/computed tomography for diagnosis of prosthetic valve endocarditis: increased valvular 18F-fluorodeoxyglucose uptake as a novel major criterion. J Am Coll Cardiol. 2013;61(23):2374–82.
28. Erba PA, Sollini M, Conti U, Bandera F, Tascini C, De Tommasi SM, et al. Radiolabeled WBC scintigraphy in the diagnostic workup of patients with suspected device-related infections. JACC Cardiovasc Imaging. 2013;6(10):1075–86.
29. Rouzet F, Chequer R, Benali K, Lepage L, Ghodbane W, Duval X, et al. Respective performance of 18F-FDG PET and radiolabeled leukocyte scintigraphy for the diagnosis of prosthetic valve endocarditis. J Nucl Med. 2014;55(12):1980–5.
30. Schouten LR, Verberne HJ, Bouma BJ, van Eck-Smit BL, Mulder BJ. Surgical glue for repair of the aortic root as a possible explanation for increased F-18 FDG uptake. J Nucl Cardiol. 2008;15(1):146–7.
31. Pizzi MN, Roque A, Fernandez-Hidalgo N, Cuellar-Calabria H, Ferreira-Gonzalez I, Gonzalez-Alujas MT, et al. Improving the diagnosis of infective endocarditis in prosthetic valves and Intracardiac devices with 18F-fluordeoxyglucose positron emission tomography/computed tomography angiography: initial results at an infective endocarditis referral center. Circulation. 2015;132(12):1113–26.
32. Valeyre D, Prasse A, Nunes H, Uzunhan Y, Brillet PY, Müller-Quernheim J. Sarcoidosis. Lancet. 2014;383(9923):1155–67.
33. Ardehali H, Howard DL, Hariri A, Qasim A, Hare JM, Baughman KL, et al. A positive endomyocardial biopsy result for sarcoid is associated with poor prognosis in patients with initially unexplained cardiomyopathy. Am Heart J. 2005;150(3):459–63.
34. Ishida Y, Yoshinaga K, Miyagawa M, Moroi M, Kondoh C, Kiso K. Recommendations for (18) F-fluorodeoxyglucose positron emission tomography imaging for cardiac sarcoidosis: Japanese Society of Nuclear Cardiology recommendations. Ann Nucl Med. 2014;28:393–403.
35. Birnie DH, Sauer WH, Bogun F, Cooper JM, Culver DA, Duvernoy CS, et al. HRS expert consensus statement on the diagnosis and management of arrhythmias associated with cardiac sarcoidosis. Heart Rhythm. 2014;11(7):1305–23.
36. Momose M, Kadoya M, Koshikawa M, Matsushita T, Yamada A. Usefulness of 67Ga SPECT and integrated low-dose CT scanning (SPECT/CT) in the diagnosis of cardiac sarcoidosis. Ann Nucl Med. 2007;21(10):545–51.
37. Nakazawa A, Ikeda K, Ito Y, Iwase M, Sato K, Ueda R, et al. Usefulness of dual 67Ga and 99mTc-sestamibi single-photon-emission CT scanning in the diagnosis of cardiac sarcoidosis. Chest. 2004;126(4):1372–6.
38. Treglia G, Annunziata S, Sobic-Saranovic D, Bertagna F, Caldarella C, Giovanella L. The role of 18F-FDG-PET and PET/CT in patients with sarcoidosis: an updated evidence-based review. Acad Radiol. 2014;21(5):675–84.
39. Nishiyama Y, Yamamoto Y, Fukunaga K, Takinami H, Iwado Y, Satoh K, et al. Comparative evaluation of 18F-FDG PET and 67Ga scintigraphy in patients with sarcoidosis. J Nucl Med. 2006;47(10):1571–6.
40. Mana J, Gamez C. Molecular imaging in sarcoidosis. Curr Opin Pulm Med. 2011;17(5):325–31.
41. Blankstein R, Osborne M, Naya M, Waller A, Kim CK, Murthy VL, et al. Cardiac positron emission tomography enhances prognostic assessments of patients with suspected cardiac sarcoidosis. J Am Coll Cardiol. 2014;63(4):329–36.
42. Ahmadian A, Brogan A, Berman J, Sverdlov AL, Mercier G, Mazzini M, et al. Quantitative interpretation of FDG PET/CT with myocardial perfusion imaging increases diagnostic information in the evaluation of cardiac sarcoidosis. J Nucl Cardiol. 2014;21(5):925–39.
43. Juneau D, Inacio JR, Dwivedi G, Dennie C. Cardiac involvement in rheumatoid arthritis mimicking sarcoidosis on FDG PET-CT and MR imaging. J Nucl Cardiol. 2018;25(1):348–50.
44. Blankstein R, Waller AH. Evaluation of known or suspected cardiac sarcoidosis. Circ Cardiovasc Imaging. 2016;9(3):e000867.
45. Tuominen H, Haarala A, Tikkakoski A, Kahonen M, Nikus K, Sipila K. FDG-PET in possible cardiac sarcoidosis: right ventricular uptake and high total cardiac metabolic activity predict cardiovascular events. J Nucl Cardiol. 2021;28(1):199–205.
46. Waller AH, Blankstein R. Quantifying myocardial inflammation using F18-fluorodeoxyglucose positron emission tomography in cardiac sarcoidosis. J Nucl Cardiol. 2014;21(5):940–3.
47. Slart R, Glaudemans A, Lancellotti P, Hyafil F, Blankstein R, Schwartz RG, et al. A joint procedural position statement on imaging in cardiac sarcoidosis: from the Cardiovascular and Inflammation & Infection Committees of the European Association of Nuclear Medicine, the European Association of Cardiovascular Imaging, and the American

Society of Nuclear Cardiology. J Nucl Cardiol. 2018;25(1):298–319.

48. Wada K, Niitsuma T, Yamaki T, Masuda A, Ito H, Kubo H, et al. Simultaneous cardiac imaging to detect inflammation and scar tissue with (18) F-fluorodeoxyglucose PET/MRI in cardiac sarcoidosis. J Nucl Cardiol. 2016;23(5):1180–2.
49. Schneider S, Batrice A, Rischpler C, Eiber M, Ibrahim T, Nekolla SG. Utility of multimodal cardiac imaging with PET/MRI in cardiac sarcoidosis: implications for diagnosis, monitoring and treatment. Eur Heart J. 2014;35(5):312.
50. Patel MR, Cawley PJ, Heitner JF, Klem I, Parker MA, Jaroudi WA, et al. Detection of myocardial damage in patients with sarcoidosis. Circulation. 2009;120(20):1969–77.
51. Gillmore JD, Maurer MS, Falk RH, Merlini G, Damy T, Dispenzieri A, et al. Nonbiopsy diagnosis of cardiac transthyretin amyloidosis. Circulation. 2016;133(24):2404–12.
52. Asif T, Gomez J, Singh V, Doukky R, Nedeltcheva A, Malhotra S. Comparison of planar with tomographic pyrophosphate scintigraphy for transthyretin cardiac amyloidosis: perils and pitfalls. J Nucl Cardiol. 2021;28(1):104–11.
53. Singh V, Dorbala S. Positron emission tomography for cardiac amyloidosis: timing matters! J Nucl Cardiol. 2022;29(2):790–7.
54. Dorbala S, Vangala D, Semer J, Strader C, Bruyere JR Jr, Di Carli MF, et al. Imaging cardiac amyloidosis: a pilot study using (1)(8)F-florbetapir positron emission tomography. Eur J Nucl Med Mol Imaging. 2014;41(9):1652–62.
55. Bravo PE, Fujikura K, Kijewski MF, Jerosch-Herold M, Jacob S, El-Sady MS, et al. Relative apical sparing of myocardial longitudinal strain is explained by regional differences in total amyloid mass rather than the proportion of amyloid deposits. JACC Cardiovasc Imaging. 2019;12(7 Pt 1): 1165–73.
56. Ehman EC, El-Sady MS, Kijewski MF, Khor YM, Jacob S, Ruberg FL, et al. Early detection of multiorgan light-chain amyloidosis by whole-body (18)F-florbetapir PET/CT. J Nucl Med. 2019;60(9):1234–9.

Clinical Cases of Hybrid Cardiac Imaging

11

Kenji Fukushima and Michinobu Nagao

11.1 Introduction

Cardiovascular disease remains the leading cause of death worldwide, despite advances in early diagnosis and intervention [1]. Over the past few decades, accumulated evidence has proved that evaluating organic stenosis by invasive coronary angiography was not a gold standard for managing angina [2, 3]. Nuclear cardiology (NC) had already established substantial evidence particularly in predicting cardiovascular events [4]. However, recent technological innovation has enabled the use of other noninvasive imaging modalities such as coronary computed tomography angiography (CTA), and cardiac magnetic resonance imaging (CMR) to demonstrate equivalent diagnostic accuracy to NC in coronary artery disease [5]. Furthermore, technical developments in time and spatial resolution allows these modalities to detect stress-induced ischemia [5, 6]. However, in coronary circulation, it is quite evident that there is a fundamental difference in the kinetics of contrast media and radionuclide tracers. CTA and CMR offer a first-pass quantification or visual comparison of contrast agent concentration in arterial capillaries, while NC demonstrates the quantitative or relative accumulation of tracer reflecting both arterial capillary flow and myocardial cell membrane or mitochondrial integrity [7]. Thus, hybrid cardiac imaging plays a pivotal role to enhance diagnostic confidence and comprehension incrementally compared to a single imaging modality [8, 9]. Hybrid assessment is commonly performed to obtain both anatomical and functional information and is also capable of identifying the relationship of those such as the regional ischemia and the culprit vessel, or irreversible myocardial fibrosis and metabolic damage. Latest investigation suggests that cardiac hybrid imaging of CTA and myocardial perfusion imaging (MPI) may have predictive value for future cardiovascular events [10]. In a routine clinical setting, the assessment of multimodality imaging of cardiac disease is mostly made by side-by-side interpretation, and it is often relatively challenging and time-consuming to obtain the image fusion through accurate alignment [11]. Thus, good operability and full-automatic image fusion tool are eagerly awaited including artificial intelligence assis-

K. Fukushima (✉)
Department of Nuclear Medicine, and Cardiology, Saitama Medical University International Medical Center, Saitama, Japan
e-mail: kfukush4@saitama-med.ac.jp

M. Nagao
Department of Diagnostic Imaging and Nuclear Medicine, Tokyo Women's Medical University, Tokyo, Japan
e-mail: nagao.michinobu@twmu.ac.jp

F. Nudi et al. (eds.), *Hybrid Cardiac Imaging for Clinical Decision-Making*,
https://doi.org/10.1007/978-3-030-99391-7_11

tance [12]. In this chapter, we briefly summarize and present several typical cases of cardiac disease assessed using hybrid imaging.

11.2 Hybrid Assessment for Coronary Artery Disease

CTA is known as one of the first-line modalities to detect coronary atherosclerosis in leading countries. The latest guidelines from the UK National Institute for Health and Care Excellence included CTA as a first-line investigation for newly onset typical or atypical stable angina [13]. The coronary anatomy and atherosclerotic burden derived from CTA provide useful information in diagnosing coronary artery disease. Recent technical developments have enabled the performance of dynamic perfusion CTA with minimized radiation, which can visualize vasodilator-induced ischemia. To date, FFRct, CTA-derived computational fluid dynamics has emerged as a useful tool to detect flow-limiting stenosis, except after revascularization [14]. However, stress-induced ischemia as true functional testing including flow and contractile response is widely known as an essential strategy for managing ischemic heart disease. CMR has been developed as a useful tool in the evaluation of cardiomyopathy and more recently become a promising technique to detect myocardial ischemia using vasodilatory stress for dynamic perfusion study [15]. Combining coronary MR angiography and delayed enhancement, CMR has the potential to be an ideal, comprehensive noninvasive imaging technique without radiation exposure [16]. However, CMR still has a significant time-consuming issue in clinical practice. Furthermore, both CTA and CMR have a considerable risk of causing adverse effects on image acquisitions under irregular heart rhythm, while NC does not. Additionally, contraindication of the contrast media, including chronic kidney disease and allergic reaction remains as a significant limitation and is frequently encountered in routine clinical practice. There is very little possibility of adverse effect on renal function or allergic reaction using radionuclide agent. NC has established its diagnostic utility and clinical usefulness for ischemic heart disease over the past decades [17]. Since NC firstly reported the relation between the extent of myocardial ischemia and poor outcome, a number of the studies have proved the usefulness of evaluating threshold of ishcaemic burden in determining the relative benefits of revascularization and optimal medical therapy [18, 19]. Furthermore, a number of the studies also proved the evidence for risk stratification combined with various risk factors, i.e., diabetes, dyslipidemia, and chronic renal disease including end-stage disease which has been impossible for CTA and CMR to detect [20, 21]. Of note, there is a distinctive physiological property between the contrast media and the myocardial perfusion tracers. A contrast media can visualize anatomy by filling coronary artery and enhance the microvascularity by passing through capillary vessels, while myocardial perfusion agents are delivered into myocardial cells surrogating vascular function from large vessels to a microcirculation level including the interstitial fluid flow and the cell membrane integrity [22]. Therefore, CTA is employed to detect epicardial coronary atherosclerosis, and myocardial perfusion imaging is used to evaluate regional ischemia on myocardial cells supplied by the downstream vascular bed which can be affected by functional stenosis and coronary vascularity [8]. Thus, hybrid assessment is mostly performed by the combination of coronary CTA and NC in clinical routine. The strength of multimodality assessment is not only in side-by-side interpretations but also in compensation among various imaging techniques which may capture a different aspect of the disease because there is poor agreement between epicardial coronary stenosis and reversible ischemia [23]. Simultaneous hybrid positron emission tomography (PET)-CT or single photon emission computed tomography (SPECT)-CT is the best-suited system for multimodality imaging. However, cardiac CT imaging requires higher machine specification (i.e., 64 slices at minimum and faster gantry rotation), and the specification of CT mounted in most hybrid systems is lower than that of a stand-alone system because CT-based attenuation correction is the primary purpose [23]. Thus, software image fusion has emerged as the most available technique for hybrid assessment. In the process of image fusion, the registration of different images is occasionally challenging with the increased risk of misalignment due to the motion-related effects, the inter-modality resolution, or the extensive perfusion defect [24]. Recent technological innovation has introduced high-resolution imaging such as time-of-flight PET or SPECT with cadmium–zinc–telluride detectors which might enable us to perform image fusion more accurately and less challenging [23].

Additionally, nuclear cardiology has been a long-standing player in hybrid analysis using dual or multi-tracer imaging. NC enables to visualization of the disease heterogeneity in a patient using multi-tracer imaging of different molecular targets [25]. The concordance and discrepancy between multi-tracers imaging have been widely used for risk assessment in coronary artery disease. For instance, as shown in the following cases, a hot spot uptake of acute infarction and corresponding perfusion defect provide the location and extent of acute myocardial infarction, and perfusion-metabolism mismatch is helpful in identifying viable myocardium in patients with chronic myocardial infarction.

Case 1
In routine clinical practice, a significant multivessel disease is frequently encountered. Figure 11.1 shows a 73-year-old man with significant coronary artery disease. CTA showed severe atherosclerosis in the large diagonal branch and the left circumflex artery (LCX). He was referred for stress myocardial perfusion imaging to assess the need for coronary angioplasty. Stress-rest cardiac SPECT revealed significant transient ischemia in the postero-lateral wall, and image fusion of CTA and SPECT demonstrated the regional ischemia corresponding to the LCX territory. No significant ischemia was detected in the anterior wall. The image fusion contributed as a reclassifying tool to determine the relation between the severity of lesional ischemia and the culprit artery.

Case 2
Image fusion of CTA and NC offers an incremental information. Figure 11.2 shows a case of a 66-year-old man after stenting in the left main tract for unstable angina. Follow-up CTA showed negative for in-stent stenosis. However, CTA showed broad endomyocardial low enhancement in the anterior wall which indicated myocardial

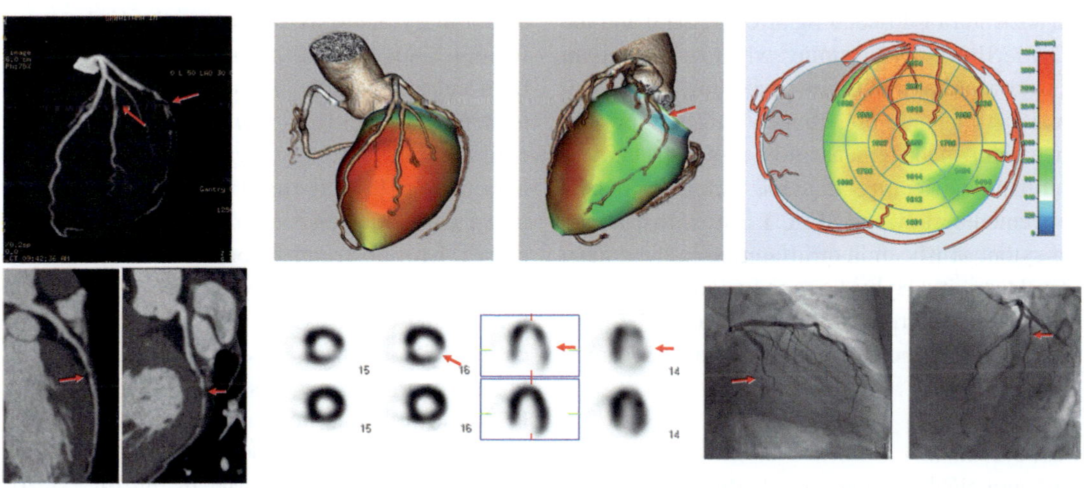

Fig. 11.1 A 73-year-old male was referred for angina. A CTA showed significant organic stenosis in LCX and diagonal branch. Stress-rest myocardial perfusion SPECT showed a significant transient defect in the lateral wall, but not in the anterior wall. Anterior and posterolateral view of 3D CTA-SPECT Image fusion clearly demonstrated the culprit region of ischemia which corresponds to the LCX territory. Invasive coronary angiography revealed total occlusion in distal LCX and significant stenosis in diagonal branch which was approximately similar findings to CTA

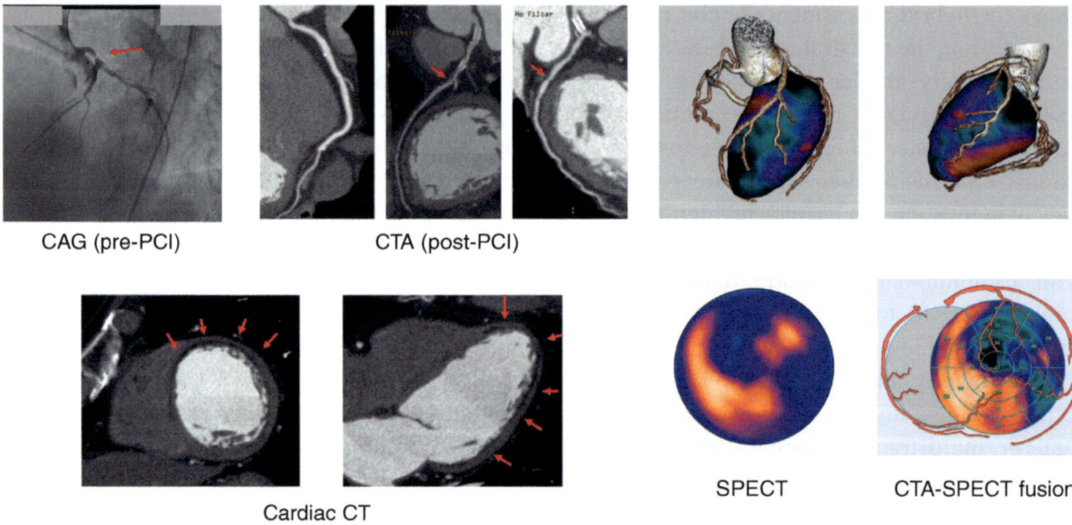

Fig. 11.2 A 66-year-old male after PCI to the left main coronary artery for acute myocardial infarction underwent follow-up CTA and MPI. Left upper panel showed coronary angiography at emergency PCI. Follow-up CTA showed mild to moderate stenosis with a mixed plaque in LAD and LCX, while no restenosis was observed in left main. Rest MPI showed a significant defect in the anterior and lateral wall, which indicated myocardial infarction without viability. Contrast-enhanced Cardiac CT derived from CTA demonstrated a significant thinned wall with hypo-enhanced contrast in the anterior and lateral area which also indicated myocardial infarction. 3D fused and 2D polar map output of CTA-SPECT fusion revealed a broad anterior myocardial infarction including diagonal territory and the posterolateral branch territory of LCX

infarction. The patient underwent a rest myocardial perfusion study which revealed a severe defect in the anterior and lateral wall. CTA-SPECT fusion demonstrated broad infarction in the left anterior descending artery (LAD) and the LCX territory. Determining whether the patient has myocardial infarction including periprocedural such as side-branch stent jail is important for patient management and follow up. CTA is useful for detecting in-stent stenosis or new obstructive lesion, and SPECT is used to evaluate the extent of ishcemia or infarction in the culprit vessel territory. Hybrid image fusion allows us to analyze and interpret information from the multiple images of the multivessel complex coronary artery disease.

Case 3

CTA and NC have a potential advantage for territorial analysis. Myocardial perfusion PET can provide quantitative myocardial blood flow and contractile reserve, while CTA can mostly provide anatomical information in coronary artery disease. Coronary territorial analysis in myocardial perfusion imaging has significant limitation due to difficulty of presumption in the variation of coronary anatomy of each individual. Image fusion allows simultaneous interpretation of both a coronary path and the location of regional Ischemia. Recently, a Voronoi diagram which can simulate coronary territorial segmentation has emerged [26]. Figure 11.3 shows a representative case of hybrid cardiac imaging by CTA and PET for obstructive coronary artery disease. A 56-year-old man was referred to our hospital for cardiac exams. CTA showed severe calcification in all three vessels which indicated obstructive disease. Rest-stress ^{13}N ammonia PET showed significant transient ischemia in the lateral region, and flow reserve map demonstrated reduced flow reserve in the LCX territory. Territorial analysis revealed the area of transient ischemia and reduced flow reserve corresponding to distal site of the LCX territory.

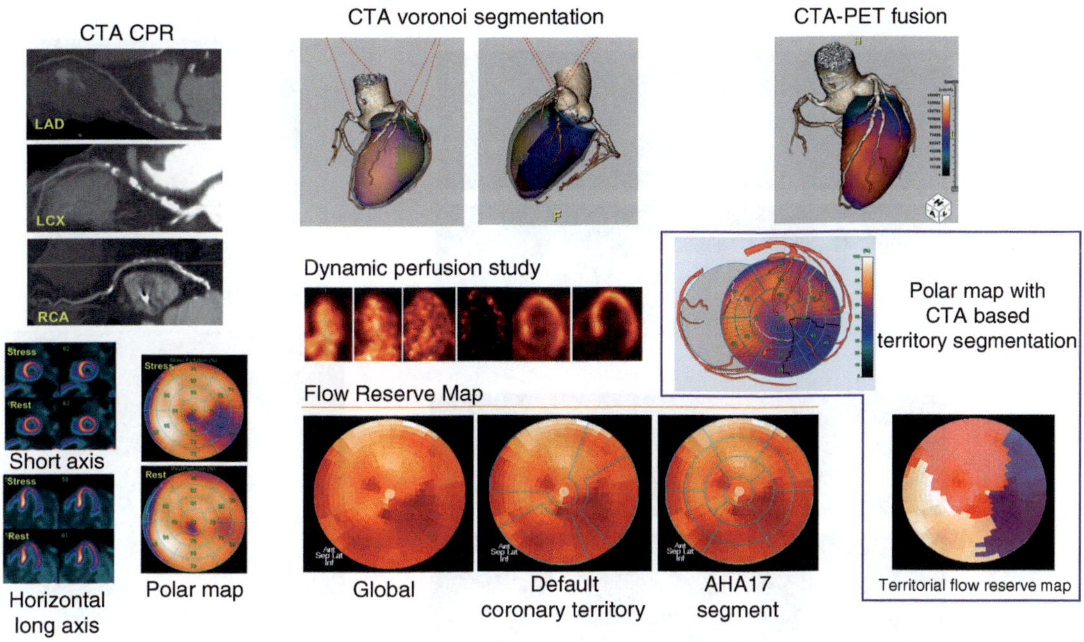

Fig. 11.3 A 56-year-old male after pacemaker implantation referred for chest discomfort. CTA showed significant coronary atherosclerosis and organic stenosis which was strongly suspected of three vessel disease (left upper). Rest—pharmacological stress ^{13}N ammonia PETCT showed transient ischemia in the lateral region with relatively preserved global myocardial flow reserve 2.0 mL/mg/min, middle lower. 3D volume rendering and 2D polar map display of the CTA-PETCT fused image revealed that the regional ischemia corresponds to the territory of the posterior descending artery from LCX (right upper). A voronoi-based coronary territorial segmentation helps to visualize the relationship between coronary anatomy and myocardial flow over the default coronary territory or AHA segment-based polar map display (right middle and lower)

This technique is promising potential in performing further assessment of atherosclerotic burden and vascular function in individual coronary arteries.

Case 4

Identifying the area of myocardial infarction is also valuable in a patient with acute myocardial infarction (AMI). A patient with AMI in the lateral wall is shown in Fig. 11.4. Emergency coronary angiography showed significant coronary stenosis in LCX and RCA. Dual isotope SPECT with ^{201}thallium (TL) and ^{99m}Tc pyrophosphate (PYP) was performed in acute phase (day 2). TL showed a severe defect in the lateral to inferior wall, and %uptake was remarkably low (30–40%) which indicated myocardial stunning. PYP uptake corresponded to the region where TL showed the defect in culprit vessel territory. Hybrid analysis confirmed the concordance of the localization of AMI and perfusion defect. Two weeks later, CMR was performed and revealed typical subendomyocardial LGE without transmural extent (less than 50% wall) which indicated residual viability. CMR is recognized as a useful modality to evaluate myocardial infarction. However, during acute phase of AMI, CMR is not used as a first-line modality due to the MRI safety issue particularly while the patients undergo infusion therapy or an intra-aortic balloon therapy in coronary care unit. NC is available for those patients under intensive care.

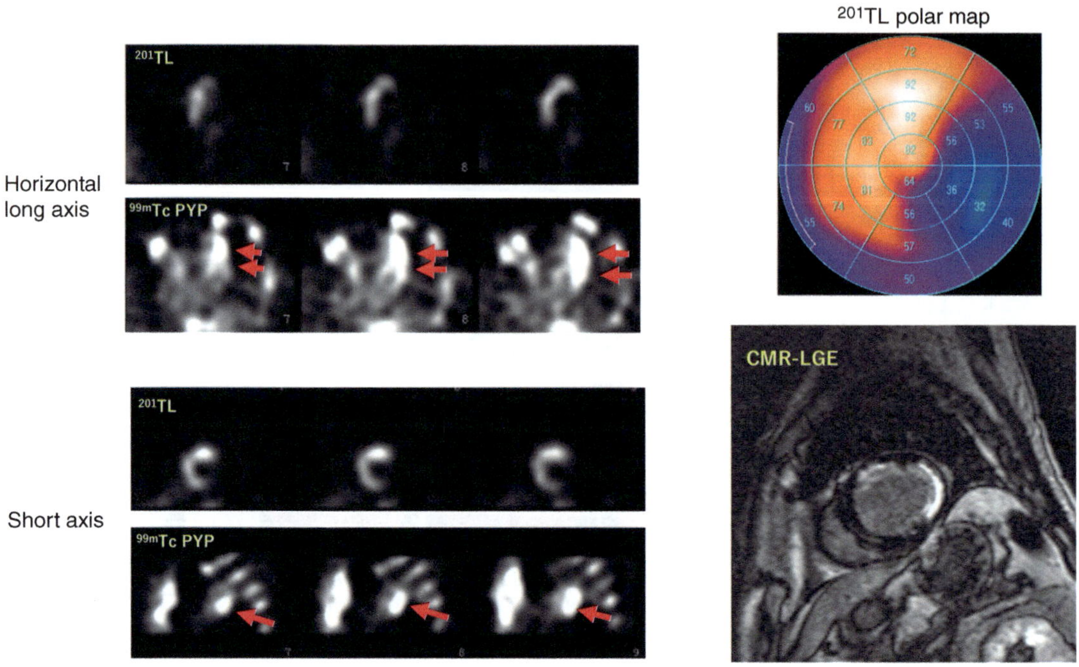

Fig. 11.4 A 54-year-old male with significant sudden onset of chest pain and ST elevation on electrocardiogram was transferred to the emergency catheter lab. Emergency coronary angiography revealed no significant stenosis with moderate atherosclerosis. ^{99m}Tc pyrophosphate (PYP) and ^{201}thallium (TL) dual SPECT were performed the next day. TL demonstrated significant perfusion defect in the lateral wall, and hot spot PYP uptake was observed corresponding to defect in TL which indicated acute myocardial infarction in LCX territory

11.3 Hybrid Assessment for Nonischemic Heart Disease

CMR is widely known as a useful modality to diagnose nonischemic cardiomyopathy. CMR has been initially utilized for imaging myocardial infarction, and it is also capable of interrogating nonischemic myocardial deformations with a multiparametric imaging technique, such as balanced cine-MRI, tagging cine, feature tracking, T2-related (dark blood, STIR), gadolinium perfusion, and delayed enhancement (LGE). A myocardial LGE has been the most common technique in the differential diagnosis of cardiomyopathy because there are distinctive enhancement patterns and extents as well as myocardial wall abnormalities among various cardiac diseases. Although the LGE imaging simply identifies regional or diffuse replacement fibrosis with any etiology, it reflects the pathological variation of the myocardial disease. For instance, cardiac sarcoidosis typically shows a sub-epicardial layer of LGE in the basal site of the ventricular wall, while ischemic cardiomyopathy shows subendocardial to transmural extent consistent with coronary distribution. To date, the most commonly used hybrid assessment is the combination of MRI and ^{18}F fluorodeoxyglucose PET-CT (FDG) for cardiac sarcoidosis (CS). FDG plays a pivotal role in imaging patients with cancer. In recent years, FDG has been used successfully to visualize myocardial inflammation and monitor the therapeutic effect of anti-inflammatory drugs in patients with CS. More recent investigations suggested the usefulness of therapeutic monitoring using quantitative measurement (i.e., SUVmax, SUV volume, and cardiac metabolic activity) beyond conventional visual grading for the activity of inflammation [27].

Cardiac amyloidosis is a disease characterized by diffuse deposition of amyloid fibrils in the myocardium clinically manifesting restrictive cardiomyopathy with conduction abnormality and poor prognosis. In noninvasive imaging, CMR plays a key role in differentiating CA from hypertrophic cardiomyopathy or hypertensive heart disease [28]. Furthermore, quantitative T1 mapping and extracellular volume (ECV) measurement have emerged and shown promising results in diagnosing CA. However, implantable devices including cardioverter defibrillators may influence the magnetic field, and occasionally metal artifact resulted in failing to detect myocardial fibrosis [29]. Additionally, using the gadolinium enhancement is not appropriate for patients with chronic kidney disease (CKD) due to the increased risk of having future nephrogenic systemic fibrosis. NC is accessible either for chronic kidney disease or after device implantation. Cardiac PET with ^{11}C and ^{18}F-labeled amyloid tracers has been extensively studied and confirmed a high affinity for cardiac amyloid deposits. Several investigations indicated the prognostic value of amyloid-PET, and also the usefulness as a monitoring tool for therapeutic effects [30]. Technetium-99m bone avid tracers have demonstrated high diagnostic performance approaching 100% for ATTR-type CA [31]. In particular, the diagnosis of ATTR CA has been established using visual grading comparing bone uptake or myocardial uptake ratio to the contralateral site [32].

Except for CA and CS, the utility of NC for nonischemic cardiomyopathy seems to be less frequent. In particular, the diagnostic value of myocardial perfusion or metabolic imaging (MPI) for nonischemic cardiomyopathy has not been well investigated, while the evaluation of cardiac autonomic dysfunction using ^{123}I-MIBG has been extensively studied [33–35]. Although MPI can mostly contribute as functional and volumetric information for monitoring nonischemic cardiomyopathy, several investigators have reported on the clinical utility of MPI [36]. Wu et al. reported that the differentiation of nonischemic from ischemic cardiomyopathy was feasible using MPI in patients with left ventricular (LV) dysfunction [37]. Tadamura et al. reported that myocardial fatty acid metabolism was remarkably reduced in patients with hypertrophied cardiomyopathy, and was related to functional impairment [38]. Furthermore, MPI can be a useful alternative tool for diagnosis and monitoring when the patients are with CKD or after device implantation which is frequently encountered in clinical routine.

Case 5

Figure 11.5 shows a typical case of cardiac sarcoidosis. Cardiac sarcoidosis is commonly diagnosed and evaluated using CMR and FDG. Hybrid and simultaneous assessment using integrated PET-MR scanner as ideal equipment for one-stop shop, while the scanner is quite limited in prevalence. Thus, a software image fusion technique has been developed and introduced in clinical routines. However, there is a possible challenge and limitation in the image alignment and fusion due to a significant difference in the image acquisition between CMR and FDG. CMR is usually obtained by breath-hold acquisition, while FDG image is obtained by free breathing. Co-registration of LGE and FDG images can be occasionally challenging, and the alignment along the X-Y-Z axes can be difficult either automatic or manually. Additionally, CS frequently shows focal FDG uptake which makes the alignment further challenging. One of the potential solutions is to merge similar morphologic images to switch functional images [39]. First, CMR-LGE and attenuation correction CT (acCT) is merged in advance and followed by switching acCT to FDG. CMR and acCT demonstrate similar anatomical information and are quite feasible to perform image fusion. The right panel demonstrated image fusion of CMR-LGE and FDG using a dedicated fusion tool (Intuition server®, TeraRecon Inc. Foster, CA). Hybrid assessment occasionally needs image fusion for precise interpretation. Figure 11.5 represents a case of cardiac sarcoidosis. A 77-year-old female presented with heart failure without significant coronary artery disease. CMR showed extensive LGE of mid-wall to epicardial-wall distribution LGE with dilated LV cavity. FDG showed significant abnormal uptake in the inferior wall, and maximum intensity projection (MIP) image demonstrated abnormal uptake in the bilateral hilar to the mediastinum. In CS, multimodality image

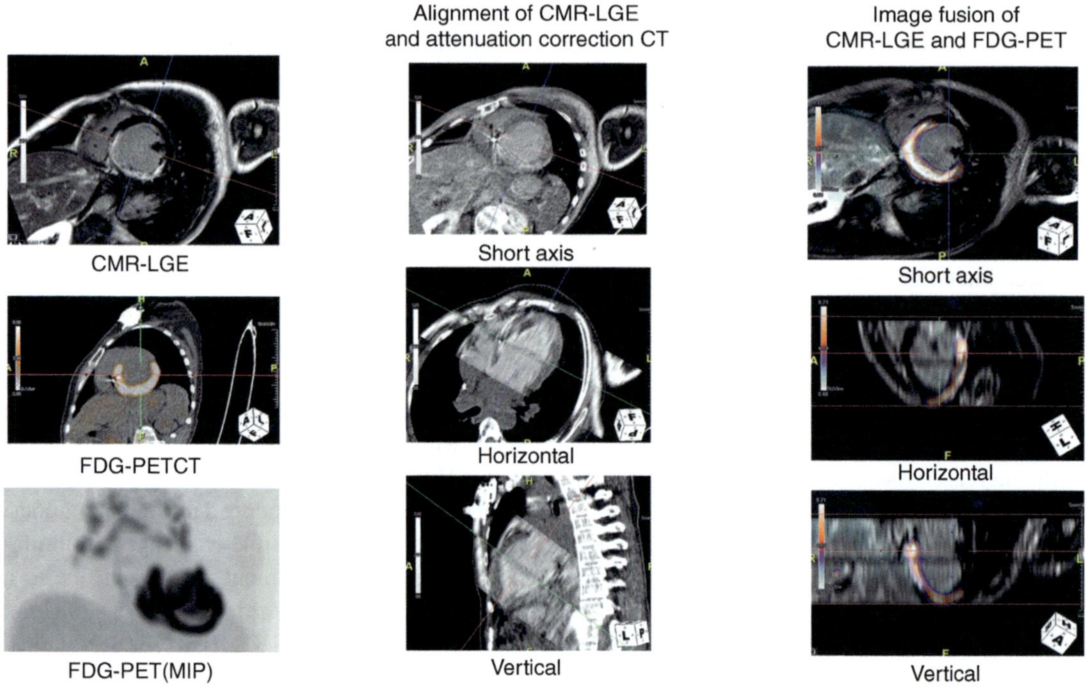

Fig. 11.5 A case with cardiac sarcoidosis (CS) is shown. CMR showed extensive mid to epicardial-wall LGE with an enlarged LV cavity. FDG-PETCT demonstrated significant abnormal uptake in the inferior wall (left upper panel). MIP image demonstrated abnormal uptake in bilateral hilar to mediastinum which indicated active extracardiac sarcoidosis (left lower). To perform precise image fusion, the alignment of CMR-LGE and attenuation correction CT (acCT) was done in advance before performing CMR-LGE and FDG-PET image fusion. As shown in the right panel, the image fusion succeeded to reveal the area of fibrosis was corresponding to active inflammation

fusion can be challenging due to the difficulty of performing precise alignment of focal FDG uptake and CMR-LGE. The alignment of CMR-LGE and attenuation correction CT was done on performing CMR-LGE and FDG image fusion, and image registration succeeded to reveal the area of fibrosis was corresponding to active inflammation.

Case 6

Figure 11.6 shows the hybrid assessment of a patient with cardiac transthyretin amyloidosis. CMR showed significant asymmetric septal hypertrophy, and LGE demonstrated diffuse hyperintensity in LV. ^{99m}Tc pyrophosphate scintigraphy showed remarkable myocardial uptake (myocardium-contralateral ratio = 2.4). SPECT/CT demonstrated the heterogeneous myocardial uptake despite diffuse myocardial disease.

Case 7

Dilated cardiomyopathy (DCM) is characterized by reduced cardiac function with an enlarged LV cavity. In clinical practice, the noninvasive approach to determine the etiology is quite pivotal due to various subtypes of DCM. To date, the etiologic assessment using delayed enhancement by CMR is the most common technique for nonischemic cardiomyopathy. However, delayed enhancement is not adequate for patients with CKD. MPI can be one of the alternative approaches to determine the etiology by evaluating the pattern of perfusion defect [37]. Figure 11.7 shows a case with idiopathic dilated cardiomyopathy. A 40-year-old female was hospitalized for acute heart failure. Coronary angiography showed normal coronary without atherosclerosis. MPI demonstrated patchy hypo uptake without significant defect. CMR revealed

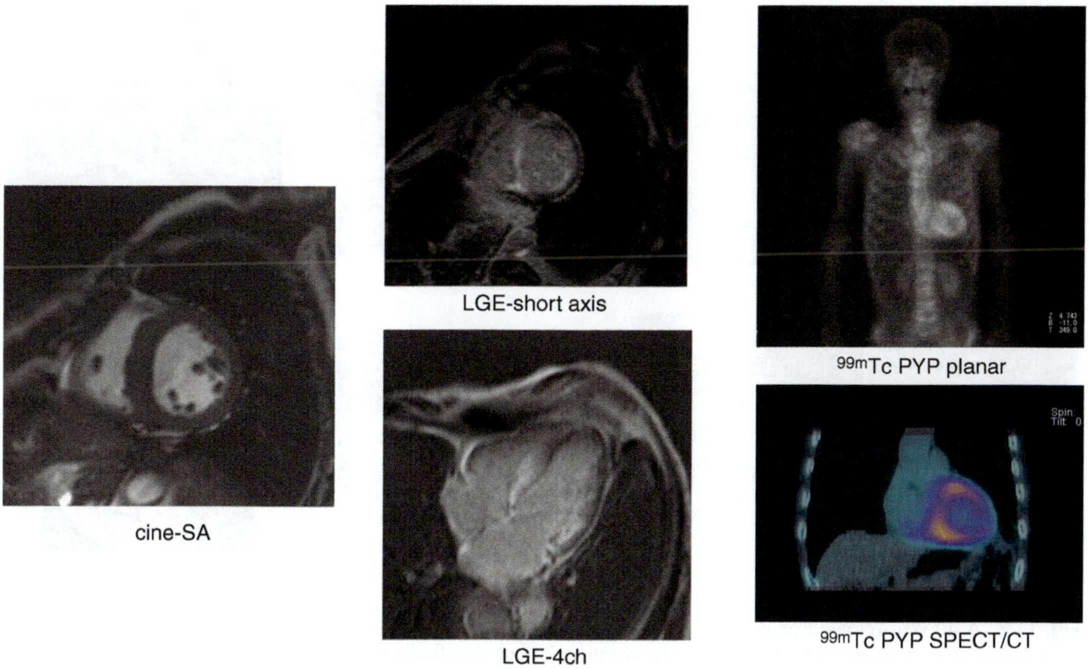

Fig. 11.6 A case of ATTR-type cardiac amyloidosis (CA) is shown. A 84-year-male with heart failure underwent a cardiac exam. Cine MRI showed significant asymmetrical septal hypertrophy, and delayed enhancement revealed diffuse but partially high signal intensity in the septal and lateral wall in the left ventricle (left and middle). Myocardial PYP scintigraphy showed remarkable uptake in the myocardium, and myocardial/contralateral lung ratio was calculated over 2.0 which strongly indicated ATTR-type CA (right upper). Cardiac PYP SPECT/CT revealed heterogeneous myocardial uptake in the left ventricle as shown in CMR delayed enhancement (right lower)

diffuse hypokinesis in LV motion, without significant delayed enhancement.

Case 8

Several HCM cases reveal cardiac failure with significant systolic dysfunction, known as dilated phase of HCM (dHCM), and mostly show asymmetrically hypertrophied myocardium with impaired wall performance. Significant delayed enhancement is observed in hypertrophied myocardium. In comparison of myocardial perfusion (^{201}TL) and fatty acid metabolism (^{123}I-β-methyl-P-iodophenyl-pentadecanoic acid [BMIPP]) imaging, significant perfusion-metabolism mismatch can be observed in the area of hypertrophied and damaged myocardium. A myocardial perfusion-metabolism mismatch is frequently observed in nonischamic cardiomyopathy [38, 40]. Figure 11.8 represents a typical case of dHCM. A 45-year-old male with heart failure underwent CMR. CMR showed remarkable asymmetrical septal hypertrophy with reduced global function and enlarged LV cavity. LGE demonstrated extensive patchy and layer patterns of LGE with mid-wall distribution. TL-BMIPP dual SPECT revealed a patchy perfusion defect and BMIPP showed a more severe defect in the anterior and inferior region were corresponding to fibrosis, indicating perfusion-metabolism mismatch.

11.4 Closing Remarks

The utilization of multimodality imaging and hybrid assessment continues to be a promising technique for a comprehensive approach to manage cardiac disease, including accurate diagnosis

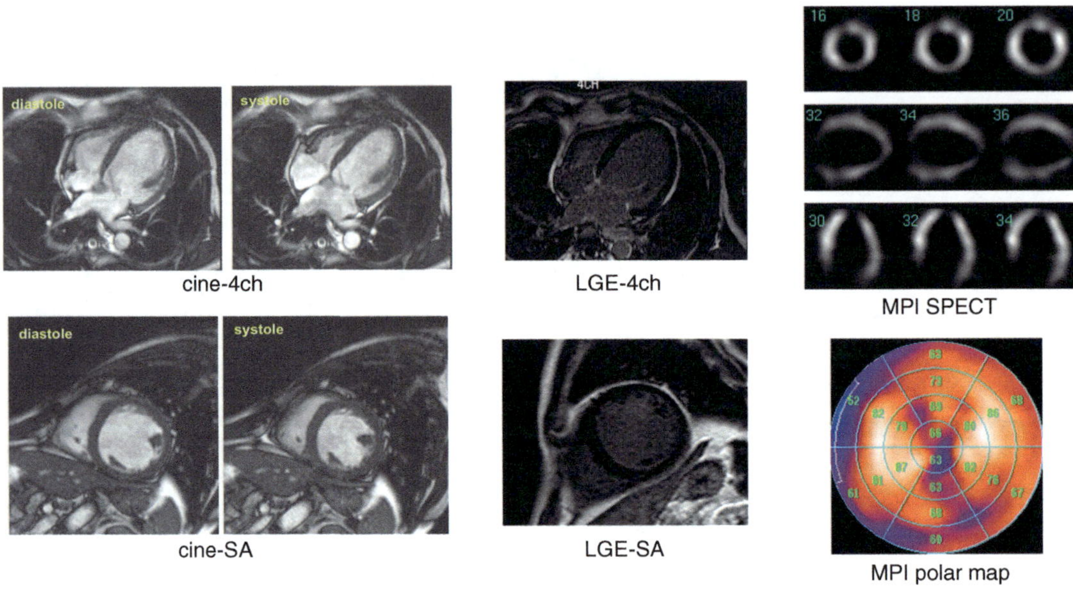

Fig. 11.7 A 40-year-female was hospitalized with acute heart failure. Coronary angiography showed no coronary atherosclerosis with reduced cardiac function. CMR revealed diffuse hypokinesis in LV motion, without delayed enhancement (middle). Myocardial perfusion SPECT demonstrated patchy and mild hypo uptake without significant defect with dilated LV cavity (right). This case was histologically diagnosed as idiopathic dilated cardiomyopathy

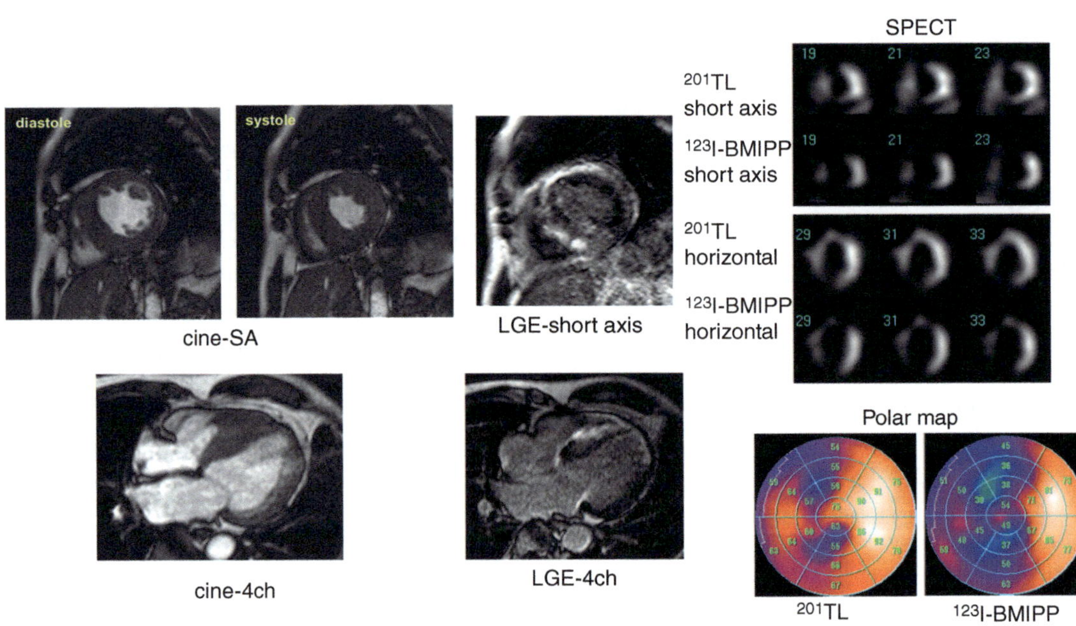

Fig. 11.8 A 45-year-old male with heart failure underwent CMR. CMR showed remarkable asymmetrical septal hypertrophy with reduced global function and enlarged LV cavity (left). LGE demonstrated extensive patchy and layer patterns of LGE with mid-wall distribution (middle). TL-BMIPP dual SPECT revealed patchy perfusion defect and BMIPP showed a more severe defect in the anterior and inferior region were corresponding to fibrosis (right upper and lower)

and prediction, and technological innovation has the promising future potential for personalized care.

Acknowledgments We thank Shintaro Nakano M.D., Takatomo Nakajima M.D., Atsushi Yamamoto M.D., and Risako Nakao M.D. for significant assistance with clinical images.

References

1. Mensah GA, Wei GS, Sorlie PD, Fine LJ, Rosenberg Y, Kaufmann PG, Mussolino ME, Hsu LL, Addou E, Engelgau MM, Gordon D. Decline in cardiovascular mortality: possible causes and implications. Circ Res. 2017;120:366–80.
2. Al-Lamee R, Jacobs AK. The ISCHEMIA trial: was it worth the wait? Circulation. 2020;142(6):517–9.
3. Tonino PA, De Bruyne B, Pijls NH, Siebert U, Ikeno F, van't Veer M, Klauss V, Manoharan G, Engstrom T, Oldroyd KG, Ver Lee PN, MacCarthy PA, Fearon WF, FAME Study Investigators. Fractional flow reserve versus angiography for guiding percutaneous coronary intervention. N Engl J Med. 2009;360:213–24.
4. Shaw LJ, Narula J. Risk assessment and predictive value of coronary artery disease testing. J Nucl Med. 2009;50:1296–306.
5. Rizvi A, Han D, Danad I, Ó Hartaigh B, Lee JH, Gransar H, Stuijfzand WJ, Roudsari HM, Park MW, Szymonifka J, Chang HJ, Jones EC, Knaapen P, Lin FY, Min JK, Pena JM. Diagnostic performance of hybrid cardiac imaging methods for assessment of obstructive coronary artery disease compared with stand-alone coronary computed tomography angiography: a meta-analysis. JACC Cardiovasc Imaging. 2018;11;589–99.
6. Chen MY, Rochitte CE, Arbab-Zadeh A, Dewey M, George RT, Miller JM, Niinuma H, Yoshioka K, Kitagawa K, Sakuma H, Laham R, Vavere AL, Cerci RJ, Mehra VC, Nomura C, Kofoed KF, Jinzaki M, Kuribayashi S, Scholte AJ, Laule M, Tan SY, Hoe J, Paul N, Rybicki FJ, Brinker JA, Arai AE, Matheson MB, Cox C, Clouse ME, Di Carli MF, Lima JAC. Prognostic value of combined CT angiography and myocardial perfusion imaging versus invasive coronary angiography and nuclear stress perfusion imaging in the prediction of major adverse cardiovascular events: the CORE320 multicenter study. Radiology. 2017;284:55–65.
7. Klein R, Celiker-Guler E, Rotstein BH, deKemp RA. PET and SPECT tracers for myocardial perfusion imaging. Semin Nucl Med. 2020;50:208–18.
8. Andreini D, Conte E, Mushtaq S. Cardiac hybrid imaging for the management of patients with known or suspected coronary artery disease. Int J Cardiol. 2018;261:236–8.
9. Even-Sapir E, Keidar Z, Bar-Shalom R. Hybrid imaging (SPECT/CT and PET/CT)—improving the diagnostic accuracy of functional/metabolic and anatomic imaging. Semin Nucl Med. 2009;39:264–75.
10. Pazhenkottil AP, Benz DC, Grani C, Madsen MA, Mikulicic F, von Felten E, Fuchs TA, Moch BH, Stehli J, Luscher TF, Gaemperli O, Buechel RR, Kaufmann PA. Hybrid SPECT perfusion imaging and coronary CT angiography: long-term prognostic value for cardiovascular outcomes. Radiology. 2018;288:694–702.
11. Piccinelli M. Multimodality image fusion, moving forward. J Nucl Cardiol. 2020;27:973–5.
12. Huang B, Yang F, Yin M, Mo X, Zhong C. A review of multimodal medical image fusion techniques. Comput Math Methods Med. 2020;2020:8279342.
13. Moss AJ, Williams MC, Newby DE, Nicol ED. The updated NICE guidelines: cardiac CT as the first-line test for coronary artery disease. Curr Cardiovasc Imaging Rep. 2017;10:15.
14. Conte E, Sonck J, Mushtaq S, Collet C, Mizukami T, Barbato E, Tanzilli A, Nicoli F, De Bruyne B, Andreini D. FFRCT and CT perfusion: a review on the evaluation of functional impact of coronary artery stenosis by cardiac CT. Int J Cardiol. 2020;300:289–96.
15. Kiaos A, Tziatzios I, Hadjimiltiades S, Karvounis C, Karamitsos TD. Diagnostic performance of stress perfusion cardiac magnetic resonance for the detection of coronary artery disease: a systematic review and meta-analysis. Int J Cardiol. 2018;252:229–33.
16. Poon M, Fuster V, Fayad Z. Cardiac magnetic resonance imaging: a "one-stop-shop" evaluation of myocardial dysfunction. Curr Opin Cardiol. 2002;17:663–70.
17. Underwood SR, de Bondt P, Flotats A, Marcasa C, Pinto F, Schaefer W, Verberne HJ. The current and future status of nuclear cardiology: a consensus report. Eur Heart J Cardiovasc Imaging. 2014;15:949–55.
18. Hachamovitch R, Berman DS, Kiat H, Cohen I, Friedman JD, Shaw LJ. Value of stress myocardial perfusion single photon emission computed tomography in patients with normal resting electrocardiograms: an evaluation of incremental prognostic value and cost-effectiveness. Circulation. 2002;105:823–9.
19. Hachamovitch R, Berman DS, Shaw LJ, Kiat H, Cohen I, Cabico JA, Friedman J, Diamond GA. Incremental prognostic value of myocardial perfusion single photon emission computed tomography for the prediction of cardiac death: differential stratification for risk of cardiac death and myocardial infarction. Circulation. 1998;97:535–43.
20. Golzar Y, Doukky R. Stress SPECT myocardial perfusion imaging in end-stage renal disease. Curr Cardiovasc Imaging Rep. 2017;10:13.
21. Yoda S, Nakanishi K, Tano A, Kasamaki Y, Kunimoto S, Matsumoto N, Sato Y, Hirayama A. Risk stratification of cardiovascular events in patients at all stages of chronic kidney disease using myocardial perfusion SPECT. J Cardiol. 2012;60:377–82.

22. Driessen RS, Raijmakers PG, Stuijfzand WJ, Knaapen P. Myocardial perfusion imaging with PET. Int J Cardiovasc Imaging. 2017;33:1021–31.
23. Gaemperli O, Kaufmann PA, Alkadhi H. Cardiac hybrid imaging. Eur J Nucl Med Mol Imaging. 2014;41(Suppl 1):S91–S103.
24. Livieratos L. Technical pitfalls and limitations of SPECT/CT. Semin Nucl Med. 2015;45:530–40.
25. Manabe O, Kikuchi T, Scholte A, El Mahdiui M, Nishii R, Zhang MR, Suzuki E, Yoshinaga K. Correction to: radiopharmaceutical tracers for cardiac imaging. J Nucl Cardiol. 2018;25:1237–41.
26. Kurata A, Kono A, Sakamoto T, Kido T, Mochizuki T, Higashino H, Abe M, Coenen A, Saru-Chelu RG, de Feyter PJ, Krestin GP, Nieman K. Quantification of the myocardial area at risk using coronary CT angiography and Voronoi algorithm-based myocardial segmentation. Eur Radiol. 2015;25:49–57.
27. Montalto S, Better N. Assessing severity of cardiac sarcoid: is SUV the answer? J Nucl Cardiol. 2020;27(6):2011–6.
28. Ruberg FL, Grogan M, Hanna M, Kelly JW, Maurer MS. Transthyretin amyloid cardiomyopathy. JACC state-of-the-art review. J Am Coll Cardiol. 2019;73:2872–91.
29. Sasaki T, Hansford R, Zviman MM, Kolandaivelu A, Bluemke DA, Berger RD, Calkins H, Halperin HR, Nazarian S. Quantitative assessment of artifacts on cardiac magnetic resonance imaging of patients with pacemakers and implantable cardioverter-defibrillators. Circ Cardiovasc Imaging. 2011;4:662–70.
30. Lee SP, Lee ES, Choi H, Im HJ, Koh Y, Lee MH, Kwon JH, Paeng JC, Kim HK, Cheon GJ, Kim YJ, Kim I, Yoon SS, Seo JW, Sohn DW. 11C-Pittsburgh B PET imaging in cardiac amyloidosis. JACC Cardiovasc Imaging. 2015;8:50–9.
31. Rapezzi C, Quarta CC, Guidalotti PL, Pettinato C, Fanti S, Leone O, Ferlini A, Longhi S, Lorenzini M, Reggiani LB, Gagliardi C, Gallo P, Villani C, Salvi F. Role of (99m)Tc-DPD scintigraphy in diagnosis and prognosis of hereditary transthyretin-related cardiac amyloidosis. JACC Cardiovasc Imaging. 2011;4:659–70.
32. Bokhari S, Shahzad R, Castaño A, Maurer MS. Nuclear imaging modalities for cardiac amyloidosis. J Nucl Cardiol. 2014;21:175–84.
33. Agostini D, Verberne HJ, Burchert W, Knuuti J, Povinec P, Sambuceti G, Unlu M, Estorch M, Banerjee G, Jacobson AF. I-123-mIBG myocardial imaging for assessment of risk for a major cardiac event in heart failure patients: insights from a retrospective European multicenter study. Eur J Nucl Med Mol Imaging. 2008;35:535–46.
34. Jacobson AF, Travin MI. Impact of medications on mIBG uptake, with specific attention to the heart: comprehensive review of the literature. J Nucl Cardiol. 2015;22:980–93.
35. Nakajima K, Scholte AJHA, Nakata T, Dimitriu-Leen AC, Chikamori T, Vitola JV, Yoshinaga K. Cardiac sympathetic nervous system imaging with 123I-metaiodobenzylguanidine: perspectives from Japan and Europe. J Nucl Cardiol. 2017;24:952–60.
36. Hassan N, Escanye JM, Juilliere Y, Marie PY, David N, Olivier P, Ayalew A, Karcher G, Stolz JF, Bertrand A. 201Tl SPECT abnormalities, documented at rest in dilated cardiomyopathy, are related to a lower than normal myocardial thickness but not to an excess in myocardial wall stress. J Nucl Med. 2002;43:451–7.
37. Wu Y-W, Yen R-F, Chieng P-U, Huang P-J. Tl-201 myocardial SPECT in differentiation of ischemic from nonischemic dilated cardiomyopathy in patients with left ventricular dysfunction. J Nucl Cardiol. 2003;10:369–74.
38. Tadamura E, Kudoh T, Hattori N, Inubushi M, Magata Y, Konishi J, Matsumori A, Nohara R, Sasayama S, Yoshibayashi M, Tamaki N. Impairment of BMIPP uptake precedes abnormalities in oxygen and glucose metabolism in hypertrophic cardiomyopathy. J Nucl Med. 1998;39:390–6.
39. Fukushima K, Nagao M, Yamamoto A, Serizawa N, Ishizaki U, Suzuki A, Sakai A, Watanabe E, Momose M, Abe K. Discrepancy between significant fibrosis and active inflammation in patients with cardiac sarcoidosis: combined and image fusion analysis of cardiac magnetic resonance and 18F fluorodeoxyglucose positron emission tomography. Eur J Hybrid Imaging. 2019;3:9.
40. Momose M, Fukushima K, Kondo C, Serizawa N, Suzuki A, Abe K, Hagiwara N, Sakai S. Diagnosis and detection of myocardial injury in active cardiac sarcoidosis—significance of myocardial fatty acid metabolism and myocardial perfusion mismatch. Circ J. 2015;79:2669–76.

12 Hybrid Cardiac Imaging: The Role of Machine Learning and Artificial Intelligence

Jan-Walter Benjamins, Ming Wai Yeung, Alvaro E. Reyes-Quintero, Bram Ruijsink, Pim van der Harst, and Luis Eduardo Juarez-Orozco

12.1 Introduction

The concept of hybrid imaging has long lingered in the minds of cardiovascular and imaging physicians. The benefit of combining imaging modalities has been increasingly demonstrated as it enhances the diagnostic and prognostic value of individual techniques. This synergistic effect could be due to various anatomical features being detected between modalities, but more often complementary anatomical information helps in the evaluation of the imaging results at the functional and molecular levels. Hybrid imaging has become an increasingly popular concept in cardiac imaging in the last decades. Predominantly, hybrid imaging has been evaluated in the combination of myocardial perfusion data from single photon (SPECT) and positron-emission computed tomography (PET) with coronary artery anatomy from computed tomography (CT), and myocardial metabolism imaging with PET with tissue characterization through cardiac magnetic resonance (CMR). On the other hand, invasive imaging has evolved to deliver complex anatomical-functional mapping for arrhythmia detection and modern analysis in angiographic images is on its way to deliver functional parameters with increasing ease. Ultimately, it is expected that the expanding hybrid imaging gamut will provide high-quality information to improve clinical decision-making.

While the technical feasibility is established, the time and labor consumed in processing and interpretation of the vast and increasing volume of data remains the major challenge of this era. It is within this landscape that the implementation of modern machine learning (ML)-based artificial intelligence (AI) has gravitated towards medical image analysis. ML offers the possibility to explore, integrate, and analyze massive amounts

J.-W. Benjamins
Department of Cardiology, University of Groningen, University Medical Center Groningen, Groningen, The Netherlands

M. W. Yeung · P. van der Harst · L. E. Juarez-Orozco (✉)
Department of Cardiology, Heart and Lung Division, University Medical Center Utrecht, Utrecht, The Netherlands

Department of Cardiology, University of Groningen, University Medical Center Groningen, Groningen, The Netherlands

A. E. Reyes-Quintero
Electrocardiology, National Institute of Cardiology "Ignacio Chávez", Mexico City, Mexico

B. Ruijsink
Department of Cardiology, Heart and Lung Division, University Medical Center Utrecht, Utrecht, The Netherlands

Department of Adult and Paediatric Cardiology, School of Biomedical Engineering and Imaging Sciences, King's College London, London, UK

F. Nudi et al. (eds.), *Hybrid Cardiac Imaging for Clinical Decision-Making*, https://doi.org/10.1007/978-3-030-99391-7_12

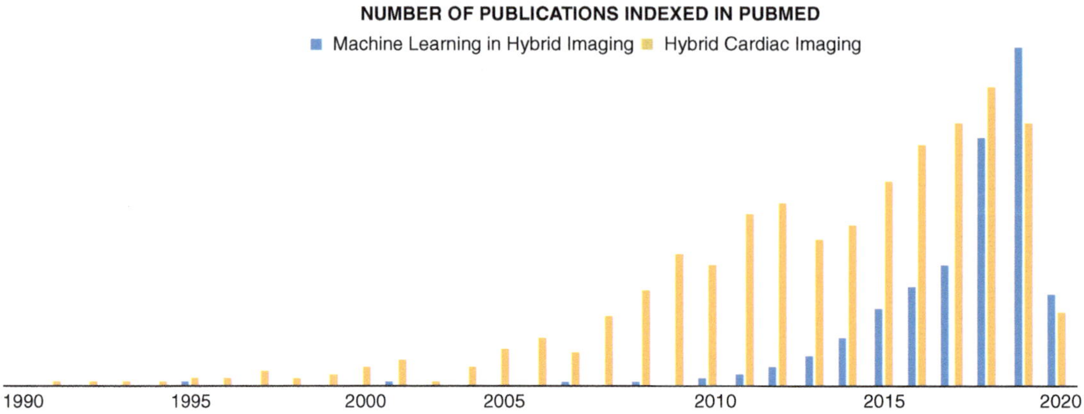

Fig. 12.1 Number of publications per year found in Medline. Mesh Terms and Keywords "Hybrid Cardiac Imaging" (yellow) and "Machine Learning in Hybrid Imaging" (blue). Both topics have witnessed an increase in publications, but more rapid growth has been seen in hybrid cardiac imaging

of data through its complex nonlinear dependencies, which notably are generally not fully exploited by traditional statistical modeling. In this sense, (cardiovascular) imaging represents a logical target for such analytics, given the gauge of its information stream. Figure 12.1 shows the number of publications indexed with the topics "Hybrid Cardiac Imaging" or "Machine Learning in Hybrid Imaging" in the last three decades in the literature database PubMed.

In this chapter, we present core concepts in modern machine learning-based AI. Further, we discuss recent advances with respect to data processing, image analysis, result interpretation, and clinical decision support within the context of (hybrid) cardiovascular imaging through a selected body of scientific work. Finally, we summarize the applicability and the envisioned potential of machine learning-based AI in daily clinical practice.

12.1.1 Machine Learning-Based AI

Machine learning (ML) is a field in computer science that involves the generation of computer systems (algorithms) that are capable of iteratively learning by exploring and utilizing patterns within data to act specifically, without being explicitly programmed. This process of system adaptation in order to optimize the task at hand (e.g., classification or prediction) mimics biological learning. In contrast, AI refers to the application of such systems with a practically orientated tasks that commonly would require at least human-level intelligence (e.g., driving, playing Go, or making a medical diagnosis).

Notably, neither of these terms is particularly new. In fact, the previous surfacing of AI into the common interest during the 80s and 90s became dampened by the limitations of its underlying algorithms, which depended on explicit programming (i.e., rule-based instead of learning-based). The original roots of ML and AI, as well as the concept of programmable learning, date to half a century ago and have only recently resurfaced their current new era is due to the convergence of three crucial forces, namely: large amounts of available data for robust-scale learning iterations, increasing computational power with parallel processors making the necessary operations time-feasible (i.e., Current graphic processing units or GPUs), and the innovation in the architecture and complexity of dedicated ML algorithms thus the substrate, the engine, and the fuel.

ML can be divided into three main types based on how the system "experience" is acquired: supervised learning, unsupervised learning, and reinforcement learning. Supervised learning algorithms take a set of examples (training set) and ask the model to learn to pick up the features that are associated with specific labels in these examples. For instance, a classification model learns to predict skin cancer with images labeled by dermatologists [1]. In comparison, unsupervised learning algorithms do not restrict the learning trajectory with labels but instead ask the model to organize the data based on features crafted by the model itself, allowing it to identify patterns within the dataset. This approach may be particularly useful in exploring high-dimensional data for complex patterns such as nonlinear relationships that may translate novel structures previously unknown and relevant to the task at hand without the constraints of a strictly defined output. This has demonstrated value in the clustering of genomic or radiomic features in cancer samples to reveal subtype characteristics [2, 3]. Finally, reinforcement learning takes emphasis on learning through interaction within an environment. In the case of reinforcement, the model, often termed an agent, navigates in a specific environment, and performs self-initiated actions for which it is subsequently rewarded or penalized; with the aim to maximize the cumulative rewards the agent learns to solve the target task in the respective context (the predefined environment). Reinforcement learning is typically applied to tackle evolving problems, updated through interaction with environment, such as playing video or board games. In the medical field, reinforcement learning has been proposed to optimize therapeutic regimes which may be modified based on patient response [4, 5].

There is a myriad of ML algorithms that can be employed depending on task complexity and intrinsic data characteristics such as dimensionality, operationalization nature, and composition. Figure 12.2 summarizes the discussed types of learning, exemplar algorithm (see description below), and their potential application sphere in (hybrid) cardiovascular imaging.

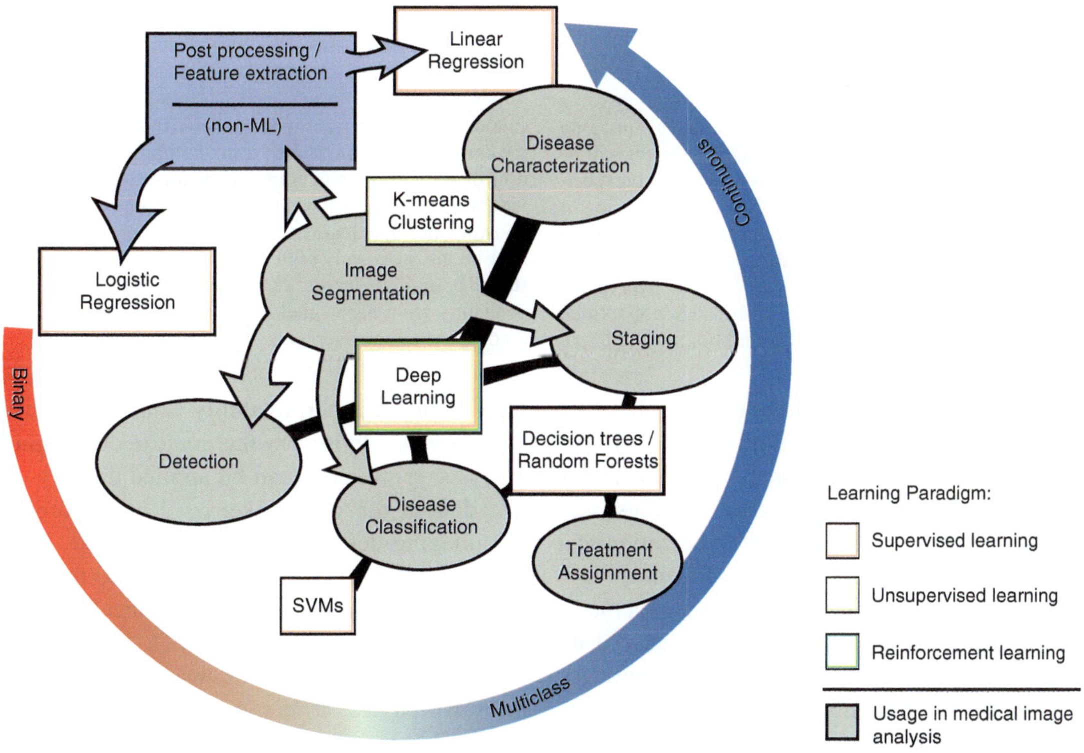

Fig. 12.2 Overview of types of ML and their usages in Medical Imaging. A wide range of ML techniques are available, each serving a narrower or broader range of purposes in medical imaging and contingent upon the type of input data. DL has a growing relevance in medical imaging processing. Segmentation represents a central task in this spectrum of DL applications, providing directly extractable automated measurements, but also functions as a first block to provide inputs for other DL models in (hybrid) chains of models for disease classification, staging, characterization, and detection of structural abnormalities

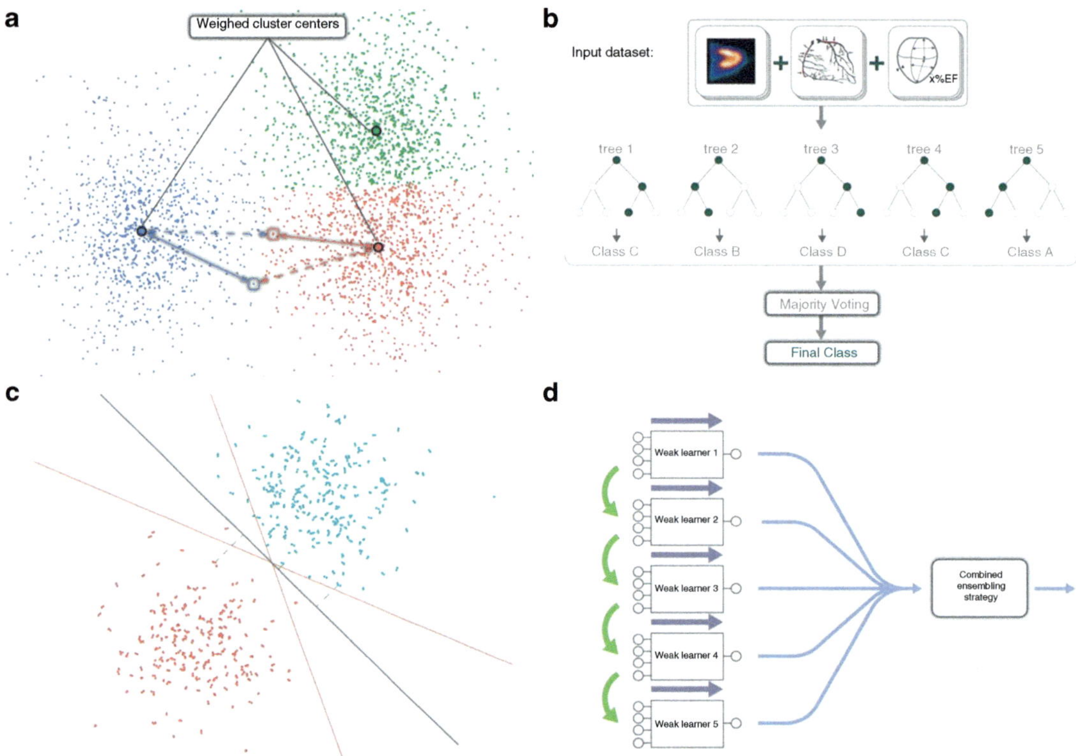

Fig. 12.3 Types of ML found in medical imaging explained. (**a**) k-means clustering: each data point will be assigned to a cluster with the closest center in a prespecified feature space such as anatomical characteristics of cardiovascular structures; (**b**) random forest: features can be submitted for construction of decision trees to arrive at an ensembled model; (**c**) SVM: an optimal hyperplane (black) that separate two classes is estimated, nonoptimal hyperplanes shown in red; (**d**) Ensembling: multiple so-called "weak learners," trained to solve the same problem, are combined into a weighed result combining the prediction of each learner to improve performance over individual ones. Different strategies can be chosen, e.g., in boosting, multiple learners are trained sequentially dependent on the previously built learner, while in bagging and stacking, multiple learners are trained in parallel and independently from each other. One strategy to combine the predictions can be averaging or voting

A distinctive commonality between ML algorithms is that they seek to minimize the error of the model expressed by some type of cost (or loss) function. Alternatively, this means that learning progresses through the optimization of a specified driving function (or set of them).

Traditional modeling techniques seen in medical imaging analysis include linear and logistic regression (which notably also represent ML approaches by definition), decision trees and its ensemble version known as random forests, support vector machines (SVM), k-means clustering (Fig. 12.3), and several types of deep neural networks (vide infra) (Fig. 12.4).

The reason behind the popularity of linear and logistic regression in medical research is their arguable interpretability and ease-of-use and implementation. In the context of imaging analysis, regressions can be applied directly on raw data at the pixel/voxel-level or performed on imaging-derived variables obtained from pre-processed data, with or without features from other data sources (e.g., clinical or biochemical profile of the patient). However, a known drawback is that as the number of features surpasses a certain threshold (which approximates 1 per 10 cases in a binary output distribution) with respect to the sample size and balance (i.e., number of positive and negative cases to the outcome variable of interest), most features are expected to be non-informative. To exemplify such situation, consider that the num-

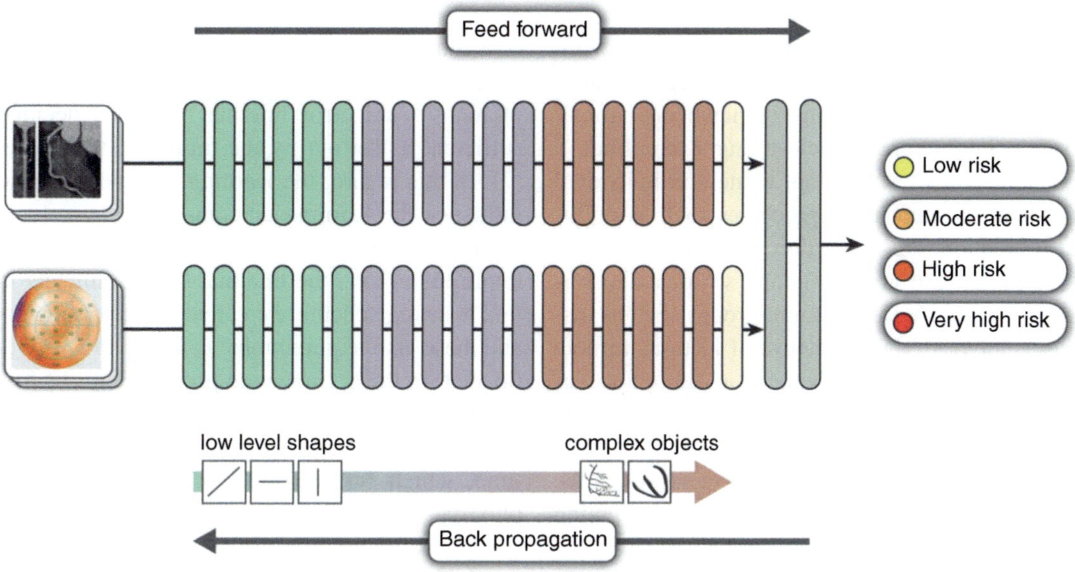

Fig. 12.4 Schematic overview of a deep convolutional neural network. Images from various modalities are submitted to the network in which spatial features on ascending levels of complexity will be learned by the network; the network then combines those features to achieve a defined task (e.g., classification of myocardial ischemia)

ber of background pixels that take up much of a given image poses an unsurmountable difficulty when trying to find the best fitting linear model that allows for flexible interpretation and later generalization to a new input set (image). In such situation, one could consider opting for a regularized form of linear model, namely Ridge, Lasso, and Elastic net regression. Both Ridge and Lasso regression shrink the coefficients of features by applying either an L1 or L2 norm (the cost function) while Elastic net regression takes a combination of both penalty terms, fine-tuned based on the data at hand. Another ML technique known as boosting can be applied to classical statistical models to obtain an improved final model from multiple weaker models or *classifiers* (ensembling).

Decision trees as well as the ensemble of decision trees, termed random forest, are supervised learning methods used to build classifiers for typically discrete outcomes. As suggested in the name, decision trees resemble a flowchart with a set of splits that can be used to determine the class label for each new incoming data point, step by step through the tree. The set of decision rules and respective positions in the tree are selected and optimized using a labeled training set. The main advantage of the decision tree is its interpretability as it mirrors the natural human decision-making process as in a differential diagnosis or clinical work-up. A random forest is an aggregate of multiple decision trees each built on random resampling of the training set. Alternatively boosting can also be applied to build an ensemble for greater performance.

Support vector machine (SVM) is another popular supervised learning method in which individual data points are first projected in a feature space based on their respective values for the selected features [6]; a hyperplane is then estimated to best separate members of different classes (typically 2 classes). In the context of medical imaging analysis, SVM may be used in disease diagnosis, staging, and prognosis. It should be noted that the performance of an SVM classifier depends substantially on the feature space thus processing and preselection of radiomic features may be necessary.

K-means clustering belongs to the unsupervised learning paradigm. With a preselected number of clusters (k), every data point will be assigned membership to one closest randomly initiated cluster center (mean of the cluster) in k-means clustering; as the cluster centers get updated with new members, the computations are repeated until convergence (i.e., no change in membership for all data points). K-means clustering exemplifies a phenomenon we should not witness in individual development-dependent processes such as political affiliation. This algorithm can be used to organize pixels into groups (image segmentation) as well as organize samples into groups such as disease subtypes. There are several features to note when applying this technique: as the choice of "k"—number of clusters will lead to a different result, an assumption on the structure of the dataset has to be made and sensitivity analyses of the resulting clusters' robustness, such as computing cluster silhouette, may be warranted.

Deep (convolutional and other types of) artificial neural networks, for which the term Deep Learning (DL) has recently been coined, are a subclass of ML which models that can be trained under every learning paradigm. A typical neural network is composed of layers of processing units (i.e., perceptrons, and consequently traditionally called multilayer perceptrons) which mimic biological neurons. In these structures, each unit receives an input from units at a previous layer and reacts to cumulative signals by activation or lack thereof and emission of a signal towards neurons at the next layer (in a feedforward network). This emission was originally controlled by nonlinear activation functions such as a sigmoid function. Due to the limited range in the gradient of the sigmoid function which results in difficulty in optimization, it is in practice replaced by alternatives such as rectified linear units (ReLU), which output the positive cumulative input and zero otherwise, or a leaky version ReLU where a negative input would be assigned a small output. The units between two neighboring layers are connected and the strength of these connections (often called weights) is adjusted during training. With sufficient data to tune the weights, typically in the magnitude of millions, a DL model learns how to transform the data and automatically extract features to solve a specific (e.g., classification) task. Unlike typical linear/logistic regression models where solution of a single global minimum error (point of convergence) is possible (with mean square error as the cost function), DL models require iterative optimization by gradient-based methods towards one of many local error minima, which is deemed sufficient as set out by the trainer of the model [7]. In this regard, the learning scheme will also influence the learning outcome, whether a local minimum (which minimum) can be reached, time required to reach the minima, etc. Parameters in this learning scheme are called hyperparameters and these also require tuning (often with a validation set) in the optimization process (Fig. 12.5).

Optimization of a DL model is hence expensive in terms of both computational resources and time, which further scales with network complexity. As mentioned previously, technological advancements in the form of GPUs has enabled relatively fast training of highly complex neural networks, and consequently DL has shown tremendous revolutionizing success in the field of computer vision since last decade. DL was shown to outperform other ML methods in image recognition. DL is now widely adapted for solving tasks in many different fields such as natural language processing, speech recognition, and bioinformatics. As medical imaging analysis shares many tasks with computer vision including object detection, classification, image segmentation, and enhancement, this field has seen an explosion in the use of DL. A selection of the body of reports available will be further discussed here.

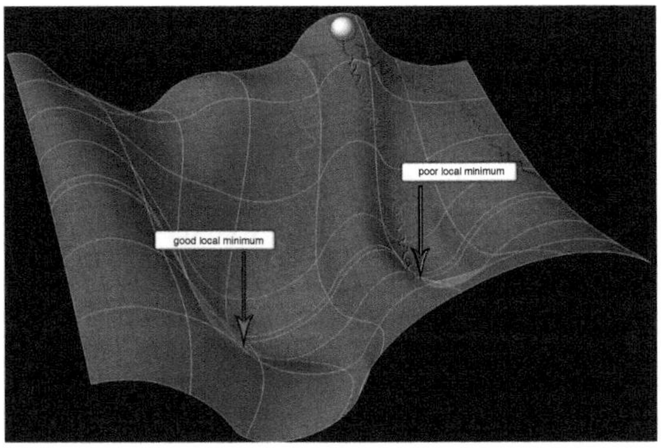

Fig. 12.5 Optimization in DL with convergent to a better or worse local minimum. Learning process of DL involves iterative reduction of the loss function until a local minimum is arrived using gradient-based algorithms. The hyperparameters in the learning scheme may have a great impact on the learning trajectory, and consequently, on which local minimum is arrived

12.1.2 ML in Cardiovascular Imaging Analysis

ML classification models have already been developed to automatically detect or differentiate between imaging views (axis). For example, Khamis et al. applied label consistent K-singular value decomposition, a discriminative learning dictionary technique [8]. This linear algebra method decomposes a complex matrix (such as a digital image) in multiple unitary matrices and a diagonal matrix that is uniquely determined by the complex matrix.

A typical example of modern ML techniques is the application of (convolutional) DL to improve time efficiency during image interpretation by humans. Zhang et al. demonstrated this approach for multiple tasks in the automated processing of ultrasound images, including view detection, chamber segmentation and detection of hypertrophic cardiomyopathy (HCM), cardiac amyloid, and pulmonary arterial hypertension [9].

Another use for ML implemented in numerical data (i.e., echocardiography-derived structured data) is exemplified by Cikes et al. They proposed an unsupervised ML algorithm that integrates both clinical and complex echocardiographic data acquired in heart failure patients, that could be used for identification of patients that are likely to respond well to cardiac resynchronization therapy [10]. Inputs for the model are combined volumetric, strain and tissue-deformation sequences extracted from 2D echo imaging and a range of variables, extracted from patient demographics, clinical variables, laboratory measurement, use of medications, and functional variables derived from ECG and echo. The algorithm uses a sequence of multiple kernel learning for dimensional reduction and k-means clustering for the eventual "phenogrouping" of patients. Cox proportional hazard analysis of the differences between left ventricular end-diastolic volume index before therapy and 1 year after treatment showed significant differences between the groups.

A wide range of variation in DL network architectures, such as ResNet [11, 12], AlexNet [13], and DenseNet [14, 15], have been implemented for medical imaging. However, a comparison of different architectures by Blaivas et al. has demonstrated that newer architectures that improve on different ML model tasks in other fields, may not always show improved performance when applied in medical imaging [16]. In their research, different types of models were compared, when trained for the classification of views in cardiac imaging. Even though hyperparameter-optimization details were not specified in this publication, (implying limitations in terms of reproducibility and verifiability common to most of the studies of the kind published in medical journals) this paper touches upon an important aspect of applying emerging novel algorithms within the space of medical imaging. With most of all medical images being constructed from tomographic image capturing and carrying a single grayscale brightness channel, medical images differ fundamentally from photorealistic images for which most network architectures have been developed. Medical images also display structures by local variations in brightness, thereby containing edges and surfaces, utilized by DL architectures. Contrarily, while image details may be limited in channel count, 3D medical imaging techniques such as CT can substantially add to the tomographic nature of more basic imaging modalities. Data contained in 3D images exceed the information flow provided by the flattened 2D photographs produced by regular cameras and smartphones. It is therefore important to select an adequate architecture with correct characteristics for capturing the target region(s) of interest (for instance, specific cardiovascular substructures) and to thoughtfully adapt architectures to accommodate the tomographic nature of medical images. The greatest lesson drawn from this research is that eager advances in DL implementations should always be balanced with sensitive deliberation of their actual adequateness and relation.

DL has also been used to classify image orientations [17], by dividing those into four classes according to 0-, 90-, 180-, and 270-degree rotations. Albeit this application may only be useful in the extraordinary absence of image metadata, as produced by imaging modality instances, this research demonstrates that DL can distinguish between differently oriented examples of the same cardiac view, a complex task in traditional computer vision that may link to improvements in hybrid image fusion.

Another approach to time-efficiency improvement in data analysis is focusing on the delineation of cardiac images, which may be quite labor-intensive as suggested by the fact that most cardiac images are ultimately never annotated if only manual delineation tools are available. Whether there is potential diagnostic gain to be sought is still an open matter.

Segmentation models have been developed for fully automatic delineation of cardiac chambers on CMR [18, 19] and to derive secondary measurements during post-processing, such as cavity volume, tissue masse, wall thickness, and ejection fraction [20, 21]. Most of these implementations are based on the U-NET architecture that was developed especially for the segmentation of medical images [22]. Further variations on this architecture have been developed, such as V-NET [23] which improves on U-NET through the implementation of residual functions, inspired by ResNet [24] or Ω-NET, which offers specific advantages in terms of improved segmentation and predictive power on multiple cardiac views within a single model, without prior knowledge about the presented view [19]. Segmentation optimization through ML has also been applied in coronary arteries and myocardium in CT angiography [25, 26] and in measurement automation for intima-media thicknesses on carotid ultrasound images [27].

Liu et al. developed a 3D DL model for the detection of malignant tumors in pulmonary CT, using multiple slices to construct a spatial representation of a nodule, to be then classified for malignancy by the network. DL-based models like these have found their way to software applications with FDA clearance for use in the clinical setting.

Similar DL designs have been proposed for the prediction of calcium scores. Wolterink et al. have reported on DL-predicted calcium scores from cardiac CT images, with a 0.944 (95% CI: 0.918–0.962) intra class correlation coefficient in comparison to traditional calcium scoring [28]. A paired DL architecture was used, where one convolutional network accounted for extraction of voxels of interest (VOI) from the source CT image and a second one was trained to predict the calcium score on the extracted VOI. Two different architectures consisting of 2.5D and 3D architectures were compared to assess volumetric cardiac structures, using triplane (axial, sagittal, and coronal) inputs for the 2.5D CNN and 3D volumetric data as input for the 3D CNN architectures, showing a slightly better sensitivity of 0.72 over 0.71 for the 2.5D architecture. Further, an improvement in either architecture was demonstrated by the implementation of ensembles of CNNs with different input sizes and dimensionalities.

Lessmann et al. proposed another combined CNN architecture for calcium scoring, in this case on low-dose chest CTs that were initially acquired for cancer research [29]. In their proposal, the first of two CNN models was not used for extraction of VOIs, but to perform preselection of smaller subregions that potentially contain calcified areas. A second CNN was then used to perform the calcium scoring on those preselected areas.

Notably, these advances in ML implementation on cardiovascular imaging have exclusively dealt in terms of single data sources/types for specific established tasks in daily imaging practice. And much in the same way that individual cardiac imaging techniques have been optimized and then introduced into the conceptual realm of hybrid imaging (vide infra), the ML horizon has arguably expanded into both the combination of algorithms applied in a single workflow and the combination of data sources (e.g., clinical and imaging) for task optimization to exploit the value of individual types of models. Expanding from basic segmentation, for instance, Zreik et al. developed a "hybrid" solution for the prediction of myocardial ischemic lesions in CT angiographic imaging by subsequently implementing a convolutional neural network, an autoencoder, and an SVM model [30].

While FFR is currently measured in an invasive procedure with the use of pressure wire and hyperemic stimulus, there has been research in estimating FFR from CTA image bypassing the invasive procedure. With coronary arteries and left ventricular mass segmented, a computational fluid dynamics (CFD) modeling-based estimation is possible. This process is however computationally expensive [31]. Consequently, with the aim to expedite the assessment of CT-derived FFR, Itu et al. synthesized 12,000 artificial coronary trees and their corresponding FFR by combining the computational blood flow model with anatomical assumptions of the cardiovascular structure [32] reflected in 28 features and variations thereof used to train a DL model to predict FFR in independent new CT data. Result from a small set of data from real patients ($n = 87$) showed an almost perfect correlation of DL-estimated FFR and the reference FFR estimated using computational fluid dynamics, indicating successful knowledge transfer to the DL model. With the knowledge structured and stored in the network, estimation of CT-FFR resulted much faster than traditional CFD approaches computing FFR de novo. Nonetheless, while there was an 80-times compression in the estimation of FFR by DL model (2.4 ± 0.44 vs 196.3 ± 78.5 s) data preparation, i.e., generation of the coronary anatomical model for features to be input to DL modeling, required 10–60 min and became a bottleneck that diminished the gained efficiency of that workflow. In this regard, Kumamaru et al. independently proposed a fully automated workflow in which the data preparation step would be replaced also by the ML model. More specifically, they proposed a hybrid of 2D convolutional generative adversarial (cGAN), a 3D convolutional ladder, and a fully connected neural network for automated estimation of minimum FFR [33]. Both (convolutional) autoencoders (CAE) and cGANs can be used to generate the desired image but they differ in the learning strategy: an autoencoder learns to convert the input to desired output with a set of mathematical operations fixed and stored in the trained network; while GAN learns to generate output that would appear to be as close as a real output that the competing discriminator network would not be able to differentiate it. One key philosophy in GANs is that the generator network must learn the underlying distribution of the data in order to perform well enough to "fool" the discriminator. The generative nature might allow GANs to potentially outperform autoencoder architectures which would be restricted by the provided training set. The authors argue their results improve on prior because their method utilizes input from coronary CT imaging, which seems to be more informational than the accumulated data from different myocardial views.

Notably, the performance of the automatic workflow may not yet be compared to simpler DL models which utilized radiomic features pre-engineered by experts [10, 32, 34]. Table 12.1 summarizes the oriented tasks for which DL has the capacity to optimize workflows and performance.

Table 12.1 Main tasks optimized through DL in cardiac imaging analysis

Task	Description	Example usage in medical image analysis
Object detection	Recognition of target objects and their location within an image	Cardiac structure identification and location
Semantic segmentation	Assignation of pixels/voxels in a 2D/3D image into a sensitive class	Segmentation of cardiovascular (sub)structures of interest for quantification and fusion
Classification	Class labeling for each data point based on the input image and its relation to the selected output	View classification in different imaging modalities Coronary artery calcium scoring Cardiovascular disease classification Differentiation of cardiovascular tissues Prognostic evaluation for adverse outcomes from aggregative imaging
Characterization	Feature extraction and pattern exploration from the datasets	Radiomic feature generation

12.2 ML in the Current Context Hybrid Imaging

12.2.1 Data Pre-processing in Hybrid Imaging

Combining information from two different imaging sources, often not directly overlapping in space, time, or dimensions is challenging. The ability to identify complex, nonlinear relations between data is bound to make ML a valuable tool to provide better image preparation, processing, and data fusion in hybrid imaging.

12.2.1.1 Attenuation Map Generation

PET imaging requires attenuation correction (AC) for a reliable quantification of tracer activity. A photon attenuation map for this purpose can be generated by co-registered data from CT or CMR. In simultaneous PET/MR imaging, the MR imaging-based AC (MRAC) is currently generated through a segmentation-based method—with the use of ultrashort echo time (UTE) sequences the image is segmented into soft tissues groups or air for which specific coefficients are then assigned to construct the attenuation map. While some performance gain can be obtained through the addition of bone information (atlas-based) to this method, ML has been recently implemented to this end. Liu et al. explored the utilization of DL for the construction of magnetic resonance-based AC maps [35]. With concurrent PET/CT data in addition to PET/MR data, they trained a fully convolutional autoencoder (CAE) network to generate a pseudo-CT image from an MR image with the true CT image as reference. Thereon, PET images were comparatively reconstructed based on the true CT-based AC, the segmentation-based AC with MR, the atlas-based AC with MR, and the AC based on pseudo-CT produced by DL. The DL model was trained on scans from 30 subjects and all methods were tested on a hold-out set of 10 subjects with the co-registered CT assigned as the reference. DL-based AC resulted in the least construction error among all MR AC methods, while the segmentation-based method was outperformed by all the other methods.

Further, it has been suggested that DL may also be useful in scenarios where other methods are expected to have suboptimal performance. For instance, in the absence of suitable references for the atlas-based method. This was explored in a study by Ladefoged et al. on a group of pediatric patients with cerebral tumors [36] since atlas-based AC was expected to perform poorly as it is based on adult subjects with normal anatomy for which sufficient age-matched pediatric references may not be available. Once again, a DL model was trained to generate a pseudo-CT image for AC which demonstrated better performance than the vendor-provided segmentation-based one, not only on the agreement with the reference AC (by co-registered CT) but also in the clinical metrics characterizing the brain tumors. These results hint at the potential clinical benefit of optimizing a basic processing step in advanced imaging (AC) by means of powerful ML analytics such as DL.

Notably, the aforementioned studies were conducted on neurological imaging, while the same approach can be adapted for cardiovascular purposes. The transferability and relevance DL-based AC requires validation in the context of cardiac imaging. And a recent study by Shi et al. has explored the notion of directly generating attenuation maps for SPECT by encapsulating the complementary information across modalities gathered in cardiac SPECT/CT [37]. Taking the CT-based attenuation map as labels and SPECT scans (from photopeak window and scatter window), the authors trained two types of DL architectures, a fully CAE as well as GAN by addition of a competing discriminator network. In the current study by Shi et al., no significant difference was found between the autoencoder and GAN in the generation of attenuation, i.e., SPECT reconstructed using AC from both architectures using both primary and scatter window inputs were consistent with the CT-based AC, but there was a substantial bias for the autoencoder architecture if only primary window input was supplied which might be related to a limited mapping capacity resulted from the reduced input space. Albeit the promising results in the study, it is important to note that these DL models are sensitive to training set such that biases created/existing in the training set could propagate to the model which was also evident in the current study—the slightly worse performance in female subjects might be attributed to a difference in sex ratio between the training set and test set and there exists indeed an anatomical difference between sex. This suggested extensive finetuning with local data to adapt to the target distribution will be required for such DL models to be useful in clinical practice.

12.2.1.2 Full-Dose Image Estimation from Low Dose Image

Generation of CT image with DL is not limited to AC for emission data. As image denoising using autoencoder is an extensively researched task in the field of computer vision, there is also an interest to transform low-dose CT scan into high-resolution image that would be equivalent to a high dose CT, as dose reduction generally leads to a higher signal-to-noise ratio. There is a clear benefit to patients if the high-resolution CT image could be constructed with lower exposure to radiation. In this regard, it is worthy to point out the potential incremental value of hybrid imaging for image reconstruction with the additional information collected. This was supported by a study by Xiang et al. who estimated normal dose PET image using low-dose PET/MRI data [38]. In this study, the authors trained a relatively simple CNN which is composed of a stack of three blocks of 4 convolutional layers (total depth = 12) on scans from 16 patients. Compared with training on losing dose PET scan alone, training on both low-dose PET and T1 images from MRI resulted in better estimation in all subjects, as assessed in leave-one-out cross-validation. Often, DL-based methods could be easily modified to accept images of different modalities offering an easy way to process data; additionally, the processing time of feedforward networks, the type of network commonly used in computer vision, is often very short. Notably, in the aforementioned study the DL model performed comparably with the state-of-the-art method for standard-dose PET estimation but took only close to 2 s to process each sample and output the estimated PET image as opposed to the state-of-the-art method which took 1008 s in average. In another study by Chen et al., multiple co-registered MR images were combined with a pseudo ultra-low-dose PET image to reconstruct the full-dose image of the brain for amyloid plaque detection (ground truth); the ultra-low-dose images in this study were artificially created through sub-setting the events (100-fold) of the original full-dose image [39]. Again, a fully CAE architecture was used, and the model was trained on a dataset consisting of 32 patients under a fivefold cross-validation setup. Consistent with the previous study, image reconstructed using both MRI and ultra-low-dose PET scan showed the highest similarity to the original PET scan as measured by three typically used metrics (peak signal-to-noise ratio, root mean square error, and structural similarity index measure) among submitting the ultra-low-dose PET scan alone for training and the scan without reconstruction. But perhaps more importantly, the reconstructed image using both MRI and ultra-low-dose PET scan offered higher agreement in clinical assessment with the original full-dose image by the same clinician; in particular, almost all positive cases (22/23 subjects) could be recovered from the reconstructed images using combined input as compared with 20/23 subjects from the reconstructions from PET scan alone. The results from this study showed improvement in the hybrid imaging protocol, in this case lower radiation exposure, which may be optimized with the aid of ML.

12.2.2 ML in Data Integration and Analysis in Hybrid Imaging

Medical images often require post-processing and review by experts to ensure their diagnostic and prognostic role in clinical practice. At the same time, this need also conveys a workload that scales with the number of incoming patients and the complexity of the modality. While expert revision is an important gatekeeper for the quality of the result, parts of the clinical workflow are very much suitable for automation. This allows on the one hand for more efficient use of time and human resources, while on the other it increases reproducibility due to potential interobserver differences.

Within current mainstream hybrid imaging, manual contour adjustment is often required for an accurate estimation of the perfusion values in SPECT/CT. Betancur et al. reported an ML model built with the aim to automate, for example, the localization of the mitral valve plane (VP) during left ventricle segmentation [40]. In their study, a total of 22 plausible features, some derived from the scan while some describe clinical characteristics of the subject (sex), were considered and finally selected based on the ranking in information gain for the construction of an SVM model. Learning from the manual contours by two experts the model, in general, achieved higher correlations with the experts' VP localization in stress images (AC/non-AC) than rest image (AC/non-AC) (Person correlation 0.79–0.90 vs 0.66–0.80); Notably, there was no significant difference regarding the diagnostic values—the SVM model achieved comparable performance in classification of obstructive stenosis with the two experts with a value of 0.8 in AUC by tenfold cross-validation. This showed the potential of ML methods in condensing knowledge and experience from multiple experts and they could be used to aid the clinical practice.

In PET/CT, the acquisition protocol for the CT component is often not optimized for the estimation of calcium score. This implementation could avoid extra radiation if the calcium scoring is estimated directly from the CT images. Išgum et al. investigated such a possibility in a cohort of 133 patients who underwent both myocardial perfusion PET/CT and calcium scoring dedicated CT [41]. After standard imaging processing steps to remove noise, features characterizing candidate calcified lesion describing shape, intensity, and location of the lesion, were computed using the processed CT scans originally for attenuation correction (CT-AC) during PET/CT; an extremely randomized trees model (a decision tree based ensembling method) was then trained on these features to classify each lesion. To examine the model performance in a clinical context, patients were assigned to CVD risk category using the resulting Agatston scores. They reported a high correlation between calcium scores manually estimated from CT-AC by expert and those from the automatic ML-based method (two-way mixed intraclass correlation coefficient: 0.77 at rest and 0.83 at stress, by tenfold cross-validation) with larger disagreements in high calcium scores. Comparing the reference manual scoring with CSCT, both manual and automatic scoring methods using CTAC were underestimated and were statistically different from the reference, indicating the acquisition as the limiting difference. The differences in agreement between the manual and automatic methods were smaller in the assignment of five CVD risk categories—both with over 80% of patients assigned to the correct category. However, the random forest model struggled in patients with high Agatston score and tended to misclassify in the two highest risk groups. The higher variability might account for the weaker performance of the extreme randomized trees model.

Cardiac MR is steadily becoming more present in cardiovascular imaging. It offers comprehensive imaging of the heart over the full cardiac cycle. More importantly, it allows for tissue and blood flow characterization. The latter makes hybrid imaging an appealing prospect in the cardiovascular realm. In hybrid PET/MR, anatomical information and myocardial tissue characteristics are used in to provide a better assessment of PET imaging. Similar to PET/CT, ML techniques can significantly improve image acquisition and analysis in PET/MR. DL algorithms have mostly been applied to provide attenuation maps, in a way similar to the previously described methods for PET/CT. A smaller but interesting branch has focused on joint PET and CMR image reconstruction in order to reduce radiation dosages. Chen et al. [39] used a U-net architecture to synthesize a full-dose PET image from its low-dose priors. By considering the anatomical information of simultaneously acquired MR images, they showed net U-net was able to reconstruct images of similar quality to full-dose PET acquisitions.

Another field of hybrid CMR is the combination of cardiac MR and invasive angiography (XMR). XMR allows for scar-guided atrial ablations [42] and radiation-free assessment of complex hemodynamics in congenital heart diseases [43, 44]. A main challenge of XMR is fast and reliable registration of catheter position or fluoroscopy imaging to the CMR images. Similar to the other image analysis problems, ML techniques can provide significant improvement of the current workflows of image registration. Deep learning registration algorithms have been proposed to learn new similarity metrics for image registration [45, 46] that can be used in conventional registration algorithms, or even perform the full registration process through a DL architecture [47, 48]. Implementation of such techniques for registration in XMR is likely to follow soon.

Emerging visualization techniques such as augmented-, merged-, and virtual-reality that can arguably relate to an updated concept of hybrid imaging, offers the possibility to render information for clinical operators on a screen, a pair of glasses, or a headset. Depending on the exact implementation, information may be presented in combination, or as an overlay of the environment the image information is viewed within. These advancements in visualization techniques may enhance the workflow and tools available in a clinical setting, e.g., in the catheterization lab, providing a 3D representation of the heart while performing an invasive procedure. The use of ML may be crucial to optimally use the data made available synchronously by multiple modalities, by rendering a mapped projection of the perfusion of the coronary arteries or a projection of the exact position of catheters on a real-time, patient-specific 3D rendering of the heart [49].

Notably, electroanatomic mapping (EAM) represents an area where developments in hybrid imaging, in its traditional sense, have continued parallelly to those in the cardiovascular imaging areas more logistically related to radiology. Three-dimensional EAM systems have become the cornerstone for safe and efficient ablation of complex tachyarrhythmias. Briefly, parting from a reference electric signal (i.e., QRS), electrograms obtained at a specific site are stored and the activation time is defined, the activation time is then compared point by point with a reference signal on the 3D geometry of the chamber of interest allowing a projection of its activation mode. Further, voltage maps can also be projected to display scar regions which in some cases correlate with the arrhythmogenic substrate [43]. State-of-the-art software with increasing ML groundwork allows for the integration of various imaging modalities such as CMR or CT in the 3D reconstruction of ablation targets (Fig. 12.6a). This technology can reduce the exposure of both patients and operators to ionizing radiation and improve clinical outcomes [50, 51]. In the same regard, intracardiac echocardiography (ICE) can be applied and integrated for 3D reconstructions of complex structures, such as coronary cusps or papillary muscles, that often prove difficult ablation targets (Fig. 12.6b). Based on corporate interests it remains relatively unknown to the scientific community how ML implementation has been incorporated or is to fuel consumer-grade EAM. Nevertheless, individual novel applications continue to develop rapidly. Undoubtedly, the major limitation for cardiac arrhythmia ablation is determining the location of its substrate. Proposed sites from rotors to drivers failed to provide a 100% efficacy in treatment even when all the potential sites are ablated. This opens the possibility for ML algorithm to accurately identify the ablation target and maybe model mechanistic paths for recurrence. Mahnood et al., used spatiotemporal features extracted from electrograms to train a Kera's based DL for organized spatial site identification, that displayed an accuracy of 95.2% to detect relevant ablation targets for atrial fibrillation with a sensitivity and specificity of 97.7% and 93.0%, respectively [52]. For local abnormal ventricular activities (LAVA), Cabrera-Lozoya et al. used image features from delayed-enhanced CMR to describe local tissue heterogeneities then fed them into a random forest classification framework with a five-fold nested cross-validation scheme in order to identify potential ablation targets. Based model feature augmentation was then carried out by applying a cell-

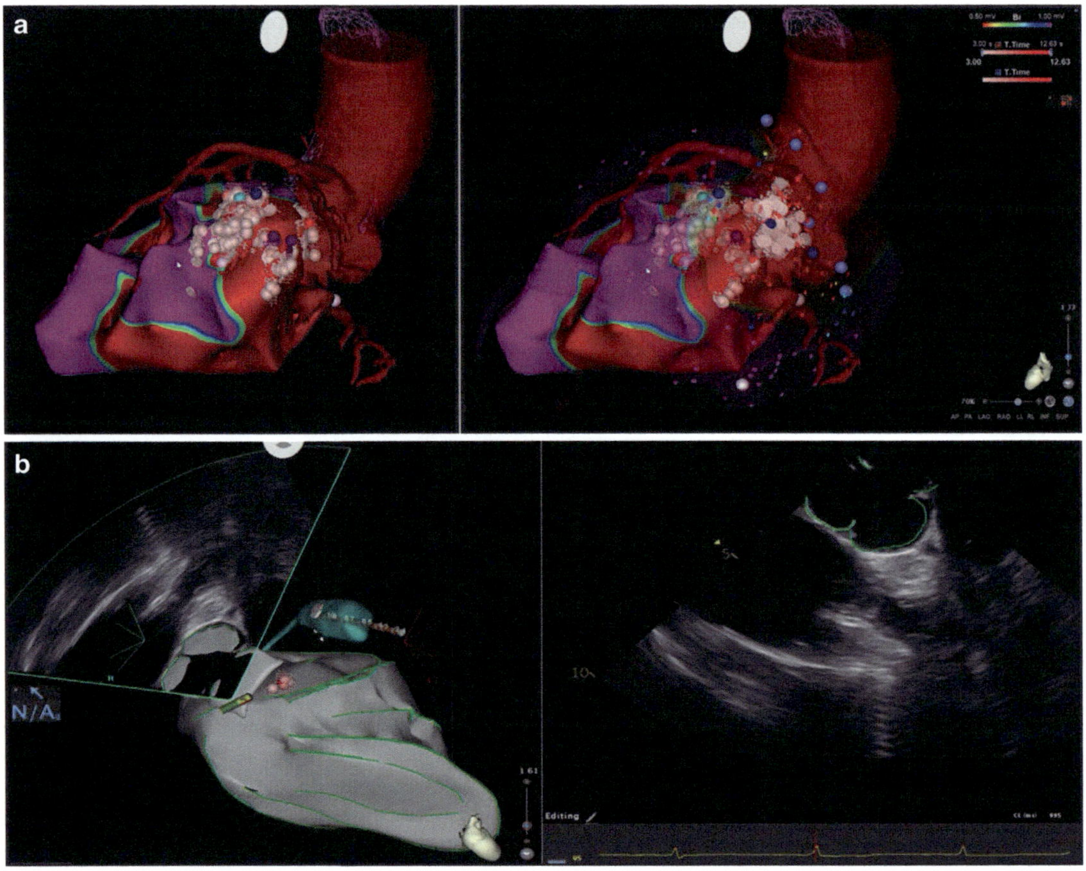

Fig. 12.6 3D Electroanatomical mapping system integration options. (**a**) Left ventricle 3D CT/EAM reconstruction for endocardial/epicardial ablation of ventricular tachycardia in a patient with Chagas disease. (**b**) ICE reconstruction of coronary cusps for targeted radiofrequency ablation of persistent premature ventricular contractions. Performed with CARTOSOUND® Module. (Images provided by Dr. Santiago Nava, Electrophysiology Department, National Institute of Cardiology, Mexico City)

specific cardiac electrophysiologic model as well as a tissue and electrogram recording model. This resulted in an algorithm with an overall accuracy of 98.9% across five patients with a LAVA-specificity of 99.4% and a LAVA-positive predictive value of 96.4%. Whether these models can generalize adequately to the larger population of patients in need for and that may benefit from ablation is yet to be demonstrated [53].

Although ML has clearly taken decisive steps into the essential components of cardiovascular hybrid imaging through the optimization of data-preprocessing, image orientation, structural delineation, and functional quantification, the landscape of clinical implementation remains underdeveloped. ML optimization of hybrid image fusion or data integration is currently being explored. Integration of other data, such as clinical characteristics with advanced imaging (a novel look into what hybrid imaging can entail), may compensate for information loss such as lower image resolution resulting from reduced dosage of radioactive tracer or lower image resolution due to less optimal acquisition protocol. For example, radiomic features extracted from the CT scans in CT/PET scan may be submitted to the ML model along with demographics such as age, sex, and cardiovascular risk factors like type 2 diabetes, hypertension, and presence of dyslipidemia to determine if the patient would be likely to suffer from myocardial ischemia. In a retrospective study by Juarez-Orozco et al. aiming to refine the prognostic value of hybrid PET/CT, CTA outputs were combined with clinical variables in a LogitBoost model (a boosting algorithm which combines weaker logistic regression predicters into a final model) to determine if a patient had suffered ischemia and would undergo early revascularization, respectively [54]. In a cohort of around a thousand patients with low and intermediate risk of CAD, they observed models taking expert-curated CTA variables outperformed models which directly took in raw CTA outputs in identifying patients who suffered from ischemia and eventually underwent early revascularization, respectively; notably, integration of clinical variables consistently improved the performance of all models. The results demonstrated feasibility of ML in data integration which could expand to various sources, such as radiomics features from different modalities, clinical information, and biochemical profiles.

It is likely that observational and retrospective evidence (based on big-data sets) will continue to gather while the necessary structures and trust in the performance of ML's novel analytics become increasingly present in the minds of cardiovascular scientists and physicians. Ultimately, it is expected that further prospective research will put the real-world performance of ML-derived to the test. In the next section, the envisioned paths of clinical implementation and the potential role of ML-based AI in the clinical reality of hybrid imaging will be discussed.

12.3 ML in Decision-Making and Clinical-Evaluation Support

ML implementations in wearable biosensors have taken the spotlight in the clinical implementation of AI as they offer the potential of large-scale screening for a vast range of both chronic and acute diseases. Recently, the Apple Heart Study provided evidence of an algorithm capable of detection of previously undiagnosed atrial fibrillation from pulse irregularity and variability [55]. However, the rate of detection triggers the question of cost-effectiveness viability. The potential of ML-based algorithms to identify patterns from a constant string of data gathered by easily accessible portable technologies sparked an interest in advanced continuous monitoring. For example, Green et al. demonstrated that a multi-instance classifier could be used to identify patients with obstructive HCM from photoplethysmography tracings obtained by a wearable biosensor with an AUC of 0.99 [56].

Within imaging, more explicit feature selection is expected to enhance the decision-support applicability of ML implementations. This is a clear need among clinicians even if especially scientifically oriented. Ease-of-use and interpretability therefore constitute paramount characteristics in every successfully ML-based AI implementation and should be a further promoter in due time within hybrid cardiovascular imaging of any kind. Decision-support on diagnoses and treatment paths, and direct extraction/presentation of the most relevant related data could greatly enhance the way clinicians use the individual patient data to treat their patients.

Furthermore, with the potential to improve diagnostic and prognostic probability estimation at the individual level, a clear niche for ML lies within the integral space of electronic health records and medical imaging systems. Decision support systems, patient-status alarm systems, and workflow enhancements in the form of relevant content selection, speech recognition, and on-the-go word predictions in text editors based on ML models are some examples already sparsely implemented. These tools may optimally use integrated data sources where available to the broadest extent and to extract the largest added value for patients.

Considering an inclusive take on the "hybrid" term, ML models have been developed aggregating imaging and structured data as well as structured data integrated from different data sources including imaging-derived parameters. Whether the current concept of hybrid integration allows for such inclusions is yes to be argued. As an example, Juarez-Orozco et al. developed a model for the classification of myocardial ischemia and an increased risk of adverse cardiovascular events based on clinical and functional (imaging-derived) variables using a boosting ensemble algorithm [57]. These hybridized modeling attempts have shown clear improvements over models based on single data sources, implying that aggregation of multi-source data into a hybrid model adds diagnostic value to other single-source trained models. Therefore, the development of models that employ hybrid imaging data is viable and may be considered in a flexible understanding of hybrid imaging and modeling. This holds the potential to uncover yet untapped insights from high-dimensional cardiovascular hybrid imaging data, which are essentially not yet fully exploited.

Whether aiming to improve clinical workflow efficiency or patient outcomes with respect to diagnosis and allocation of treatment strategies, a rich source of information lies in the aggregation of data originating from multiple imaging modalities. This designates hybrid imaging as the ultimate area to harvest from these investments as portrayed over the recent years in ML in different individual imaging modalities.

Thischapter was written in the midst of the SARS-CoV-2 (COVID-19) pandemic, which has proven to pose a challenge for medical and populational sciences. These times have brought forward the systemic weaknesses that require attention to front expectable circumstances. For instance, delays in the development of PCR-based diagnostic tools have resulted in counterproductive for the adequate detection of infected individuals at the individual level. In this regard, the creation and deployment of ML-based AI systems that facilitate clinical- and image-based diagnostics tools can prove crucial to optimize detection and estimate prognosis. For example, Singh et al. developed a multi-objective differential evolution (MODE)-based DL model that applies chest CT images and provided good performance for the classification of COVID-19 infected patients [55]. Further research into whether hybridization of these models and potential integration with other imagining modalities such as echocardiography can improve cardiac involvement in the disease and its relevance for the patient-based prognosis is warranted.

12.4 Future Perspectives and Challenges in ML-Based AI for Cardiovascular Hybrid Imaging

While studies discussed here suggest a promising path for the incorporation of ML into the common handlings of cardiovascular hybrid imaging, many have been performed on small datasets and hence should be viewed with cautious optimism. There are still tasks in medical imaging analysis, such as motion correction, where ML is yet to achieve performance on par with the status quo. Moreover, there are and will continue to be cases in which ML may not provide a better solution than the alternative, even more traditional, analytics [32, 33]. Rather, it is important to explore and identify the scenarios in which such implementations are bound to translate into clear benefits at the subject-, patient-, health professional-, and population-level.

As presented in this chapter, DL can provide powerful tools for image acquisition, reconstruction, and analysis in hybrid imaging. However, with the complexity of modeling correlations, the interpretability and accuracy of the models are suffering. Criteria on which decisions are made cannot readily be extracted from the models, and small nearly imperceptible perturbations in data can lead to significant errors in predictions [58]. Especially in medical imaging, such unreliability can be dangerous. To allow the integration of DL in medicine two main issues need to be addressed: (1) there needs to be a degree of model interpretability and (2) models need to be quality-controlled by independent algorithms that do not rely on the input of the original task, but use indirect data (for example, model outputs or priors based on existing medical knowledge). Models interpretability is challenging, and still a largely unsolved problem. Clough et al. used a "concept activation vector" technique to associate known medical concepts (such as low ejection fraction) to certain vectors in the latent space of a VAE-based classifier [59]. This approach provides some degree of explanation to the models' decisions but does not allow to fully interpret decisions made in the model. Another approach is to raise awareness about potential mistakes of a DL model using prediction uncertainty metrics [60, 61] or attention maps [62]. Apart from efforts to prevent errors in one network, providing a comprehensive pipeline for DL analysis that includes quality control measures independent of the main DL algorithm can provide a robust solution for the application of DL in clinical practice. In recent work, Ruijsink et al. proposed a comprehensive cluster of algorithms for quality-controlled CMR image analysis. Similar to conventional medical practice, this pipeline consisted of a pre-analysis image-quality check (a CNN-based image classification and several hard-coded conventional clinical rules), a segmentation network, and a quality check of the output (using SVM classification and hard-coded rules based on basic cardiac physiology). As shown by their work, using such a multilayer approach to medical analysis problems assures the levels of error detection/prevention needed for the implementation of DL models in daily clinical practice. With growing initiatives for open-access and medical image repositories such as the Cancer Imaging Archive and UK biobank cohort, it will become increasingly possible to extensively test, validate, and perhaps certify novel ML models with reference datasets that required before clinical deployment. It should be noted that data heterogeneity as well as veracity (incompleteness and inconsistency in record) may have huge impact on final performance of ML models in practice. While this issue may be mitigated by careful curation of a representative training dataset for calibration of the model, it should still be taken account when assessing the utility of ML for certain tasks in the actual clinical context. This is especially important in advanced hybrid imaging given the known nuances and disparities in deployment across medical centers and countries.

12.5 Conclusion

Machine learning constitutes the modern underpinning of AI. Its implementation is beginning to play a substantial role in accelerating solutions to technical and practical limitations currently constraining the full-blown use of hybrid cardiovascular imaging.

Process automation is crucial and often time-intensive data processing steps, such as quality control, image registration, segmentation, and analysis for diagnostic and prognostic purposes are some of the areas in which ML has gained popularity based on results optimization. The evolving concept of hybrid imaging may prove adequate elasticity to contemplate not of complementarity and synergy between imaging modalities but also between data sources and even ML-based image analysis models. At this moment, full operational ML implementation in traditional cardiovascular hybrid imaging (SPECT/CT, PET/CT, and PET/MR) are still lacking, but we find ourselves on the brink of accelerated development of clinical applications that are contingent upon acceptance and comfort with these novel analytics. The development of interpretable, quality-controlled, robust, and trustworthy ML-based models is essential to further optimize data processing, insight generation, and clinical decision support in cardiovascular hybrid imaging. Thereon, the future is open.

Acknowledgments J. W. B and M. W. Y are supported by the Research Project CVON-AI (2018B017). The CVON-AI project is financed by the PPP Allowance made available by Top Sector Life Sciences & Health to the Nederlandse Hartstichting to stimulate public private partnerships. This work reflects only the author's view, not that of the funders. Stichting LSH-TKI or Hartstichting or the Ministry of Economic Affairs is not responsible for any use that may be made of the information it contains.

References

1. Esteva A, Kuprel B, Novoa RA, Ko J, Swetter SM, Blau HM, Thrun S. Dermatologist-level classification of skin cancer with deep neural networks. Nature. 2017;542:115–8.
2. Kandoth C, McLellan MD, Vandin F, et al. Mutational landscape and significance across 12 major cancer types. Nature. 2013;502:333–9.
3. Huang S, Franc BL, Harnish RJ, et al. Exploration of PET and MRI radiomic features for decoding breast cancer phenotypes and prognosis. npj Breast Cancer. 2018;4:24.
4. Tseng HH, Luo Y, Cui S, Chien JT, Ten Haken RK, El Naqa I. Deep reinforcement learning for auto-

mated radiation adaptation in lung cancer. Med Phys. 2017;44:6690–705.

5. Liu N, Liu Y, Logan B, Xu Z, Tang J, Wang Y. Learning the dynamic treatment regimes from medical registry data through deep Q-network. Sci Rep. 2019;9(1):1495. https://doi.org/10.1038/s41598-018-37142-0.
6. Cortes C, Vapnik V. Support-vector networks. Mach Learn. 1995;20:273–97.
7. Goodfellow I, Bengio Y, Courville A. Deep learning. Cambridge: MIT Press; 2016.
8. Khamis H, Zurakhov G, Azar V, Raz A, Friedman Z, Adam D. Automatic apical view classification of echocardiograms using a discriminative learning dictionary. Med Image Anal. 2017;36:15–21.
9. Zhang J, Gajjala S, Agrawal P, et al. Fully automated echocardiogram interpretation in clinical practice. Circulation. 2018;138:1623–35.
10. Tesche C, De Cecco CN, Baumann S, et al. Coronary CT angiography-derived fractional flow reserve: machine learning algorithm versus computational fluid dynamics modeling. Radiology. 2018;288:64–72.
11. Mazo C, Bernal J, Trujillo M, Alegre E. Transfer learning for classification of cardiovascular tissues in histological images. Comput Methods Prog Biomed. 2018;165:69–76.
12. Han SS, Kim MS, Lim W, Park GH, Park I, Chang SE. Classification of the clinical images for benign and malignant cutaneous tumors using a deep learning algorithm. J Invest Dermatol. 2018;138:1529–38.
13. Hashemi S, Veisi H, Jafarzadehpur E, Rahmani R, Heshmati Z. Multi-view deep learning for rigid gas permeable lens base curve fitting based on Pentacam images. Med Biol Eng Comput. 2020;58(7):1467–82. https://doi.org/10.1007/s11517-020-02154-4.
14. Khan MA, Kwon S, Choo J, Hong SM, Kang SH, Park I-H, Kim SK, Hong SJ. Automatic detection of tympanic membrane and middle ear infection from oto-endoscopic images via convolutional neural networks. Neural Netw. 2020;126:384–94.
15. Kholiavchenko M, Sirazitdinov I, Kubrak K, Badrutdinova R, Kuleev R, Yuan Y, Vrtovec T, Ibragimov B. Contour-aware multi-label chest X-ray organ segmentation. Int J Comput Assist Radiol Surg. 2020;15:425–36.
16. Blaivas M, Blaivas L. Are all deep learning architectures alike for point-of-care ultrasound?: evidence from a cardiac image classification model suggests otherwise. J Ultrasound Med. 2019;39(6):1187–94.
17. Joshi U, Guerzhoy M. Automatic photo orientation detection with convolutional neural networks. In: Proc.—2017 14th Conf. Comput. Robot Vision, CRV 2017. IEEE; 2018. pp. 103–108.
18. Atehortúa A, Zuluaga MA, García JD, Romero E. Automatic segmentation of right ventricle in cardiac cine MR images using a saliency analysis. Med Phys. 2016;43:6270.
19. Vigneault DM, Xie W, Ho CY, Bluemke DA, Noble JA. Ω-Net (Omega-Net): fully automatic, multi-view cardiac MR detection, orientation, and segmentation with deep neural networks. Med Image Anal. 2018;48:95–106.
20. Ruijsink B, Puyol-Antón E, Oksuz I, Sinclair M, Bai W, Schnabel JA, Razavi R, King AP. Fully automated, quality-controlled cardiac analysis from CMR. JACC Cardiovasc Imaging. 2020;13:684–95.
21. Bai W, Sinclair M, Tarroni G, et al. Automated cardiovascular magnetic resonance image analysis with fully convolutional networks. J Cardiovasc Magn Reson. 2018;20:65.
22. Ronneberger O, Fischer P, Brox T. U-Net: convolutional networks for biomedical image segmentation BT—medical image computing and computer-assisted intervention—MICCAI 2015. In: Navab N, Hornegger J, Wells WM, Frangi AF, editors. Cham: Springer International Publishing; 2015. pp. 234–241.
23. Wang Y, Lu X, Zhang Y, et al. Precise pulmonary scanning and reducing medical radiation exposure by developing a clinically applicable intelligent CT system: toward improving patient care. EBioMedicine. 2020;54:102724.
24. He K, Zhang X, Ren S, Sun J. Deep residual learning for image recognition; 2015.
25. Baskaran L, Maliakal G, Al'Aref SJ, et al. Identification and quantification of cardiovascular structures from CCTA: an end-to-end, rapid, pixel-wise, deep-learning method. JACC Cardiovasc Imaging. 2020;13(5):1163–71. https://doi.org/10.1016/j.jcmg.2019.08.025.
26. Jun Guo B, He X, Lei Y, Harms J, Wang T, Curran WJ, Liu T, Jiang Zhang L, Yang X. Automated left ventricular myocardium segmentation using 3D deeply supervised attention U-net for coronary computed tomography angiography; CT myocardium segmentation. Med Phys. 2020;47:1775–85.
27. Zhou R, Fenster A, Xia Y, Spence JD, Ding M. Deep learning-based carotid media-adventitia and lumen-intima boundary segmentation from three-dimensional ultrasound images. Med Phys. 2019;46:3180–93.
28. Wolterink JM, Leiner T, de Vos BD, van Hamersvelt RW, Viergever MA, Išgum I. Automatic coronary artery calcium scoring in cardiac CT angiography using paired convolutional neural networks. Med Image Anal. 2016;34:123–36.
29. Lessmann N, van Ginneken B, Zreik M, de Jong PA, de Vos BD, Viergever MA, Isgum I. Automatic calcium scoring in low-dose chest CT using deep neural networks with dilated convolutions. IEEE Trans Med Imaging. 2018;37:615–25.
30. Zreik M, Lessmann N, van Hamersvelt RW, Wolterink JM, Voskuil M, Viergever MA, Leiner T, Išgum I. Deep learning analysis of the myocardium in coronary CT angiography for identification of patients with functionally significant coronary artery stenosis. Med Image Anal. 2018;44:72–85.
31. Min JK, Leipsic J, Pencina MJ, et al. Diagnostic accuracy of fractional flow reserve from anatomic CT angiography. JAMA. 2012;308:1237.

32. Itu L, Rapaka S, Passerini T, Georgescu B, Schwemmer C, Schoebinger M, Flohr T, Sharma P, Comaniciu D. A machine-learning approach for computation of fractional flow reserve from coronary computed tomography. J Appl Physiol. 2016;121:42–52.
33. Kumamaru KK, Fujimoto S, Otsuka Y, et al. Diagnostic accuracy of 3D deep-learning-based fully automated estimation of patient-level minimum fractional flow reserve from coronary computed tomography angiography. Eur Heart J Cardiovasc Imaging. 2020;21:437–45.
34. Coenen A, Kim Y-H, Kruk M, et al. Diagnostic accuracy of a machine-learning approach to coronary computed tomographic angiography–based fractional flow reserve. Circ Cardiovasc Imaging. 2018;11(6):e007217. https://doi.org/10.1161/CIRCIMAGING.117.007217.
35. Liu F, Jang H, Kijowski R, Bradshaw T, McMillan AB. Deep learning MR imaging–based attenuation correction for PET/MR imaging. Radiology. 2018;286:676–84.
36. Ladefoged CN, Marner L, Hindsholm A, Law I, Højgaard L, Andersen FL. Deep learning based attenuation correction of PET/MRI in pediatric brain tumor patients: evaluation in a clinical setting. Front Neurosci. 2019;12:1005.
37. Shi L, Onofrey JA, Liu H, Liu Y-H, Liu C. Deep learning-based attenuation map generation for myocardial perfusion SPECT. Eur J Nucl Med Mol Imaging. 2020;47(10):2383–95.
38. Xiang L, Qiao Y, Nie D, An L, Lin W, Wang Q, Shen D. Deep auto-context convolutional neural networks for standard-dose PET image estimation from low-dose PET/MRI. Neurocomputing. 2017;267:406–16.
39. Chen KT, Gong E, de Carvalho Macruz FB, et al. Ultra-low-dose 18F-Florbetaben amyloid PET imaging using deep learning with multi-contrast MRI inputs. Radiology. 2019;290:649–56.
40. Betancur J, Rubeaux M, Fuchs TA, et al. Automatic valve plane localization in myocardial perfusion SPECT/CT by machine learning: anatomic and clinical validation. J Nucl Med. 2017;58:961–7.
41. Išgum I, de Vos BD, Wolterink JM, Dey D, Berman DS, Rubeaux M, Leiner T, Slomka PJ. Automatic determination of cardiovascular risk by CT attenuation correction maps in Rb-82 PET/CT. J Nucl Cardiol. 2018;25:2133–42.
42. Chubb H, Harrison JL, Weiss S, et al. Development, preclinical validation, and clinical translation of a cardiac magnetic resonance—electrophysiology system with active catheter tracking for ablation of cardiac arrhythmia. JACC Clin Electrophysiol. 2017;3:89–103.
43. Velasco Forte MN, Pushparajah K, Schaeffter T, et al. Improved passive catheter tracking with positive contrast for CMR-guided cardiac catheterization using partial saturation (pSAT). J Cardiovasc Magn Reson. 2017;19:60.
44. Ruijsink B, Zugaj K, Wong J, Pushparajah K, Hussain T, Moireau P, Razavi R, Chapelle D, Chabiniok R. Dobutamine stress testing in patients with Fontan circulation augmented by biomechanical modeling. PLoS One. 2020;15:e0229015.
45. Dori Y, Sarmiento M, Glatz AC, Gillespie MJ, Jones VM, Harris MA, Whitehead KK, Fogel MA, Rome JJ. X-Ray magnetic resonance fusion to internal markers and utility in congenital heart disease catheterization. Circ Cardiovasc Imaging. 2011;4:415–24.
46. Haskins G, Kruecker J, Kruger U, Xu S, Pinto PA, Wood BJ, Yan P. Learning deep similarity metric for 3D MR–TRUS image registration. Int J Comput Assist Radiol Surg. 2019;14:417–25.
47. Sheikhjafari A, Noga M, Punithakumar K, Ray N. Unsupervised deformable image registration with fully connected generative neural network. Med. imaging with deep learn; 2018.
48. Krebs J, Mansi T, Mailhé B, Ayache N, Delingette H. Unsupervised probabilistic deformation modeling for robust diffeomorphic registration. 2018. pp. 101–109.
49. Silva JNA, Southworth M, Raptis C, Silva J. Emerging applications of virtual reality in cardiovascular medicine. JACC Basic Transl Sci. 2018;3:420–30.
50. Fernández-Gómez JM, Moriña-Vázquez P, Morales EDR, Venegas-Gamero J, Barba-Pichardo R, Carranza MH. Exclusion of fluoroscopy use in catheter ablation procedures: six years of experience at a single center. J Cardiovasc Electrophysiol. 2014;25:638–44.
51. Casella M, Dello Russo A, Pelargonio G, et al. Near zerO fluoroscopic exPosure during catheter ablAtion of supRavenTricular arrhYthmias: the NO-PARTY multicentre randomized trial. Europace. 2016;18:1565–72.
52. Alhusseini M, Abuzaid F, Clopton P, Rogers A, Rodrigo M, Baykaner T, Wang P, Rappel W-J, Narayan S. Machine learning identifies sites where ablation terminates persistent atrial fibrillation. J Am Coll Cardiol. 2019;73:301.
53. Lozoya RC, Berte B, Cochet H, Jais P, Ayache N, Sermesant M. Model-based feature augmentation for cardiac ablation target learning from images. IEEE Trans Biomed Eng. 2019;66:30–40.
54. Juarez-Orozco LE, Maaniitty T, Benjamins JW, Niemi MA, Van Der Harst P, Saraste A, Knuuti J. 10Refining the long-term prognostic value of hybrid PET/CT through machine learning. Eur Hear J Cardiovasc Imaging. 2020; https://doi.org/10.1093/ehjci/jez151.
55. Turakhia MP, Desai M, Hedlin H, et al. Rationale and design of a large-scale, app-based study to identify cardiac arrhythmias using a smartwatch: the Apple Heart Study. Am Heart J. 2019;207:66–75.
56. Green EM, van Mourik R, Wolfus C, Heitner SB, Dur O, Semigran MJ. Machine learning detection of obstructive hypertrophic cardiomyopathy using a wearable biosensor. npj Digit Med. 2019;2:57.
57. Juarez-Orozco LE, Knol RJJ, Sanchez-Catasus CA, Martinez-Manzanera O, van der Zant FM, Knuuti J. Machine learning in the integration of simple variables for identifying patients with myocardial isch-

emia. J Nucl Cardiol. 2020;27(1):147–55. https://doi.org/10.1007/s12350-018-1304-x.
58. Finlayson SG, Bowers JD, Ito J, Zittrain JL, Beam AL, Kohane IS. Adversarial attacks on medical machine learning. Science. 2019;363:1287–9.
59. Clough JR, Oksuz I, Puyol-Anton E, Ruijsink B, King AP, Schnabel JA. Global and local interpretability for cardiac MRI classification; 2019.
60. Anton EP, Ruijsink B, Baumgartner CF, Sinclair M, Konukoglu E, Razavi R, King AP (2020) Automated quantification of myocardial tissue characteristics from native T1 mapping using neural networks with Bayesian inference for uncertainty-based quality-control.
61. Sander J, de Vos BD, Wolterink JM, Išgum I. Towards increased trustworthiness of deep learning segmentation methods on cardiac MRI. In: Angelini ED, Landman BA, editors. Med. imaging 2019 image process. SPIE. p. 44.
62. Heo J, Lee HB, Kim S, Lee J, Kim KJ, Yang E, Hwang SJ. Uncertainty-aware attention for reliable interpretation and prediction. In: Bengio S, Wallach H, Larochelle H, Grauman K, Cesa-Bianchi N, Garnett R, editors. Advances in neural information processing systems, vol. 31. Curran Associates; 2018. p. 909–18.

GPSR Compliance

The European Union's (EU) General Product Safety Regulation (GPSR) is a set of rules that requires consumer products to be safe and our obligations to ensure this.

If you have any concerns about our products, you can contact us on ProductSafety@springernature.com

In case Publisher is established outside the EU, the EU authorized representative is:

Springer Nature Customer Service Center GmbH
Europaplatz 3
69115 Heidelberg, Germany

Batch number: 10732801

Printed by Printforce, the Netherlands